Finding Hope When Doctors Say There is None

Surviving Cancer in the Harsh World of HMO Medicine

By
F.H. Scribner

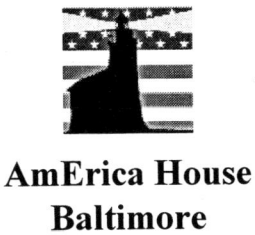

AmErica House
Baltimore

Copyright 2000 by J. M. Scribner
All rights reserved. No part of this book may be reproduced in any form without written permission from the publishers, except by a reviewer who may quote brief passages in a review to be printed in a newspaper or magazine.

First printing

ISBN 1-58851-818-3
PUBLISHED BY AMERICA HOUSE BOOK PUBLISHERS
www.publishamerica.com
Baltimore

Printed in the United States of America

Dedicated to

Jane and Susan—my living inspirations

In Memory of

My father, John, Bronson, Patrick, Caron, Lisa, Ida, Donna, MJ and Muriel,
—all of whom fought heartbreakingly well

"This is a particularly lethal and aggressive form of cancer. I want to be sure you understand that, Mr. Scribner."

—A specialist assessing the patient at
M.D. Anderson Cancer Center in Houston

Heaven and HMOs

Two doctors and an HMO manager died and are lined up at the pearly gates. The first doctor, stepping forward: "I was a pediatric spine surgeon and helped kids overcome their deformities."

St. Peter: "You may enter."

The second doctor: "I was a psychiatrist. I helped people rehabilitate themselves." St. Peter also invites him in.

Stepping forward, the third applicant says, "I was an HMO manager. I helped people get cost-effective health care."

After a moment's thought, St. Peter responds, "You too can come in." As the HMO manager walks by, St. Peter adds, "However, you can only stay three days. After that you can go to hell."

TABLE OF CONTENTS

Introduction: Today's Real World of Cancer Care 15
Chapter 1: A Rude Initiation—My First Visit with a Cancer Doctor 19
Chapter 2: Reversal of Fortune—From Nothing to the Knife 25
Chapter 3: Fear . . . and Frazzled Nerves—Getting Ready for Surgery 31
Chapter 4: Away from Innocence—Unnecessary Post-surgical Pain 35
Chapter 5: A Time of Reckoning—The Rookie Patient Strikes Out 41
Chapter 6: Ugly Words—Reading of the Pathology Report 47
Chapter 7: The Oncologist—An Eye-opening First Visit 51
Chapter 8: It's All in Your Mind—How the Mind and Body Interrelate 57
Chapter 9: The Second-opinion Mirage 63
Chapter 10: Boy on The Beach—The Second Opinion Confirms the First . . 67
Chapter 11: That First Taste of Chemo 71
Chapter 12: The Longest Journey—Phase One of My Research 77
Chapter 13: Not So Clear And Present Danger—
A Shadow Appears on the CT Film 83
Chapter 14: A Step Backward—In the Hospital Again 87
Chapter 15: More Questions Than Answers—
Many Antibiotics, Few Reasons 91
Chapter 16: Psychology as Voodoo—Dr. Drake's Label for Psychotherapy . 97
Chapter 17: An Old Foe Rears Its Head—The Shrink Turns Traitor 101
Chapter 18: A Break in The Clouds—New Doctors Take Control 107
Chapter 19: The First of Three Trips to Houston 111
Chapter 20: At Home in Houston—Sitting with the *Real* Specialists 115
Chapter 21: Bad News Is Good News—Trading One Disease for Another . 121
Chapter 22: My Typical Day—This Is Rocket Science? 125
Chapter 23: That Feeling of High Anxiety—
How Our Fight-or-Flight Response Effects Our Daily Lives 129
Chapter 24: Unexpected Twists—Two New Doctors Enter the Scene 133
Chapter 25: Strange Twists of Human Nature—
A Racing Heart Lands Me Back in the Hospital 139
Chapter 26: Little Did We Know—An Inept Doctor Reveals Himself 143
Chapter 27: Undone by Surprise—A CT Reveals *More* Bad News 147
Chapter 28: Upon Us Like Thunder—
Another New HMO Doctor and Further Delays 151
Chapter 29: An Unfortunate Concern—A Questionable Surgery 157
Chapter 30: Winning The Battle, Losing The War—
The Surgery's a Success, but The News Is Not Good 163

Chapter 31: Getting All Too Familiar With Disappointment—
   The Difficulty of Disposing of an HMO Doctor 167
Chapter 32: The Tangled Web We Weave—
   Telling the Most Negative Doctor Where to Get Off 173
Chapter 33: As Aliens and Sojourners—
   Learning That Radiation Will Destroy a Working Kidney 177
Chapter 34: Abandoning The Straight Road—
   Saying Goodbye to a Kidney 183
Chapter 35: The First Prophetic Sign—A Mystifying Falcon Appears 187
Chapter 36: Condemned in The Flesh—
   Dr. Crandle Says My Days Are Numbered 191
Chapter 37: My First IV Chemo—Shattering Myths 195
Chapter 38: With Knowledge ... Comes Doubt—
   Learning the Unsettling Rationale for My Chemo 201
Chapter 39: Bad Medicine—The Doctor Administers Chemotherapy 205
Chapter 40: Depths of The Abyss—
   Two Months into Chemo and a CT Shows a New Mass 211
Chapter 41: The Solution's the Problem?
   Source of the Testosterone Headaches Is Found 217
Chapter 42: As Children Fear Darkness—
   The Heel Pain's Found to Be a Blood Clot 221
Chapter 43: Of Doubt And Sorrow—
   Dr. Goetz Declares the Mass to Be Scar Tissue 227
Chapter 44: The Music They Played—
   Another Questionable Area Turns Up on a CT 233
Chapter 45: Let Us Not Pretend—How Am I Better Off *After* Chemo? 237
Chapter 46: Renewal of The Mind—
   A New Radiation Oncodoc Agrees to Review Uncertain CT Films 241
Chapter 47: A New Doctor Presents the Most Impossible of Conclusions .. 245
Chapter 48: Moving on Toward a Biopsy 251
Chapter 49: Flight of Fantasy—Back to Houston for Reassurance 257
Chapter 50: As Smoke Becomes Fire—Surgery's Scheduled ... *Again* ... 261
Chapter 51: And We Shall Be Changed—
   My First Meeting with Another ACC Patient 267
Chapter 52: Talk Not of Others' Lives 271
Chapter 53: A Shaft of Light—Biopsy First Impressions Look Good 275
Chapter 54: Fight Till The Last Gasp—A New Shrink, a New Approach .. 279
Chapter 55: Time: That Endless Song—Finding Relief in Music 285
Chapter 56: Houston: The Final Trek—
   The Hard Realities of Cancer Surgery 289
Chapter 57: Drink, For Tomorrow—Purging the System Prior to Surgery .. 295
Chapter 58: Into The Dim Unknown—
   Malignancy Halts the Second Surgery 301
Chapter 59: Let Us Not Pretend—A Clergyman Offers a Solution 305

Chapter 60: Strange Encounters—
    The Disappearing Old Man and the Blunt Oncologist 313
Chapter 61: Progeny of Light—
    The Identity of the Old Man Begins to Emerge 319
Chapter 62: The Good, the Bad, and HMOs 325
Chapter 63: In Giving, We Receive—The New Oncodoc and I Hit it Off . . 331
Chapter 64: A Day in the Life 337
Chapter 65: Twisted News—Good CT Results, Poor Blood Work 341
Chapter 66: Let The Dance Begin—
    The First Chemo Session Goes Smoothly 347
Chapter 67: When Weakness Becomes Strength—
    Working Through the Chemo Fatigue 351
Chapter 68: This . . . Couldn't Be—My Hair's Falling Out! 355
Chapter 69: Till Thou Return Unto The Ground—
    Becoming a Catholic Again 361
Chapter 70: Betrayed—The Things Cancer Does to Your Psyche 367
Chapter 71: Is Life an Illusion? 371
Chapter 72: Ecstasy in Such as Me—A Mysterious Blue Light in the Night 375
Chapter 73: To Work or Not to Work—
    Pondering Again a Major Change in Lifestyle 381
Chapter 74: No Stone Unturned—The Radiologist and I Meet Face to Face 387
Chapter 75: Forgiveness = Inner Peace 391
Chapter 76: An Exciting Discovery—A New Chemo! 397
Chapter 77: Change and Mitigation of the Soul—
    Chemo Is Unexpectedly Halted 403
Chapter 78: Into Fields of Light—Dr. Sloan Agrees to My Retirement 409

Today 415
Epilogue 417
Thoughts to Help You Survive. 421

Appendix A: No-cost Telephone Resources For Cancer Patients 423
Appendix B: Preparing Your Portable Medical History 425
Appendix C: The Perfect Doctor 427
Appendix D: Food as Medicine 429
Appendix E: The Internet as a Medical Resource 437
Appendix F: Meditation—How To 441

INTRODUCTION

TODAY'S REAL WORLD OF CANCER CARE

Though this is the story of one rookie cancer patient's years-long successful struggle with the life-threatening disease, it's easy to see my plight as that of any naive cancer patient in today's peculiar and often-brutal world of HMO-dominated medicine.

You'll follow an exasperating labyrinth as I seek and finally realize the correct diagnosis for my unusual cancer . . . where and how I finally accomplish this none-too-easy feat . . . what the ensuing treatments entail (including all side-effects endured) . . . and the successful payoff.

You'll see how I credit my own tenacity, various otherworldly "encounters"—and conventional and alternative treatments (meditation, spirituality, diet, lifestyle changes, and yes, the ubiquitous Internet)—for my recovery and survival today.

Also touched upon will be the fact that a cancer diagnosis can bring with it an element of good news. Butting heads with a life-threatening disease has, in many cases, forced sometimes-selfish patients—not unlike myself—to step back, to re-evaluate their lives . . . for the better.

Cancer, according to the National Cancer Institute, will kill 563,000 Americans this year. An inconceivable 1.2 million of us will be diagnosed with the disease. Almost all of us have felt the suffering, the hysteria, of this silent killer . . . in our families . . . affecting those we love. Today, the disease is more prevalent than ever—even among our children. It is projected to be America's No. 1 killer in the near future, replacing heart disease as our major cause of death.

The word cancer, by definition means 'a malignant and invasive growth or tumor.' But, by its very nature, the word also means 'unpredictability.' The disease doesn't necessarily follow a predictable growth pattern, as some statistics would have us believe. Cancer can transform its growth pattern for the better—or worse—at any given time, for unknown reasons. It can go from being very aggressive to indolent or vice versa.

In lay terms, a malignancy has a mind of its own, so to speak. And therein lies our hope. We can, through an integration of mind-body, spirituality, diet, lifestyle changes, and traditional medicine alter cancer's random and destructive course.

Science is still trying to unravel the many mysteries of the disease—is it or is it not initiated by forces outside or inside the body? Or both? Is cancer one mechanism, or is it several hundred separate forms of the disease, as some doctors insist?

Through cell renewal and growth our bodies are capable of existing for 80 to 100 years. In this renewal process, billions of our cells duplicate themselves every day. Old cells disintegrate as new daughter cells take their place.

In most cases cancer occurs when a single cell, at the genetic level, somehow loses its capacity to regulate its own replication. This process alone, however, does not degrade the body.

The wondrous human body has hundreds of genes within each cell that watch over and guide cell replication—so a single mutation doesn't result in a malignancy. It's when there are recurring mutations, passed on from daughter cell to daughter cell, that a cancer is created.

A replicating cell must flawlessly remake billions of bits of coded DNA. In this ongoing, enigmatic process, coding errors occur. These errors can be magnified through the actions of free radicals, sunlight, numerous chemicals agents, radiation, poor diet, viruses, smoking, and lifestyle stresses.

There is no predestined growth rate, but it's said that one cancer cell is capable of multiplying into a mass of 100 billion malignant cells—roughly the size of an egg—in about three years. For a tumor to propagate to that extent, it must acquire a blood supply to nourish itself. This ability, by a burgeoning tumor, to give birth to supplementary blood vessels, is known as angiogenesis.

Primary cancers—e.g., prostate, lung, and breast—aren't invariably what bring about the demise of a patient. More perilous complications arise when these primary tumors discharge malignant cells into the blood and lymph system, which travel to unaffected regions of the body and establish invading colonies of malignant cells, called metastases. It is this spreading of cancer that most often causes death by eventually destroying the function of the newly invaded site—say the liver, for example.

A selfish disease cancer is, a suicidal disease . . . one that, confoundingly, if left untreated, brings about its own demise . . . through the wasting of its human host.

Simple as it sounds, it's cancer's ability to make a cell replicate ceaselessly that science, since its earliest days, finds so puzzling. When the scientific world does identify the cure for the disease—and I believe that will come very soon—also unraveled will be many intriguing explanations as to why our bodies age as well.

Successful treatment of cancer encompasses both body and mind. Unfortunately in today's western medicine nearly all physicians are educated to see their duties mechanically—zeroing in on one area of the body as needing treatment. Other cultures see disease as affecting the whole body . . . not just a single, isolated component. Thus, to be most effective, you as a patient in today's western world must take it upon yourself to embrace the whole body—including the mind—in your treatment.

With the growing threat that more and more of us—and our children—will contract this murderous disease, it's incumbent upon us as a nation, as human beings, to stop accepting this epidemic as inescapable: something we all struggle with as a result of aging. We must take every occasion to push for a cure, a halting to cancer's dreadful wasting of innocent human life.

Whether you're a newly diagnosed cancer patient or one who's been dealing with the disease for some time or a caregiver or the friend of a friend with cancer, there's a world of stimulating information . . . and hope here.

You may at times, see some of the incidents as being too explicit—different therapies, the encounter with the elderly 'angel,' the ghostly B-25 fly-by, for example—but it's intended they be presented this way . . . to express A-Day-In-The-Life sort of representation of what it's really like being a cancer patient—both mentally and physically.

The described events will introduce the cancer patient—indeed anyone remotely caught up in the disease—to an explicit perception of what's involved, from the patient's point of view, in today's cancer treatments . . . the mental and physical sides surgery, chemotherapy, radiation . . . dealing with unfeeling doctors in the oftentimes brutish world of HMO medicine.

Prepare yourself to take an instructive, and sometimes unpleasant, trek through the confusion that is today's cancer care . . . .

One final thought: While this is a factual narrative, actual names have been replaced . . . not, however, to safeguard the innocent. The exasperating mistakes, the lousy doctors described, are unquestionably authentic. Litigative turmoil is not something I want to introduce to my now-peaceful, now cancer-free life.

CHAPTER 1

A RUDE INITIATION—
MY FIRST VISIT WITH A CANCER DOCTOR

A cool, blustery day on California's central coast. Sunny, but long-sleeve weather. Christmas season, 1989. My wife and I are sitting in an oncologist's office—our first of many visits. Seated across the desk, this completely demoralizing doctor's flashing a Xeroxed graph, running his finger along a declining line, describing how, in no uncertain terms, he doesn't expect me to be among the living in a year and a half.

This disturbing and unexpected revelation takes place within minutes of our being seated, after our initial introduction.

Sitting across from this cold-blooded cancer specialist, a man resembling a lanky Groucho Marx, my introduction to the ghastly and often contradictory world of cancer treatment and prognoses is like being struck in the chest time and again with an ice pick.

My father died eight years earlier of prostate cancer. With me I carry heavy baggage—guilt, fear. I hadn't attended his funeral in Florida for a number of family-squabble reasons—all silly now. Vivid images of how he must've looked on his deathbed still menace my late-night thoughts.

Now, at age 47, here I am, a terrified, medically naive cancer rookie, listening to this oncologist predict my soon-to-be demise . . . not knowing that doctors often make profound blunders . . . scoot arrogantly out onto shaky statistical limbs. Having been raised from childhood to revere doctors, all doctors, and their opinions, I was thoroughly indoctrinated in the belief that in every case, THE DOCTOR KNOWS BEST (TDKB: an acronym I'll use occasionally for brevity). Whatever a doctor does or says is gospel.

Thus, to me, it's time to start looking for a headstone.

Making our way down the steps from the clinic, I have to physically assist Jane, my weeping wife . . . that crushed is she by this doctor's off-hand remarks.

Physicians, I've since learned the hard way, are only humans—flesh and blood—who possess a bit more education than most of us, but often far less compassion. This discovery, and how to successfully cope with the many fearful aspects of cancer, are the guideposts of this book. Despite what some callous doctor says about your fate, there is hope—always. You must persevere even in the face of any doctor's most dire predictions.

Medical schools don't bestow on these people any special insight. Doctors aren't prophets, aren't psychics, aren't seers, aren't fortunetellers. The person delivering an annulling decree is usually basing it upon statistics. And those statistics, as they relate to much of today's medicine, are more often than not, old news. There's so much happening so fast in the world of cancer research and treatment—so many medical breakthroughs—that the quoted statistics are quite often obsolete. And, the stats definitely don't take into account details of *you.*

As you can guess, Christmas of 1989 was not a happy occasion for me. Throughout the holidays, knowing 'I had a cancer that was going to kill me,' I was overwhelmed by a sense of aloneness, isolation. This couldn't be happening to me!

The everyday complacency of my former life was gone forever. Despair locked onto me like the rusty jaws of an iron trap. Festive Yuletide hymns, carols . . . the fragrance of fondly remembered treats . . . the percolating multi-hued Christmas tree lights . . . the pine-tree scent only served to more sharply drive home feelings of finality.

Four weeks earlier: I'd undergone a six-hour exploratory surgery to remove an unknown mass from the left upper quadrant of my abdomen—a vaguely defined area just below the left rib cage. Still I was experiencing considerable post-surgical discomfort in the area.

Pre-Cancer . . . Five Months Earlier

Bumper-to-bumper traffic on the 101 Freeway. The sun: an exploding disk in the windshield. Friday morning. My eyes, blurry with distress. Like any other workday, I'm making the 40-mile commute to my office at Rockwell International in the San Fernando Valley. The wetness in my eyes isn't brought about by the sun or anything as romantic as a tune on the radio . . . though perhaps the music's underscoring a feeling I've had of late. A belief something's really physically wrong with me, really, deep-down wrong. (Other cancer patients have said they too knew instinctively they had cancer before it was diagnosed.)

Yesterday, Thursday, I'd undergone a cat scan—a CT of my abdomen. I'd been feeling some discomfort in upper abdomen for several weeks; months, actually. Various medical exams began after I complained of a set of symptoms that wouldn't go away. My primary-care HMO doctor, a General Practitioner, an uneffusive middle-aged woman, listened to my lungs, my heart, checked my blood pressure and so forth. If these 'flu-like' symptoms didn't go away in a couple of weeks, she said, return and see her.

Weeks later I returned with the identical symptoms. Again she sent me on my way, saying I should return once more if the symptoms persist beyond two weeks. In all, I saw her three times in three months with the same symptoms. No diagnosis.

Earlier that year, without realizing it, I'd made a blunder of sorts when my employer opened annual medical insurance enrollment. To save money—because Jane and I and my teenage stepchildren had never really been sick—I decided to take the family off the existing indemnity plan and go with a temptingly inexpensive HMO, a Health Maintenance Organization. The HMO's monthly premium was significantly less than my former policy.

HMOs aren't inherently bad, once you learn how to 'work' them, as we'll see later. But you quickly realize that a lot of HMO employees, including physicians, become inured by a civil-service approach to life, business, medicine. The Hey, It-Ain't-My-Job approach to everything frequently rears its familiar head. Often it's difficult to find *anyone* within an HMO to whom you can plead your case.

As an HMO patient, you are allowed to choose your primary-care doctor, also known in HMO jargon as a Gatekeeper. He or she is your first line of defense against disease, illnesses of all sorts. Conflictingly, he or she is also the HMO's first line of defense—against spending.

Within a month, give or take, the symptoms were back, full force: an unpleasant feeling of bloatedness following each meal, an overall feeling of weariness, prolonged constipation, unexplained chills, instant fevers, night sweats, facial paleness, elevated blood pressure, throbbing headaches lasting days at a stretch—and, strangest of all, unnerving recurring nightmares. (Only one doctor—a psychologist—has ever attached any significance to these dreams. Seems MDs don't put much credence in what our minds are telling us about our bodies.)

This time, after listening to my lungs, the GP orders a chest x-ray, more to appease me than anything. Days later, she calls, saying the radiologist who reviewed the films noticed a dark shadowy shape below the rib cage. He wants another x-ray. Can I come back?

Positioning me for a follow-up x-ray, a fleshy young female technician seems overly reticent regarding the need for this follow-up.

"Is this 'shadowy' thing he's concerned about," I persist, still not too troubled, "the real reason I'm back?"

Glancing at me, she's got that I-Know-More-Than-I'm-Allowed-to-Tell-You look. Shaking her head, she smiles. "They don't like us explaining things. Sorry."

Days later: I'm at work, yet another doctor telephones. The radiologist. "There's definitely something there," he offers soberly, after quickly identifying himself. "We need to get a better look. We've got you scheduled for a CT in two days. Come in tomorrow and pick up your CT prep kit." In his curt, doctoral fashion, he throws out an appointment, an address. He doesn't, however, give me a chance to question him. Like, what's a CT or a CT prep kit?

FINDING HOPE WHEN DOCTORS SAY THERE IS NONE

Three days after my first-ever abdominal CT: It's Friday and I'm again at work. I'm in a conference with a very demanding vice president. The phone interrupts us.

"According to their report, things are still pretty much up in the air," I hear the GP's voice saying quickly, as if, out of the blue, I'll know who she is, what she's talking about. "They're still . . . not sure. Two different radiologists have looked at your pictures. They don't *think* it's cancer."

This evil word, coming from out of nowhere, with remoteness of a steel-tipped arrow, strikes with convincing impact. *"C-a-n-c-e-r?"* I echo powerlessly, feeling my breath leaving me.

The vice president's eyes come up from the mound of vu-graphs in his lap.

"Correct," she goes on. "They say there's some evidence of calcification. Toward the center of the mass, but—"

"Wait a minute, doctor—what mass?"

"The one we picked up on your scan, Mr. Scribner," she fires back almost indignantly as if I'm supposed to already know this.

Once the word cancer's been mentioned in reference to you, *by an authority figure like a physician,* your mind sucks it up like water poured on sand, conjuring up every sort of horror . . . because you know with certainty: You now have this vicious killer. With this gut-wrenching news having been dumped upon me, over the phone, on Friday, Jane and I spend a portentous weekend—alone, with no one knowledgeable to turn to—in the terrifying, but undeniable world of cancer diagnosis.

A week later: I'm lying on a hard Formica table in the nuclear medicine department at the community hospital. I've been injected with a radioactive substance that's supposed to further define the liver, the spleen. Both or either of these organs is thought to be 'the mass,' or involved with the mass seen on the CT films. Radiologists are trying to rule out certain conditions with this test.

"Hey!" the gregarious girl operating the scanner whispers in staccato fashion, positioning my torso just so. *"You're—the—one!"*

"I'm the one . . . *what?*" I respond cheerlessly.

"The one nobody knows what to do with. They're *all* talking about you."

These remarks, probably made in innocence, are like tiny drops of acid on the flesh, startling. "So, you're saying what? I'm some kind of anomaly?"

"Heavens, no. I didn't mean it that way. Usually these guys—the doctors—get a bunch of other radiologists together and come up with something. But with you—" she pauses, watching a flickering image on her screen, "they're all saying different things. I hear them talking. If you ask me," she continues studying her screen, "it's your spleen. That's what's out of whack."

At this point in my medical history, I know I have something called a spleen. I don't know exactly what it's for. Within a day or so, I get a reading on these nuclear tests in a face-to-face meeting with a disheveled, gray-haired radiologist.

"Your spleen . . ." he comments, clearing his throat, wrinkled hands gesticulating awkwardly, "you can live without. Yours, it looks like, is enlarged. For whatever reason." He's now shaking his head, emphasizing the lack of reason. "This happens. We're not sure why. The good news is: It's not serious. You have nothing to worry about. It'll go back to normal in time . . . your spleen."

Still a firm believer in TDKB, I don't question his learned findings. He's the specialist, the expert—remember? An instantaneous implosion of relief, of euphoria, fills me. I'm home free—no stinking cancer! Time to get out the confetti and celebrate!

Little did I know . . . . This was to be my first experience with misdiagnosis.

FINDING HOPE WHEN DOCTORS SAY THERE IS NONE

CHAPTER 2

REVERSAL OF FORTUNE—
FROM NOTHING TO THE KNIFE

This meeting with the radiologist, then, ends on a positive note. Clearly there's a little something to be concerned about, but nothing that won't rectify itself. Go away on its own. No reason to fret.

Jane and I crack a bottle of frosty champagne; revel a bit in this wonderful news.

"This radiologist, doctor something-or-other," I'm clarifying as Jane empties her second glass, "said in time the spleen will repair itself. Go back to regular size. I don't need to do anything."

"I'm so delighted," she sighs, touching her glass to mine, an expression of relief on her face. "You had me worried."

Weeks later: A recurrence of the now-familiar flu-like symptoms occurs. The after-meal bloatedness and swelling now begins cropping up more often. The other, more unspecific indications—including the freakish nightmares—return as well. This damn spleen business isn't righting itself like it should!

A Friday night bowl of chili and crackers leaves me suffering miserably, feeling acutely bloated. It's around nine o'clock.

"I'm feeling really lousy again. Like I'm going to explode," I lament to Jane. "Why don't we go to Urgent Care so somebody there—somebody new—can check this out?"

I'd resolved to take this strategy principally to get a fresh set of doctor's eyes on the problem. Deep down, I wasn't really satisfied with the disheveled radiologist's findings. They just didn't ring true. Inherent pessimism, call it. Or maybe it's because when a physician speaks of cancer and you in the same sentence, you don't lightly put the perception aside.

At the HMO's Urgent Care office I'm examined by a thoroughgoing, young nurse practitioner. Initially I take offense at being downgraded to someone less than a doctor. But as this very precise nurse checks my vital signs, she's inquiring about my general fitness. Next, she's palpating (feeling) my stomach. Remarkably, this hands-on exam is something none of the physicians prior to her had done.

Lying there, keeping an eye on this nurse as she explores my midsection with skillful, persuasive fingers, I catch her eyes flaring for just an instant as she bears down on the area beneath my left ribcage.

"Find something?" I inquire, rising up on one elbow.

"Please, Mr. Scribner, do not move," she cautions, motioning for me to remain positioned exactly as I am. "I'm going to get a doctor. We'll be right back."

Glancing at me, Jane closes her magazine. "What was that all about?"

"Did you see her? When she pushed in here—her eyes?"

"I was reading. Sorry."

"She shoves in right here and gets this weird, wide-eyed Uh-Oh look. Like something scared her."

"Well, sure. It's that spleen thing again. You told her, right?"

Before I can reply, the nurse practitioner re-enters, doctor close behind. A spirited, polished-faced guy, Dr. Jones has a sound handshake, a charitable smile. Appearing unduly composed, yet methodical, he's behaving as though he's been forewarned of some serious abnormality. Feeling my belly—no telltale flash appears in his eyes—he invites me to talk about my recent medical history.

"So, doctor," I ask, after filling him in, "it's the spleen again, right?" He'll agree, I anticipate, informing the nurse to relax—nothing's out-of-sorts here.

"I'd have to hypothesize differently," he replies, staring straight forward, still groping deeply in the tissue of my gut. "In fact, I want you to see your primary-care doctor tomorrow. We're going to request further x-ray studies."

"I just had a CT. The radiologist said I had a distended spleen. No big concern. It'll go back to normal in time—by itself."

"All the same," this young doctor urges, folding his arms tightly, "I'd like to see you have another exam. We'll ask for more coverage this time."

"Another scan?"

"At this point, Mr. Scribner, while we can't say for sure," Dr. Jones is smiling affably, "I'd like to have another. I'm going to request both abdomen and chest."

"So," I continue, now quite uneasy, "you're saying then . . . it could be more than just the spleen?"

"I'm not saying anything explicitly, Mr. Scribner. But promise me you'll comply. It's absolutely vital that we eliminate certain things."

With some nervousness, the subsequent day I call my GP. She squeezes me in two days later. By then she's spoken with the Urgent Care doctor. Another CT's been ordered for the following week, she tells me without fanfare. She doesn't have time to embellish. Again I'm blindly following directions—still in the grasp of TDKB.

Three days after this CT, the phone in my office rings.

"This is Dr. Sydney, the radiologist you spoke with earlier this month. I want you to know we sent your new films out and had them reviewed by various other doctors."

"But," I acknowledge with all the suspicion, all the impatience I can muster, "everything's already been decided—I have an enlarged spleen."

"Not quite. Some things we still can't nail down."

"It was you who told me it was my spleen, right?"

"—And most of us still think it is."

"So, what's the point in sending the films to other doctors?"

"Because, Mr. Scribner," he replies, pausing only briefly, "they want to operate."

"What? Who wants to operate?" A nervous flow of blood's streaming into my now—cramping stomach.

"They want to go in and see unequivocally what we're dealing with. Exploratory surgery. In all actuality, you should be appreciative of our catching this."

"—Appreciative, doctor? My brain isn't even registering any of this. My spleen's screwed up, I thought. Now all that's out the window?"

"This, I know, is catching you off guard, Mr. Scribner. Dr. Lutes will be the surgeon. I strongly endorse your meeting with him. Tomorrow. Here at the clinic. He's very proficient."

One minute the radiologist tells me this, the next he's gone. Phone's dead. No one seems willing to extend a hand, saying, 'Here's what we're dealing with . . . and here's what we want to do and why.' HMO doctors, it seems, just don't function that way.

That evening, after a full day's work, I'm feeling enormously washed out, lying on the carpeted floor by the bedroom window that overlooks the Pacific, recounting for Jane the radiologist's call. "—And, the doctor tells me all of this over the phone. Can you believe that? Like can we get any more impersonal? Do doctors do anything face-to-face anymore?"

"But . . . how can he be saying this?" Jane's wondering, sitting on the bed, above me, peering down. "This is the same guy who told you not to worry, right? Are these people on the same page—or are they all this incompetent?"

"Evidently there's more to it than I was first told," I reply, watching the soothing Pacific lap the shoreline. "Guess I knew there would be, all along."

Jane's ordinarily—not always—more placid, more reflective than me: "Are you, since all this is new to us, blowing this out of proportion?"

Rolling over, transferring my stare to the white ceiling: "Not actually. Something fairly ominous is going on inside me. I can feel it. Sixth sense kind of thing."

"Just because one of these bone-heads brought up cancer. You're not thinking—"

"I'm getting panicky, hon. A person can tell when something's really wrong . . . . You just know."

"Eric," Jane says, assuming a kind of sudden standoffishness, "you know how you get sometimes."

"C'mon, let's stay together on this . . . I can honestly say something's wrong."

That night, as I had many a night before and thereafter, I get little, if any, sleep. The word cancer is all consuming, poised like a neon sign in the expansive gloom. Obsessive mental pictures . . . my father . . . the cancer that destroyed him. I see myself fading in a sustained, slow death . . . .

My former father-in-law, a robust individual one day, a fragile cancer patient the next, passed away of colon cancer some 23 years back. Just 44 years old, he was. Me, an innocent 24-year-old. More discerning family members had retreated from the hospital room . . . to stand, peering through an eight-inch slice of window in the door. My father-in-law's weak fingers were clutching mine. Never had I experienced mortality—life slipping from one's body.

The moon, a bluish gaunt sliver, arcs across one windowpane then the next, till it vanishes in the Pacific. In the violet light of daybreak, I crawl cautiously from bed, heavy with a feeling of bleakness. The remainder of my life seems now proscribed. Shaving, I visualize the surgeon—a devil-like little man—sitting cross-legged on the bathroom counter, sneering, telling me how and where he's going to slice me.

"Better this morning?" Jane asks sprightly, punching me gently, reaching around my waist to snag some personal cosmetic.

"Here I am, 47 freakin' years old," I reply, looking at my reflection in the mirror. "My health ain't supposed to be an issue."

"Want I should be there—at the surgeon's?"

"Nothing I can't handle," I hear the macho side of me reply.

"Don't forget—call as soon as you know."

Dr. Lutes is systematic, a personable guy in his sixties. Of stocky build, he's about five-foot eight, sporting a crisp white shirt, knit tie, burnished wingtips; clean-shaven, both face and head; a reddish, hygienic look about him.

"Mr. Scribner . . . what it looks like we have," Dr. Lutes is saying, circling an indistinct grayish outline on my backlit CT film, "is a mass on or near your spleen. That's the reason we're recommending surgery. The issue will be resolved one way or the other. Are you aware that seven different radiologists analyzed your films? You, young man, are a celebrity. In a way you probably don't want to be, though."

"There's no way around this? You're sure?"

"A biopsy was discussed," he replies, nodding thoughtfully. "I had to decline. Too risky. Too much chance of hemorrhage. Then we'd have no choice—but to go in, right there and then."

Following his gesticulating hands, I frankly anticipate seeing something singular about them: He is, after all, a surgeon. (That caught up am I in this exalted TDKB thing.)

Feeling utterly detached, sitting there, having a doctor tell me anything but that I had a cold and had to drink lots of fluid, I somehow surrender my orientation . . .become an out-of-body bystander, asking questions for this alien being who's become me.

"An incision here," the surgeon goes on, casually running his forefinger under my left ribcage. "Ten, maybe 14 inches long. Three to four days in the hospital. A month off work, maybe."

Can he be talking about . . . *me?*

FINDING HOPE WHEN DOCTORS SAY THERE IS NONE

CHAPTER 3

FEAR... AND FRAZZLED NERVES—
GETTING READY FOR SURGERY

In a meat-locker-size examination room, I disrobe. Dr. Lutes begins a very thorough physical exam. About him there's the faint but pleasant aroma of Juicy Fruit gum. He's not chewing anything, however.

While his hands don't look special, they're quite forceful. Fingers dig painfully into my armpits, into the place where the legs join the torso, into the collar-bone area. The exam is among the most thorough I've ever undergone. He checks ears, fingers, teeth, throat, and feet—you name it. He even probes and massages my prostate. This is a fellow who doesn't like surprises.

"So how do I stack up, doc?"

"If I hadn't seen your CT, and had to go by what I see here today," he says, pulling off his latex gloves, "I'd say you were one healthy male, one *very* healthy male. Even your teeth are exceptional."

The words infuse me with confidence, hope. "So—" I jest nervously, but actually seeking a straightforward answer, "why don't we drop this whole surgery idea?"

"Seems a contradiction, doesn't it? You look good, you feel good, but we know something's not quite right," he says, putting on a medical face. "Wasn't too many years ago we didn't have CTs that allowed us to look inside people with that kind of detail."

"So..." I continue reluctantly, "what do you think it is? This thing in me?"

Dr. Lutes seems hesitant to answer. "A lot of people have looked at your films. Smart people. And nobody seems sure. Certainly, I don't want to guess."

In me is the urge to ask if he thinks it's cancer. But fear, trepidation, makes me back off.

"What if... it is cancer? Will you—" I pause, recalling a newspaper story of a patient who'd undergone some sort of surgery only to have the doctor sew him back up because of invasive cancer in the area, "—have to call in another surgeon. A cancer surgeon?"

"Mr. Scribner," Dr Lutes replies almost sarcastically, "there is no such thing as a cancer surgeon." (This is untrue. There are many surgeons who specialize in cancer surgery, especially at the large comprehensive cancer centers throughout the United States.)

A framed photo on the wall, a gleaming green and red racing car with the doctor standing next to it, catches my eye. "That yours—that car?" I ask, hoping to secure a further link, a deeper bond between him and I—something beyond this mystery disease and knife.

"Hobby of mine," he replies, his voice immediately becoming more amiable. "It's how I unwind—build and race drag machines."

A conversational pathway opens. Something Dale Carnegie said in his book. The surgeon and I talk horsepower and mechanics for a good ten minutes. At one point he laughs to himself. "When I bring this monster to the line (starting line at the drag strip), the guy opposite me frequently thinks he's going to somehow intimidate me. He doesn't know what I do for a living. Nothing panics me." As he talks, I imagine him sitting behind the wheel, bald as a newborn, grinning wildly at his opponent.

Dr. Lutes is much looser, more comfortable, now leaning against the wall. By the time I leave, we've established a thin bond of camaraderie. This is good for the patient's well being: you want to know the guy who's going to be cutting on you. (Of course at this point I didn't know I should've checked into his record, his credentials—malpractice suits, that sort of thing. Not that these issues came to matter in the long run. But again, I was lulled by TDKB.)

Afterward I call Jane.

"What about you—how did you do?" she asks.

"We talked a lot about cars and that kind of stuff. The guy smells of Juicy Fruit. Gives you a good feeling, like he's a kid someplace inside. And he doesn't have a hair on his head."

"Again, I ask: What about you? What did he say? Anything new?"

"I really am having a hard time coping with this whole business," I respond. "Doesn't seem like it's me we're talking about."

"He . . . offer any ideas? About what this thing might be?"

"Said I'm one healthy male. That he's never seen anything like me—or this thing in me, actually—in all his years. Least he was honest. One thing's for sure: he's not scared of anything. That's nice to know. Seems like a competent, decent guy. Guess he's been doing surgery since the mid-fifties."

"He's that old?"

"Maybe sixty. Lots of experience."

"Well, I'm glad you're comfortable with him. I just wish you could've gotten more answers."

"Surgery's next Tuesday. Seven a.m. They want me there at five. Oh, and four days before, I have to stick to a clear-liquid diet—nothing but water, Jell-O, apple juice. Stuff like that."

"Lucky you."

Despite all the advances in medicine in the past few decades, my case still baffled them. They were going to resort to the tried-and-true method: the knife. I had no idea what they were going to find. A guy at work told me of his friend who'd had a grapefruit-size tumor removed from his stomach that proved to be nothing—a benign growth. But I had my fears. I did, however, manage to shift my focus from cancer to the possibility that they'd find some anomaly, something as harmless as a clog in a sink, some thing that shouldn't be there. Afterward we could all chuckle about it. Then I'd get on with my life.

Most of the folks at Rockwell were aware of the mystery surgery I was scheduled to go through. My boss, a guy younger than me by some ten years, with little actual worldliness or maturity, often referred to the unnamed thing within me as 'The Alien.' Something the doctor's knife would allow to fly out of my stomach—like in the movie of the same name. Other co-workers were more sympathetic, especially the older ones. Either way, I tried to remain unaffected and maintain a sense of humor.

The day before surgery, I brought a can of Campbell's beef bullion to work for lunch. Rather than eat the stuff cold, something that didn't sound too tantalizing, I go to the neighboring engineering department and ask if I can use their secret microwave oven. Since this was a company no-no—a department having a hidden microwave—I explain to a secretary/friend the real reason I'm eating bullion.

"Oh, my God, you poor dear," she breathes, hand to her breast, leading me to the secret microwave. Her over reaction and concern rekindles fears, as I trail along behind her, about what the doctor might find.

"Frank Logan, you remember him," she goes on, "just passed on, last week." She's a small woman, fifty plus, wearing a cheap wig, too much facial powder. All and all, a very sincere but misguided lady. *"—Cancer,"* she whispers emphatically. "Only found it a month before . . . .But, hey, what am I saying," she announces perkily, suddenly aware of the gloominess of her conversation, "—yours won't be anything like that. Frank was old, retired."

This was the first time I realized that people—at least people around me—feel compelled to report to you all the gory details of the cancer deaths they're aware of. This is somehow supposed to make you feel better. You hear about aunt so-and-so who was yellow as a lemon, nothing but skin and bone, in agony for weeks—"No, months come to think of it"—before she 'passed on.'

Then of course you hear innumerable stories of the people—both young and old—who are sliced open only to be stitched back up because they're 'already too far gone.' And the whispered conclusion: "It was everywhere—the cancer."

Finally these stories, both before and after my surgery, became so commonplace, so upsetting, that the moment I see one coming I advise the storyteller to say something positive, or not say anything at all. Most people stop right there, and smile blushingly: Through some twisted sense of insight, they actually thought they were doing me a favor by relating these horror stories. Even my own mother-in-law laid a few He/She-Died-An-Untimely-Cancer-Death stories on me before I had to tell her, too, to cool it.

The night prior to the surgery I had to give myself a Fleet's enema—something I hadn't had since childhood—at precisely 10:00 p.m. My entire system, according to the surgeon, had to be purged, flushed clean. As I lay on the cold bathroom floor administering the enema, that lonely sense of isolation resurfaces—you're doing this alone—making me shiver. The rug's coarse against my side, the tile icy where it touches bare skin. For many long minutes I lay there, staring at the where the walls and the floor came together under the sink, wondering dispiritedly, "Is this truly me?"

By the time Jane and I get to bed, I feel very light, empty—both emotionally and physically.

"By this time tomorrow," she says reassuringly, "this'll all be behind you."

"Like that's supposed to cheer me up. I've never had any real surgery before—a damn tonsillectomy back in '68. I've always been so healthy."

"And you are now," she says, touching my arm, kissing me. "They won't find anything. You'll see. It'll be a big nothing."

Once the lights click off, I lay there, rethinking all of what's transpired up this point—and how, through all the tests and doctor-talk, the word cancer keeps creeping in . . . . What'll I do, I wonder, if it really is cancer?

4:00 a.m.: The alarm goes off. Pushing the button, I realize in an instant all the preliminaries are behind me now. I have to be strong, face the music. Mechanically I get up and shave, shower. The windows, still black with night. According to the surgeon's list of do's and don'ts, I'm not supposed to wear any cologne, aftershave or deodorant. I take care not to swallow any water as I brush my teeth. I tend to be an organized person, to follow directions.

Jane gets my things together in a small suitcase: robe, slippers and so forth for the stay in the hospital. Coming in the bathroom, she looks at me. We hadn't spoken thus far. She caresses softly my bare arm. "Holding up okay, babe?"

Part of me wants to open up, to cry like the scared child I really am. "Hey, I can do this."

CHAPTER 4

AWAY FROM INNOCENCE— UNNECESSARY POST-SURGICAL PAIN

Lonely gray-violet sunlight's just breaking on the distant horizon as we begin that incredibly long eight-mile drive to the hospital. No other cars on the road at this early hour. I—we—are alone. Early mornings I've always hated—this one's probably the worst. Jane is driving. Neither of us have much to say. If she has any fears, she's hiding them well.

Checking in at the admitting desk, I secretly hope there won't be anyone there, or that whoever is there will say this has been one nasty joke. We can all go home.

After check-in, Jane and I wait for the surgery prep nurse to appear. It's still not light outside. There are three other couples, equally intimidated by this process, sitting uncalmly on admissions' area couches waiting to be called: at least I'm not the only one. There's minor consolation in that.

All the others are called before me. Finally a lean, almost bony little nurse pushes open the large hallway doors and listlessly calls my name. She's reading from a clipboard.

After exchanging ritual greetings, apropos of the time of day and the hospital setting, Jane and I follow the nurse. After being weighed, having my blood pressure checked, and undressing, the nurse—Carla, by name—begins shaving my chest, whole abdomen, pelvis, and armpits.

"Least . . . " Carla offers, making small talk, rinsing her disposable razor in a plastic pan, "you don't have AIDS."

"Is that supposed to be comforting?" I reply. "—And what brought that up, anyway?"

"Nothing really. Your blood work."

"I hadn't even given that any thought at all. I already have enough to worry about."

"They check everybody. Doctors want to know. Before," she adds, whispering.

"Anything else of interest in my blood?"

"Nope. All looked pretty normal."

FINDING HOPE WHEN DOCTORS SAY THERE IS NONE

Carla turns out to be quite humane, even soothing. She wishes me well, and tells me to make sure the floor nurses are there to help me walk the day after surgery.

Donning a hospital gown, I'm told to climb on a gurney. A youngish guy, kind of reformed bad-ass-looking fellow, pushes me down the empty hallway to the elevator. He's smiling thinly, saying not to worry—sure, like he's been here. In the pre-op holding area, another nurse—this one quite serious and professional appearing—introduces herself as Dorothy, then expertly guides a needle into a vein in my arm, starting the IV. She's explaining, as she goes, that the doctors will be in shortly, if I have any questions. Jane and I have since parted company—no 'civilians' allowed in the pre-op holding area.

A very ordinary-looking middle-age man with a thin black mustache—my anesthesiologist—introduces himself sleepily, choking back a yawn, and explains his role. Into a port in the IV tubing he inserts yet another needle—something to relax me, he says.

The operating room's where I first make eye contact with Dr. Lutes, my surgeon. There's an element of comfort in seeing a familiar face in this very unfamiliar place. He seems methodical, efficient, shaking my hand, taking charge, and telling me to relax.

Last thing I remember, prior to being awakened, is a blazing white light centered directly over my body. Now, through the thick fog of anesthesia, an illogical woman's voice is whispering directly into my ear: "Mr. Scribner! ... Mr. Scribner!" Her voice was strong, direct. "Mr. Scribner, it's over. We're through. You can wake up now."

A massive, burning sensation—my first conscious perception—is ripping at my midsection. An incredible sense of shock like nothing I'd experienced before. The impaling torture's like something you might expect if someone had maliciously torn you open using a dull chain saw, with no anesthesia.

Writhing, the last thing I want to do is become more conscious. Or move. Groaning miserably is all I manage. Barely audible, through clinched teeth, I try to describe my sense of agony to the nearby nurse.

"Doctor—" I hear her say quietly, but insistently, "the patient needs more morphine. Pain's pretty severe, he's saying."

The doctor's unconcerned voice: "Give him some more—but he's close to the threshold."

Listening to them speak, hearing their words in a sort of surreal nightmare, I'm fading in and out of this gray, this impaling consciousness. This abhorrent pain, like a rabid dog, is following me relentlessly, ripping at me, growling, and remaining intolerable. Sensing Dr. Lutes' nearness, I reach out like a desperate infant, clutching his hand . . . attempting to transfer to him some of the agony I'm feeling.

My next awakening . . . hours later in a regular semi-private room. (I say 'regular' because I've since learned I should've been in Intensive Care due to the extensive surgery, blood loss). My bed is next to the window, not that it matters. An elderly gentleman in the next bed is apparently hard of hearing—TV's up loud.

Relentless pain continues emanating, nonstop, from my midsection to all points throughout my body. So massive is its grip that I can't even move or roll on my side. Opening my eyes, I see my 28-year-old son, Marc, and Jane. Despite the overwhelming pain, I feel the urge to offer a polite, upbeat greeting, but can't. The fog of surgery, the immense wash of pain, clouds all thoughts, vision, and abilities. I can't pretend all's well.

"Is it that bad, Pop?" Marc asks quietly, taking my limp hand.

"Like nothing before," I manage to mumble, trying not to move a muscle. "Rather be dead."

Morphine's only knocked the pain back a bit—it's still a rabid dog, ripping at my midsection. Surgery, I later learned, took almost six hours and required seven units of blood (pints to you and I) because of the vascularity of the 'growth.'

Jane, standing next to the bed, seems to have adopted an I've-Had-Two-Kids, Don't-Tell-Me-About-Pain attitude. "They don't know what it was yet," she's saying. "It was big, that much they know."

Despite the pain, the grogginess, part of me feels anger and wants desperately to know what this living thing was they removed from me. "Can you . . . find out . . . more?"

"Just rest now," Jane insists, putting me off. "We'll keep checking."

"Damn it," I mutter at her blasé attitude, "can't somebody find out? Now!"

A nurse, standing by quietly till now, offers, "Pathology usually takes time, Mr. Scribner. Nobody can say till then."

"What . . . about . . . this . . . awful pain?" I ask reluctantly, feeling somehow less of a man.

"We're allowed to give you an injection every two hours," the nurse replies kindly. "Doctors orders. He controls everything. Is it really that bad—the pain?"

"It'd feel better if I was dead!" I moan irritably, believing my condition should be obvious.

Jane's looking at me oddly—like I'm acting childishly, or being rude. A sense of anger festers in me—how can someone who's supposed to love me remain so aloof? She says: "We should go and let you sleep."

Now I'm in pain *and* feeling deserted.

"I can't sleep—I hurt too bad!" I moan, looking toward the blank ceiling for sympathy.

After another morphine injection, in the butt, I drop into a light, unsatisfying sleep. Not at all the kind of drugged stupor I'd hoped for. Morphine, I thought, was supposed to be powerful enough to carry you off to some blissful, dreamy state—far from it. Old war movies had painted an erroneous picture.

The massive, tormenting pain recedes only partially, into the uncarpeted hallway, it seems. Lurking there, at arm's length, laughingly, it's awaiting its next opportunity to growl, to pounce.

To add to the misery, late that night, with the hospital window open wide due to the unseasonably balmy weather, there came a riotous din from the parking area below. Car engines revving . . . . Motorcycles screaming up and down the street . . . rubber squalling on pavement . . . people laughing convulsively, yelling loudly—very loudly.

Apparently I'd been sleeping lightly, off and on. In addition to my on-going surgical pain, I now have a booming headache. My throat is bone dry, raw. The din from below brings me back to reality—a reality I don't want—as if someone's slapped me hard in the face, re-establishing that intense burning sensation below my ribs.

My finger crawls to the nurse's button. Five minutes go by. Ten. Still no nurse. After about fifteen minutes she arrives, none to happy that I'd rang several times. An older woman—heavy-set, bleached blonde—this nurse in no way pretends to be sympathetic.

"I can give you a shot, but that noise, honey, you'll have to live with. It's Yolanda's Mexican restaurant. Closing down for the night. One-forty-five on the button. You can set your watch by it." The stocky nurse stands by the open window, gazing down into the parking lot as if to confirm her words. "Happens every night. Think this is loud? You should hear it when the hospital chopper delivers somebody."

How can any human being cope, I wonder, unable to sleep. The pounding headache, the burning throat, the pain . . . the raucousness below.

After maybe five more minutes, she returns with a syringe. Roughly pulling my lower torso toward her, she causes a new level of pain to explode across my midsection. I wince badly. She swabs a spot on my rear, plunging in the needle.

"Will that get rid of . . . this headache?" I ask, thinking if morphine can't knock out a headache, nothing can. "And my throat . . . it's really dry . . . . Can I get a sip of water?"

"No fluids, sugar. Doctor's orders. Nothing orally. Your throat feels bad because of the tubes they stuck down there. Some patients are allergic to morphine. *Gives* them headaches."

The drug, once injected, seems to take a fortnight to kick in. Time drags ahead, minute by minute, on throbbing waves of pain. The clamor below continues. I ring for the nurse again.

"Are you saying . . . there's nothing you can do?" I demand weakly, angrily. "About this pain and all that damn noise?"

"Been like this for years, sugar," is her simple reply as she strolls from the room. "We can always shut the window, but then you'd roast."

Advice: Any time you're going to have surgery, be absolutely sure to talk frankly with your surgeon—*before the surgery*—about the sort of pain relief he plans to provide and how long he will provide it. Never *assume* automatically that you'll receive adequate pain relief—*be sure.* If pain relief is *not* a priority, make it one. There's no reason for you to suffer unduly following surgery—in fact, with proper pain relief you'll not only feel much better, but you'll be able to move about more freely and will heal more rapidly.

FINDING HOPE WHEN DOCTORS SAY THERE IS NONE

CHAPTER 5

A TIME OF RECKONING—
THE ROOKIE PATIENT STRIKES OUT

The raging anger in me only serves to heighten the non-stop pain. Truly, I'm feeling miserable: My head's pounding horribly, my throat's stripped raw, the incision's like a fire in my gut, and now there's a sticky film of sweat forming between me and the lower sheets. None of this can I shut out with sleep.

Throughout the night—if I am able to doze off—someone enters, nosily, flipping on the overhead lights, drawing blood, taking my temperature and blood pressure. They—the nurses' aides and young lab technicians—don't seem to care in the least that a patient's in pain, is desperately in need of rehabilitative sleep.

Some time around three or four in the morning, a couple of nurses began a boisterous conversation outside my closed door. Some party they'd attended that evening's the focus of all their hilarity. I squeeze the red call button, asking the desk nurse if she can please do something to stop all the chatter outside my room. She'll look into it. Nothing comes of it.

I go virtually all night with no sleep whatsoever. Despite the oppressive pain, the extreme discomfort of this airless room, no one seems to care.

Is it just me? Or is this modern medicine in action?

Around dawn, the real tumult begins. My throat's dehydrated, feeling as if the walls have painfully adhered to one another. I can't even swallow. I've had less painful cases of strep throat. This unfortunate realization dawns on me: *no one's going to relieve my discomfort, my misery.*

At around 7 o'clock a small, sour-puss nurse barges into the room as if she owns it, telling me it's time for a pain injection. Taking this opportunity, I unload a bit on her—about all the noise, the inattentive nurses. This doesn't sit well with her. Not at all. Her already dour demeanor changes for the worse. After rudely throwing back the sheets and pulling me roughly toward her, I watch her raised arm come down sharply. Suddenly I feel the violent, vindictive bite of the needle she's slammed angrily into my buttocks.

Now I'm ready to fight, but what to do? In cutting off my nose to spite my face, I resign to tough it out—I'll show them—no more of these pain injections;

these opportunities for the nurses to take their anger out on me. The shots always come too late, anyway, and the aggravation just isn't worth it.

Seven-thirty: Dr. Lutes appears quietly in the doorway, looking all neat and clean in a pressed white shirt, tie, and black wingtips. At seeing him, a sense of empowerment courses through me: Now there'll be some action. He'll do something about the God-awful noise, the pain, the nurses. He cares, he's my doctor . . . These damn nurses will get their come-upance now.

After a brief greeting, he lifts the sheets, then my gown, glancing at the intact dressing, feeling it coarsely here and there. "Has anyone touched this? Lifted it or done anything?" he asks suspiciously.

"Were they supposed to?"

"They better not. I left strict orders not to tamper with it."

"Generally," I say, with a good deal of strain, figuring this news will spark some ire in him or at least elicit a probing question, "the nurses did as little as possible. All night."

"Still having pain?" he asks disinterestedly, standing, placing his hands on his hips. The smell of Juicy Fruit once again follows him, but now the sugary scent—is it some kind of weird cologne—has a stomach-turning effect.

"There's never been any let up," I reply. "And all night," I go on weakly, "it was so noisy in here a dog couldn't sleep. The nurses don't come when you call them. It's way too hot. And at two in the morning, the restaurant on the street below sounded like Mardi Gras time—"

"—They've had problems with that place for years," he concedes blandly, without resolution.

"But," I ask incredulously, "you can do something, right? I really need some sleep. I'm drained. I feel really bad."

"Not much I can do," Dr. Lutes replies vacantly. "Short of having them move you to another room."

"Can we at least," I continue, now realizing he's a head-in-the-sand leader—except when it comes to his sacred bandages, "increase my pain medication? I hate to sound like a baby, but . . . ."

"—They're giving you what?" He looks at my chart. "An injection every two hours?"

"If I can convince someone to come in here."

The doctor nods, dispassionately. "Sorry. That's about the best we can do. At this point."

"Well . . . what about food? When can I eat? Or have something to drink? My throat's like an old lake bed."

"Not till we get some indication your stomach's working. I have to hear gas sounds down there." Taking his stethoscope, he listens at several spots below my ribs. Shaking his head: "Don't hear anything yet."

"What about some ice chips then?"

"Nothing till we hear some stomach action. You'll cramp up otherwise. And if you think you're in pain now . . . ."

"Any news on my pathology report?" As I say this I hate the sound of the term 'my pathology report.'

"Still no word."

Jane comes in shortly after that. She kisses me, asks how the night's gone. But remarkably, she too, like everyone else, plays down the noise, the heat and the pain. Just sleep through it, she offers.

"Well, shit, doesn't anybody give a damn if a person's hurting or gets any sleep?" I shoot back, rekindling the deep-seated anger I'd felt during last night's bout with the noise, the nurses' attitudes.

"Honey, you have a way of blowing things way out of proportion." Moving a chair nearer the bed, she sits down. "I'm sure if it's as bad as you let on, the doctor or somebody would fix it."

"Son-of-a-bitch! You're supposed to be on my side. I hurt like I just fell face down in a bed of burning embers. You think I'm dreaming this up!"

"Eric, you get carried away. This is a hospital. Their job is taking care of people. Nothing can be as bad as you say."

"Thanks. I really need all this support."

Turning away, I stare out the window—wondering what process turns normally sympathetic people into ice cubes once they enter a hospital room. A new nurse comes in and introduces herself. She looks to be in her early thirties. Her name is Liz. She'll be with me all day, she says kindly.

Liz takes my vital signs for about the fiftieth time since midnight. "How's the incision," she asks, a genuine interest in her voice, "—the pain?"

"You *really* asking?"

Grimacing a bit, Liz smiles sweetly. "Sounds like your experience hasn't been all that great so far."

"All across here—the stomach's pretty bad. The incision. If you can imagine what it feels like to have somebody hack you open with a chain saw. I can hardly move. And I'm sweating a lot against the sheets."

"What did you have done? Let's see," she says, thumbing through my chart. "—Your surgery, I mean."

"The whole thing—exploratory surgery—took about six-hours. To take out some weird mass."

"Six hours. That's about as major as you can get. You are in pain. Poor thing."

It feels remarkably uplifting to have someone listen and sympathize.

"Says here that you can have 150 milligrams of morphine. Every two hours."

"I also have a killer headache."

"Probably it's the morphine," Liz explains. "Some patients react that way. You told the doctor? I saw him in here a bit ago."

"No. I didn't connect the two. I bitched mostly about the noise. Last night."

"What do we have to do," Jane asks, "to get him moved to another room?"

"Let me check and see what's available," Liz offers, standing to leave.

Several hours later, still in the same room, two nurses' aids appear in the doorway, proclaiming they're going to get me up for a post-surgery walk—doctor's orders. I try talking them out of it, due to the profound pain, the dreadful dizziness, the sliced-open sensation I'm still experiencing. They refuse to take no for answer. I decide, vindictively, to let them shoulder my entire load—the burden of my six-foot, 185-pound frame. Positioning themselves on either side of me, the nurses place their arms under my arms, and begin straining, lifting.

After some excruciatingly painful maneuvering, I'm almost standing, but leaning heavily, almost drunkenly, on the two small nurses. My head, due to the exorbitant pain and yesterday's anesthesia, is swimming dizzily. After maybe five steps, I feel very faint.

"Tell us you're not blacking out, Mr. Scribner!" one nurse says urgently.

"I told you," I reply gruffly, "I'm not well enough for this!"

By the time I get to the door, a distance of maybe ten feet, one nurse, breathing heavily, tells the other, "That's enough. Let's get him back."

In bed, my head's woozy. I feel on the verge of passing out. My heart's beating erratically. The two nurses look at me for a moment, then leave, having done their duty.

In all, I was in the hospital for three very unrestful days. Each day was basically the same, hour upon hour of unrelenting pain, daily treks down the corridor, nurses carrying on loudly at night. The new room I was finally given, on the other side of the hallway, offered better late-night soundproofing and temperature. I did, despite all, manage to sneak in some sleep in the afternoons.

Eight a.m. day four, the day I'm scheduled to go home: There are sufficient stomach sounds. I'm allowed to consume some Jell-O, a small bowl of tasteless soup. Dr. Lutes, standing bedside my bed, is unfolding the newly generated pathology report. He's repeatedly assured me 'the thing' he took out, described as looking like a volleyball, half deflated, was totally encapsulated. He'd 'gotten it all.' Good news.

Comforting words—especially to a cancer rookie.

Advice: Do not, under any circumstances, tolerate poor service or conditions in a hospital. Recognize that a hospital is first of all a business like a car dealership, a bank, or a hotel. In none of these enterprises would you tolerate substandard treatment. But somehow we look the other way when a hospital—an integral part of the sacrosanct medical establishment—treats us like second-class citizens.

Hospitals and their employees tend to feed on our—the new patient's—vulnerability.

When you're hospitalized and you're uncomfortable for any reason, let the nursing supervisors know about it. Politely demand a resolution. If this doesn't result in immediate corrective action, demand to speak directly to the hospital administrator, either in person or on the phone. He or she will definitely react when you explain your problem *and* that you're going to contact the hospital's accreditation agency unless something's done immediately.

This is the day of dog-eat-dog HMO medicine. Many HMOs and their affiliated hospitals rely on delay and avoidance tactics when you request something—a medical service for which you've already paid—from them. Unfortunately, if you, the patient, don't speak up for yourself . . . *no one will.*

FINDING HOPE WHEN DOCTORS SAY THERE IS NONE

Chapter 6

Ugly Words—
Reading of the Pathology Report

Warm early morning sun—this is California—beams brightly through the nearby window. The day, it seems, is off to a good start. I'm feeling upbeat, albeit still horribly sore, to the point where I hate to move. (I'd refused pain medication since the evil Nurse Ratchet incident.)

Standing over me, Dr. Lutes reads aloud the pathology report: this is his first reading as well as mine. Odd way to provide a patient with his status, I'm thinking. But I have no experience with surgery, with hospitals, with pathology reports. Maybe this is a good sign, my sense of TDKB is telling me.

Dr. Lutes' reading begins without expression. The report describes the mass in clinical terms, in millimeters, in kilograms. The words go on to say the specimen possesses a gritty texture when sliced.

"I spoke directly with Dr. Cooper—the pathologist—about this," Dr. Lutes states, looking at me over his glasses, an element of trepidation entering his voice. "I knew this was going to be a tough case," he adds candidly. Continuing, after a pause: "Eric, she uses the word 'carcinoma' here." He pauses again, reading to himself. "In the end her diagnosis describes the cell structure as being suggestive of adrenal cortical carcinoma."

Carcinoma! The word strikes with the impact of a thrown cement bag. My stomach instantly recognizes the term, cramping torturously.

"What's . . . that mean?" I ask, buying time, feeling a heavy weight of emotions: isolation, loneliness, a desperate hope that I'd misunderstood.

"Well," he goes on, slowly, vaguely, "what we do next is send you to see Dr. Drake. That's his bailiwick. We'll let him explain. He's an oncologist. Best in the county, too, for my money."

"What do I do . . . now?" I ask, feeling a new hollowness enter my life.

"Go home, take it easy for a few weeks. Have a good Christmas with your family. I'll set you up to see Dr. Drake. Try not to concern yourself."

"But . . . doesn't carcinoma always mean—"

"The body, Eric, is an odd machine," Dr. Lutes explains, interrupting, as if trying to somehow soften or sidestep this issue. "I've seen all sorts of oddities in my 35 years—some good, some not so good. Well, here," he says, reopening the pathology report, "the pathologist has included photos of the dissected mass. Let me show you what we've got."

Honestly, the last thing I want to see is a photograph of whatever it is they took out of me. But as he thrusts the pictures before me, I look. Two 3x5 color Polaroids taped to a page. There, in a stainless-steel surgical dish, sliced in two equal pieces, is the large, once-living thing. Still not referred to as a 'tumor' by anyone—the circular thing is shades of blood red and pale yellow, not unlike a grotesque pizza. I grimace as the image emblazons itself into my mind . . . that was growing in me, I think, feeling oddly violated. . . . My body produced *that?*

Immediately, I try pushing the grotesque pictures out of my mind. This much I knew: I never wanted to see or think of those photos again. Their realness hits too near home.

"Before you ask, we don't have any idea of how long it'd been there," Dr. Lutes offers, folding the report. "Pathology can't tell us that. Maybe six months, maybe six years . . . maybe longer. Consider the growth of a human embryo—" He pauses a moment, seized by a wave of apparent sympathy. "It goes from nearly nothing—an egg—to seven or eight pounds in a matter of months. The body, Eric, is capable of some pretty incredible feats. Not all of them, unfortunately, desirable."

Human nature being what it is, I don't want to ask—*do I have cancer?* He hasn't used that word yet. Maybe, I'm thinking to myself, again taken by naiveté, this is an okay kind of cancer—like a mild skin cancer—not some deadly malignancy that can spread and take my life.

"You sure you got everything, doctor?" I ask redundantly instead.

"I lifted it out totally encapsulated. There were many, many small veins that had to be tied off. That's the reason for the length of surgery and most of the pain you're feeling. But you've got to remember (I can see in his face he's being too honest, too soon), a mass within the body, in order to grow and survive, must have a supply of nutrients—blood flowing into and out of it—just like any other living thing. This is where the inherent problems come in. What I'm saying is . . . that blood, just as it does in the rest of your body, was flowing to and from your growth. . . . Follow me?"

"I . . . I . . . " I stammer absently, not thinking of anything, really, except the horrors of a cancer death.

"So," he goes on, "it's a bit misleading when we proclaim, 'we got it all.' We removed all we could see . . . but this is a systemic condition, Eric. There could be cells, released by the mass, anywhere in your body."

Feeling suddenly isolated, I really need someone nearby who cares about me, someone who'll touch me. "Is there any good news here?" I ask, feeling more desperate than I had in my entire life. Literally, I can feel me heart rate growing erratic.

48

"Her report, Dr. Cooper's, concludes that the cell structure is suggestive of malignancy. The word 'suggestive' leaves room for hope. So nothing's definite. This is why I want you to see Dr. Drake. He'll sort out the pieces."

Dr. Lutes thinks a moment, then moves ahead: "When you see him—Dr. Drake—one question I want you to ask: 'Where will I be in five years?' "

My insides go hot with a whole new kind of fear. "Don't think I follow," I say, lying. The crush of ordinary life, of gravity, has suddenly tripled. Nothing registers. I don't hear or see anything.

"I'm going to let you go home today . . . but I want you to remember that question."

Once he's gone, I lay there, alone in the hospital room, consumed by a dizzying swirl of morbid thoughts. I know, without him saying as much, I have cancer.

This single fearsome word echoes within as if it's fallen into a bottomless mine shaft. My soon-to-be-released-from-the-hospital cheerfulness is now gone, bleakly crushed, replaced by the deeply disturbing news that my own body's become a renegade, turning against me, creating its own form of threatening alien life.

"The idea of Christmas, doc," I whisper simply, aloud, to no one, to the empty room, "doesn't sound so hot right now." For maybe thirty minutes I lay there, the dire news having an immobilizing effect. With arms numb, feeling incredibly heavy, I hold the phone to my ear.

"It's—ah—me . . . . Yes, he was here. Said today's the day. I can go home . . . . What do you mean—'I don't sound right'?"

When I finally tell her, there's dead silence on the other end. Immediately I regret what I've done: giving my wife life-altering news over the phone. Perhaps I've become so accustomed, so inured to doctors doling out negative or distressing news over the phone. Doctors never seem to tell you anything anymore face to face. The phone's become their bad-news buffer.

The doctors told me I'd have to have more tests—over the phone . . . they told me they had no idea what this thing in me was—over the phone . . . they told me it could be cancer—over the phone. Welcome to the age of once-removed medicine.

Jane, normally a rock-solid person, is, when she walks in, crying openly. She, without saying as much, had adopted a tacit It-Can't-Happen-To-Us approach in all this. Now here she is, about to embark on a years-long cancer battle with me.

She's been in tears, apparently, since our phone conversation. Her reddened eyes look like a child's when they get sand in them. She actually tries hiding her sorrow with an attempted smile. But it comes out all cockeyed.

Hugging me, physically merging with me in a way that's never happened before, she clears her throat: "What did he say—exactly?...Oh, why wasn't I here!"

"No one knew when the report would show up. It wasn't your fault."

Seeing her like this makes me feel all the more sorry for having told her over the phone. But would face to face have been any better—any easier?

"He stood right where you are and read me the pathology report. He hadn't read it, either. It uses the words, 'suggestive of malignancy.' So . . . " I go on uncertainly, looking out the window at the blue, problemless sky, "it's not definite."

In that it's human nature cling to anything for hope, she now attempts another smile, wiping away fresh tears. I explain about Dr. Drake—the oncologist. This is a word—a key to a whole new ugly world—I don't recall either of us ever using before.

Still in considerable pain, I'm sent home from the hospital—four days after major surgery—without pain medication. Take aspirin or Advil, I'm told, which I do on an hourly basis. Advil, I quickly learn, relieves the widespread pain more effectively than aspirin. In the days, the weeks that follow, the physical discomfort subsides. But there's always that date with the oncologist to think about.

Advice: The most important doctor on your medical team is one you'll probably never see—your pathologist. This is a physician who, through his interpretation of your slides, sets the stage for *all* treatment to follow. If this doctor's wrong, off-base in his evaluation of your condition, your treatment's going to be wrong from day one. This, of course, can lead to dire consequences, even needless death.

I recommend: (1) meeting your pathologist face to face to get a 'between the lines' interpretation of what he's written up (at least one pathologist told me he'd jump at the chance to be the one who presents his findings to you so there's no error in what he meant), and (2) always, always, *always*, get at least one more opinion on your pathology slides.

More often than not you'll be amazed at how differently different doctors interpret these. It all boils down to this: A patient improperly diagnosed, because his pathology's been erroneously interpreted, is about to set sail on the wrong course, on the wrong ocean.

Always get a second opinion on your pathology slides.

CHAPTER 7

THE ONCOLOGIST—
AN EYE-OPENING FIRST VISIT

Having had other major surgeries since this one, I can see where Dr. Lutes' crude, minimalistic approach to medicine was affected by two things. First, he may've truly been old-school, having been trained under some twisted, out-dated system that believed the patient, in order to heal properly, should suffer. The more suffering, the better. Persistent agony . . . is that supposed to make the patient appreciate the recovery process or the surgeon's skill through some contorted sense of logic?

Or, second: Perhaps my early discharge and lack of adequate pain medication were a result of HMO-mandated cost-cutting measures. This I can only guess at. HMOs will do whatever they can to hold down costs. This euphemism actually means: All money saved is distributed to our executives who already receive exorbitant salaries at the expense of your medical care. How HMO execs can sleep at night, knowing other human beings are being denied adequate medical care under the guise of cost effectiveness, continues to astound me. Today, more than ever, you must stand up for your medical rights. You, unfortunately, must act as your own medical advocate.

In the ensuing weeks I'm able, as my physical condition improves—God knows how—to channel thoughts of the surgery and its grim findings into a narrow corridor of my mind, one I seldom travel. Thus I'm able to endure—if endure is the right word—Christmas.

Dinner that day, however, ends in misery. My cramping stomach bends me in half. I've somehow pulled apart the incision, I'm thinking. In time, in hours, the discomfort passes.

Since that first surgery, my stomach's never been like the old days. I've had to relearn, re-pace my eating habits. No more overflowing plates.

After Christmas some friends drop by unexpectedly. These are my first non-family visitors. Ed and Lori are dressed up—she in a lime-green full-length dress, he in an ill-fitting black suit and tie. They've been to some obscure dinner function in L.A. I'm sitting in the TV room—something I've only been able to do for short periods because of persistent pain in my midsection—when they arrive.

Ed, having known me for a good many years, comments without forethought, saying I look undernourished. "Mostly I can see it in your hands," he adds. Well aware of this, I don't appreciate anyone calling attention to it.

Now, realizing his faux pas, an awareness, a cautiousness creeps into Ed's voice. The hour-long, seemingly obligatory visit turns out to be, overall, rather pointless and tense. Though we've been close friends over the years, my guests seem, more than anything, repelled by my situation, as are many people. As adults we tend to insulate ourselves, to become tentative in the presence of someone who's been newly diagnosed with a fearsome condition like cancer.

The reason for Ed and Lori's uneasiness becomes apparent when, as they stand to leave, they reluctantly reveal that an intimate acquaintance of theirs, 'a big, muscular sort of guy of only forty-six,' had just died a month earlier. Cancer, of course. Ed's ill-fitting suit had been his friend's bequest.

By the time I go to the oncologist, four weeks have gone by. I'm feeling quite healthy—robust, in fact. My energy level's strong, my appetite good. I've even put on a few pounds. All of this says to me—the face I see in the mirror—that all's well. It's hard seeing yourself as having a serious illness when you feel so damn good.

I'm Dr. Drake's last patient that day. He, also a member of the HMO clinic that employs Dr. Lutes, occupies a drab, gray, windowless office on the second-floor—not unlike a jail cell—with matching drab gray metal desk, cluttered shelves, crammed bookcases. Untidiness seems somehow obliquely indicative of an oncologist's bleak line of work: Things out place, no finite conclusions in sight.

Jane and I sit across from this unemotional man, at his inhospitable metal desk—this tall, balding, bespectacled, Groucho Marx-looking character of about fifty, who has only greeted us indirectly minutes before. Studying he is, some Xeroxed sheets before him.

"My first impulse," he begins, moving his round spectacles in place with an extended thumb, "when Dr. Lutes told me about you, was that we were looking at a case of lung cancer—metastasized to the adrenals. This is not uncommon. But he assured me that wasn't the case. He said he'd reviewed your chest x-rays and they were clean. This was primary adrenal. And that's unusual."

Following 'Take a seat,' these are Dr. Drake's first words to his new patient. No get-acquainted preliminaries, no niceties.

Still extremely naive in these matters, still believing doctors are the supreme authority in all matters medical (a la Marcus Welby), I ask innocently: "Is this a serious kind of cancer, doctor?"

"I assure you it is, Mr. Scribner. And—" he continues almost huffily, "yours happens to be a very rare variety."

"Is . . . that bad or good?" I want to know, thinking rarity might equal intensified medical interest.

"Usually," he replies, nodding, "not good."

Having said this, he goes back to reading the multiple sheets in his hand. I glance at Jane. Nibbling she is her lower lip—as she does when she's unconsciously nervous. Over her shoulder, on a metal bookshelf, my eye, as if drawn to flashing neon, happens upon the title, *On Death and Dying*. Rather unfeeling of this man, I think, cringing, to have those taunting words so openly exposed. Salt in the wound.

"So," I begin slowly, weakly, "where do we . . . go from here?"

"That's what I'm working at," Dr. Drake says vaguely, his eyes still scanning the separate Xeroxed sheets. "Information on your type of cancer's not easy to come by. I retrieved some data from the NCI—National Cancer Institute—and the medical library."

It may be been petty of me, but I'm feeling uncomfortable with this man talking about *your type of cancer*. This kind of exclusivity I don't need. "—And what's it say?"

"What we'll do, I think, is send your slides—your pathology—to the California Tumor Tissue Registry. See what they think."

"But doctor," I say, hoping to redirect the conversation down a more affable pathway, "I feel great. Look great!"

"As you'll see, Mr. Scribner," the doctor replies, his face still expressionless, "how you feel plays only a minor role in the diagnosis and treatment of this disease. Some patients feel good almost to the end. I won't kid you. You won't find many oncologists who set up treatment protocols based upon how you look or feel. We rely on concrete data, test results: MRIs, CTs, blood work, x-rays."

"What's this tumor place you talked about?" Jane asks, her voice almost cracking.

With Jane's question, I realize this is the first instance where anyone's used that word—tumor. Its effect is immediate, ugly.

"I'm hoping they can confirm or shed some doubt on what Dr. Copper, the pathologist over at the hospital, has written up."

"She did say," I interject, trying add a sliver of enthusiasm, "it was *suggestive of malignancy*."

Dr. Drake nods pathetically, as if talking to a child. "You'll find that's the way they talk—pathologists; mostly to cover themselves—in the event of litigation."

"How long . . . before we know?" Jane continues. She uses a Kleenex from her purse. "—About the slides?"

"Couple of weeks would be my guess."

"And then?"

"Then we decide."

"Decide what?"

"Which course of treatment to take, of course."

"You lost us, I'm afraid, doctor," I put in, feeling a sudden stab of sharp pain.

"Follow-up treatment," he responds almost irritably. "Whether it's radiation or chemotherapy, or both."

These unsettling words, used in reference to me, I never thought I'd hear. But here I am, a 47-year-old adult, flesh and blood, sitting across from an oncologist—a cancer specialist—who's looking at me, using those very frightful buzz words. I'm feeling a shortness of breath. Once more, it's hard to believe it's actually me . . . sitting here . . . hearing this.

"He has to be *treated?*" Jane asks, a definite quavering to her voice.

"Seems obvious, Mrs. Scribner," Dr. Drake replies stoically. "This type of cancer requires action. From all I've read, it can be very aggressive."

"When you say aggressive—" Jane resumes, then pauses.

I'm watching her tearful eyes, thinking of Dr. Lutes' five-year question.

"Let me show you," Dr. Drake offers, grasping tightly one of the papers in his hand as if we might attempt to rip this treasure from him and run. "According to this NCI graph, your husband—who's either a Stage III, or Stage II at best—can expect to live maybe another year and a half at best."

"People . . . die of this?" Jane persists, in obvious bewilderment, still unwilling to accept that this is us sitting before this unfeeling doctor.

"Most certainly. This is very serious business. We may, however, be able to arrest it for a time. I'd rather not go into any of that now, though, or any of your what-if questions. Until we get back results from the tumor registry."

Descending the stairs from Dr. Drake's second-story office, Jane's become so rubber-legged, so teary, that I literally have to hold her tightly: She's that shaken by the oncologist's scathing conclusions. I, too, feel the full weight of his prognostications. But my reaction—my overwhelming first reaction—is one of disbelief. This can't be me—I feel too damn good.

In the following weeks, while waiting for the tumor registry's report, I do little other than take it easy. Or try to. Perhaps my own innocence or as I've said numerous times previously, my naiveté keeps me going. Something deep within, even this early on, tells me this disease is *not* going to put me under. With that determination welling inside, I have a strong foundation on which to build my recovery.

Alas, at this point I have no idea where to start.

I've been off work now for about six weeks. I'm feeling pretty good, physically. But lying around the house, knowing I have cancer and am doing nothing about it bothers me deeply. Always I've been a grab-the-horns kind of person. At this point an idea begins to germinate. That idea, or notion, is that as my enemy's growing in real proportions—the cancer—I have to do all I can to understand it. As most of us are raised to believe: In order to overwhelm an enemy, you have to know that enemy.

Thus with name of 'my cancer' scribbled on a piece of paper I head for the local library. I live in a relatively small coastal community. Our library isn't all that large—so, once I locate the sparse collection of medical books, most of them greatly outdated, and begin looking for information on adrenal cortical carcinoma, I find zilch. Dr. Drake said this was a rare condition and as such, little is going to be available, at least locally. (I didn't yet have access to a home computer or the Internet.)

Broadening my search, I locate a good bit of information on cancer in general. Fortunate am I to stumble upon several uplifting books; books that deal with cancer in realistic, but positive terms—as an often-curable disease if treated promptly and properly. I emphasize those words: promptly and properly. There is, as the doctors will tell you, usually one window of opportunity to treat the disease and, if that window's missed, the likelihood of affecting a cure or cancer-free state is greatly diminished.

Once the diagnosis is made you can never be too prompt or too thorough in your search for new information, for treatments. Cancer's a state-of-the-art disease—by that I mean treatments are changing rapidly, day by day—and no one, doctor or otherwise, can keep up with all the rapid-fire advances, especially when we're talking about a rare or sparsely documented cancer.

Among the first books I come upon—and thank God I do—is Annette and Richard Block's *Fighting Cancer*. Before checking it out, I thumb through it a bit. A sentence in the Introduction leaps out: "Cancer is the most curable of all chronic diseases." Several pages later, "Cancer is a word, not a sentence." Yes! Yes! Yes! Reading these two simple, yet profound observations infuses me instantly. I'm uplifted, my go-get'em spirit's bolstered. I read where Richard Block had, many years earlier, beaten the cancer 'they' said was going to kill him.

I can do the same!

If someone's beaten this disease, anywhere, anytime in this world, I feel suddenly, stubbornly, that I can too. In me now—and I know it sounds simplistic—burns a desire: a desire to carry the fight to whatever extent necessary to whip 'my cancer.' That day, I take home only a small armload of books. This I can definitely say is the infancy of my years-long, endless cancer-survival quest.

In my youth, in high school football actually, I learned something I'm able to dredge up, to use in my recovery quest: Our ever-pissed-off coach told us that in order to win, in order to succeed at any given task, you had to give at least 100% effort. At the time, some 25 years ago, his words rang of mathematics and pretty much fell on defiant teenage ears. Sure, we knew if we charged ahead at 80% and the opposing team came at us 100%, they'd kick our butts. They'd win the encounter. That seemed obvious. Not something we had to think about, or learn... or could ever apply to any other areas of our lives.

I hadn't consciously employed this 100%-approach to life, outside sports, till now. As I say, I could feel myself being infused with a new sense of strength, of determination. The fact that my father and father-in-law had succumbed to this disease no longer dominated my view of the cancer's absolute power.

Realizing little or nothing was written about my type of cancer, I begin expanding another of my naive notions: Since mine's a rare cancer, I'll get special attention wherever I go. I'll be cancer's Golden Boy. Doctors will be drawn to, intrigued by this rarity... I'll have papers written about me. Doctors I don't even know will gladly get involved—probably at no cost—just to learn more about this cancer, this adrenocortical carcinoma. I even imagine passionless Dr. Drake getting on the bandwagon, presenting papers at national cancer seminars. I might even be asked to tag along as living proof, like some crude circus act, that this rare disease does indeed exist. But then I've always been a dreamer.

Cancer is one of life's detestable eventualities—like the Gestapo or the mysterious and deadly IRS—which I never joke about. Bad, bad luck. So long as cancer remains distant, I don't have to question its domain, its role in my life. Knowing that my father died of the disease, however, causes me to believe, at times, that cancer's expansion is inevitable—my day is coming. Seems some researcher's always making headlines, connecting cancer and your bloodline. The unspoken message: When cancer wants you—a la the Gestapo or the IRS—it'll reach out and take you.

CHAPTER 8

IT'S ALL IN YOUR MIND—
HOW THE MIND AND BODY INTERRELATE

Reading takes me quickly down some rather mysterious roads. I uncover some extraordinary discussions on visualization, meditation, cancer diet, and something called the mind-body relationship. Seems we Americans tend to treat disease as though it were a separate entity, something not influenced by the mind. Yet other cultures recognize a major illness for what it is—a body-wide affliction.

Just as we humans are not independent of what takes place around us, neither is the mind—or body—independent of the other. In fact, the brain's been shown to think and communicate with other cells in the body by way of chemical messengers known as neuropeptides. White blood cells, a major component of our immune systems, for example, have receptors for these neuropeptides. And amazingly, white blood cells also have the ability to produce these same chemical messengers so that they, the white blood cells, can communicate with the brain. Thus the body is the mind, and vice versa. Each of us is . . . a body-mind.

The scientific study of how our thoughts, our feelings are transferred into chemical messengers that signal various systems within the body is known as Psychoneuroimmunology. This relatively new branch of research looks at the effects of stress on the nervous system, how our thoughts influence our immune system, and how all of this can result in aberrant cell division—malignancies.

To date, scientific research has discovered that nerve fibers actually terminate on the surface of white blood cells. This is further evidence that our immune systems 'talk' directly with our brains. To paraphrase Deepak Chopra, endocrinologist and author of several best-selling works on the subject: The immune system is constantly eavesdropping on the inner dialogue of the mind.

An important conclusion, this is. For unless a cancer patient has a death wish, and I've never known one who did, he/she is facing major, continuous psychological hurdles every minute of every day. Now that we've seen how the mind and body interrelate, we can also see how this stress-driven exchange between the two can be detrimental to our health, our healing. The immune system, under perceived conditions of stress (however that stress is defined), is in a suppressed state and becomes ineffective in eliminating malfunctioning cells—cancer—from the body.

Understanding that the mind can and does influence the body, gives new meaning to the relevancy of a cancer patient's strategic beliefs—primarily the belief that he or she can and will survive this disease. In other words what we think can and does positively or negatively influence our healing process.

In my early quest for alternative measures for combating cancer, I come upon numerous references to Buddhist philosophy and the mind-body connection. This isn't something—the mind-body connection—I'd ever really considered seriously. Eventually I find myself becoming more and more curious about how these highly focused people—Buddhists—are able live fully and appreciate the present.

How can this approach to life be beneficial to a cancer patient's recovery?

In Buddhist philosophy we get a sense of how the body and mind interact, and what it's like to see and feel each moment for what it actually is. This is something we cancer patients should strive to do. But seeing and feeling each moment isn't something we Westerners do intuitively, though we may believe we do. When someone tells us we must live, truly live each moment, it's frequently perceived as so many idle words. To really live the moment—and within the moment—we must actively participate and become acutely aware of the now. No easy task.

How often have you, for instance, had a bowl of ice cream and only really tasted the first couple of bites? Or driven through an intersection and asked yourself: 'Was that light green?' This occurs because we're most often living—thinking—in the future or past. You can only truly live in the present.

To acquire the ability to be mindful of each moment, we're required to experience the essence of reality, to recognize and appreciate it. We have to distinguish that all things are connected. (Just as we now recognize how the mind and body are connected.) We have to learn to appreciate the journey, to 'see' each moment with the five senses: sight, sound, touch, taste, smell. Only then can we say we're truly living in the moment. No easy feat, as I've indicated. The mind, it seems is always running off, doing its own thing.

Living in the moment is, in the truest sense, living. No longer are we wasting time dwelling in the spoils of the past or polluting the present with false or grim thoughts of the future. Because, after all, the present is, tangibly, all there is. The present is the only real moment—it's real in a way last year or tomorrow can never be.

In some literature on cancer survival, the authors claim it's beneficial to return to a busy state, and by this they're usually referring to your routine, everyday line of work. It's my belief, however, and the belief of notable others (e.g., Drs. Bernie Siegel and Carl Simonton), that just the opposite may be true. To truly recover from cancer you must change the life, the lifestyle, the employment, whatever caused or significantly contributed to your disease.

Getting rid of negative sources of stress, of discontent, no matter what they may be—a loveless marriage, an unfulfilling job, disagreeable living conditions, etc.—is perhaps the most positive step you can take in making your recovery a successful one. It has been for me—this, and other alternative measures, including the proper cancer-fighting diet, which we'll talk more about later.

Now that I've retired, acquaintances—those who don't understand one who's made peace with life—sometimes ask if I get bored 'doing nothing.' At first I made excuses, because I thought I was supposed to say 'Yes, I miss working at a hellishly stressful job and losing sleep nightly and biting my nails.' Now, however, I respond with a smile, saying, "I occupy time doing whatever I want. I'm never bored. Boredom's a negative, self-inflicted punishment."

A realization of life's design has raised me to the point where I can appreciate very simple things with undivided satisfaction. For when a doctor looks at you and declares you have cancer, your world instantly changes forever. And nothing's more precious than this minute, this life. This too seems trite . . . unless you've experienced this ominous occasion.

Fortunate enough am I to reside near the seaside—the great-hearted Pacific's just a stone's throw away. Sitting on the breezy beach using all five senses—even on a bleak, sunless day—provides a subtle sense of triumph, a serenity the body thrives on. This type of connectedness (as any good minister or Buddhist will tell you) with your surroundings, the forces of Nature and God, is vastly more healing than any of Man's wonder drugs.

Ask any experienced negotiator and he'll tell you the hardest person in the world to negotiate for is yourself. You have too much at stake to be unbiased. Stir in the uncertainties of a life-threatening disease and you have even more at stake. This is a major reason why, I believe, it's so hard for many patients to deal frankly with their doctors. Neither of you can take what the other says lightly . . . too much hangs in the balance. Thus it's best to have a third-party negotiator working for you.

The second visit with Dr. Drake comes roughly three weeks later. He still hasn't heard from the tumor registry. He has, however, further researched adrenal cortical carcinoma (now referred to as ACC) and come up with a specialist's name.

Prior to this visit with Dr. Drake, I asked Jane to play the heavy, to be the one who requests a second opinion. At least at this point I knew enough to seek a second opinion. She'd disagreed when I said he, Dr. Drake, would be put out by the request—that I didn't want to upset him or turn him against me, the patient. Many doctors have an over-blown sense of self and pride—and, in truth, many hate being questioned, especially by us lowly, know-nothing lay people. Against her will, Jane agrees to pose the second-opinion question.

"Not much is known or written about your type of cancer, I've found, Mr. Scribner," Dr. Drake begins, again thumbing through a sheaf of papers he's apparently pulled together on ACC. He's no warmer, more cordial today than our earlier visit.

Jane and I are again sitting across the mouse-colored metal desk.

"I was thinking doctor," I begin, not knowing quite how to present my thoughts. There's quiet for a moment while I consider things. "I mean, since this case, my case, is so unusual . . . I was thinking that maybe people—doctors, I mean—would be especially interested in me. In treating me, learning more about this weird disease."

It's here that Dr. Drake says something that fairly startles me.

A thin-lipped smile, he replies: "Quite the contrary, I'm afraid, Mr. Scribner. Most physicians—myself among them—feel they're never going to encounter this condition again, so why spend a great deal of time studying it?"

"But I thought—since it's so rare . . . there'd be *more* interest."

Shaking his balding head: "We just don't have time to go chasing after every rare illness. The best we can do for our patients is treat the diseases we're familiar with—the 'common' cancers, if you will—and leave the rare ones to specialists at medical schools."

"Then there *is* someone," I ask, feeling a spark of hope, "who understands this ACC?"

"You could say that," he offers vaguely. "The M.D. Anderson Cancer Center in Houston is supposed to be the authority, if that can be said. They're part of the University of Texas Medical School. Doing a computer search last night, I came across a name. When he and I talked this morning, he recommended adjuvant therapy—a drug called Mitotane; an oral chemotherapeutic agent. He recommends starting at eight to ten grams a day. Then working your way up."

For some reason I latch onto this strange word adjuvant and, hoping this is my sought-after loop-hole, ask about its meaning.

"Essentially it's a treatment we use as insurance, for lack of a better word—something that will hopefully prevent the disease from recurring. For a time, at least."

"So . . . then," I say, caught a little skewed, "I may not have ACC, after all? If this is just insurance?"

"That's not what I said, Mr. Scribner."

"But it is possible . . . that I don't have cancer, right? Dr. Lutes got it all?"

"Possible, yes. Likely, no."

"Okay, then. Would you say chances are good," I continue, sensing the tiniest positive note in all this, "—that it's gone? That I *don't* have it?"

"I don't like speculation nor do I like 'what-if' questions," Dr. Drake replies tersely, pushing his small round glasses back on his nose with the point of his thumb.

"Would you at least say," I persist, "there's maybe . . . a thousand-to-one chance it's not there?"

"Probably much higher, Mr. Scribner, like ten million-to-one. But we're not accomplishing anything here. We have to discuss the possible use of this drug."

Disappointed, I ask: "How long would I be taking this . . . drug?"

"There's the catch: You'd have to take it the rest of your life. And there are serious considerations and complications," Dr. Drake explains, sliding a Xeroxed sheet my way. "—Like first of all, its use may be considered experimental by your HMO, and thus not paid for. . . . It can cause severe side-effects, such as permanent loss of function in your remaining adrenal gland, diminished mental abilities, nausea, diarrhea, spaciness. . . . This drug, Mr. Scribner, could even kill you. And it's rather expensive. Around a thousand dollars a month."

Glancing quickly at the sheet he's given me, I see it is information detailing the side-effects of the drug he's talking about. This thunderstorm of confusing news, like most of the alarming revelations a patient receives when struggling with cancer and its vulgar treatments, sets me back. I've been taking quite a few vitamins daily for some time at that point, megadoses some would say, so the thought of taking additional pills—even 10 grams a day—didn't really concern me so much as the other issues: insurance coverage, unpleasant side-effects, possible death.

"What's the likelihood, doctor . . . of a cure?"

FINDING HOPE WHEN DOCTORS SAY THERE IS NONE

Chapter 9

The Second-opinion Mirage

Removing his circular glasses, Dr. Drake works the hinge mechanism slowly in his reedy fingers. "Mr. Scribner," he says half-heartedly, clearing his throat, "with this type cancer, cure is not a word we use. Unlike some cancers, ACC has no five-year cure rate. Your cancer can be exceedingly fickle. It can recur—come back—even after a long period of time. Five, even ten years. So you see, we oncologists are very reluctant to use that word."

I'm beginning to feel shut off, disconnected, as if I'm the only person on earth doomed with this curse, this ACC. "Well," I ask, crestfallen, "what's the purpose, then, in taking this drug that might kill me?"

"Because that's all there is," he says, seeming ever-so-slightly to relish in the delivery of stinging news. "There are no other drugs. And radiation's not advised."

As you become more and more inundated by cancer and its crude language and treatments—maybe it's the very fact the disease can result in your death—you quickly come to feel like an alien (not visitor, mind you) in a medical no-man's land where no one speaks your tongue, no one seems to discern, or listen to, what you're saying.

When doctors are spewing their sterile and remote medicalese, you most often feel excluded, though you're frequently the center of discussion. It often seems your physical presence is, for them, merely a living example of some textbook write-up on your disease. You're not humanly there. You are: words on a page that have come to life . . . a gathering of negative statistics . . . a collection of blood, bone and tissue, without a mind, without feelings. All of this, too, while you're dueling with the brutal knowledge that you may not be here next year to see something as ordinary as Christmas.

I turn to Jane with raised eyebrows—the signal to ask about the second opinion. She's nodding passively as if someone of royal stature had decreed a new statute.

"So that's today's good news?" I go on, unconsciously contrasting the harshness of this visit with other times I'd seen doctors, usually as a child, and they patted me on the head, saying, 'Everything will be okay, Eric.'

"If that's how you wish to term it," Dr. Drake replies, a slight elevation to his chin. "The question now is, do you want to start on Mitotane and when? The sooner the better, by the way, is the consensus."

Out of his view, I press Jane's foot with mine.

"Oh! Dr. Drake!" she interjects as if startled. "We were going to ask. What about something like . . . a second opinion? We'd like to get one."

"That, Mrs. Scribner, is not called for in this case. We have everything we need already. I've checked with the experts."

"But," she persists politely, my heavy foot on hers, "I thought it was sort of, well, standard. In cases like this—and," she adds, leading with a benign smile, "we'd sure feel better."

"Mrs. Scribner, I can assure you, a second opinion's a waste of time," Dr. Drake replies, a trace of animosity in his words. An inadvertent tautness in his body position subtly underscores his annoyance. "But, if you insist," he goes on, looking for an instant as if his professionalism's been trampled upon, "I'll submit your request to UR—the HMO Utilization Review process. That's the committee that has to authorize this sort of thing. Standard HMO procedure."

"Really," Jane strains to say kindly, a bit put out herself, "we'd sure appreciate it, doctor."

"Where'd you have in mind?" Dr. Drake asks curtly, noisily removing a small note pad from his center drawer.

"We talked about it and thought . . . maybe . . . you could recommend a place."

"My recommendation is that you don't need a second opinion, Mrs. Scribner."

"In that case," Jane offers, recognizing the futility in this, "Norris Cancer Center in L.A. At USC. Fifty miles away, not that far."

Finished scribbling a note to himself, Dr. Drake looks at me once more, over his glasses: "And your decision on the adjuvant therapy? The Mitotane?"

"Wow," I say, caught off guard, feeling hard-pressed like a cornered animal, "that's something . . . it's a . . . big decision. I'm going to hold off, I think, till we see what comes of this second opinion. And, I'd like some time to myself . . . to let things settle a little. We're not exactly talking aspirin here, the way you describe this Mitotane."

He nods with an empty expression—as if to say, 'Nothing ventured, nothing gained.'

"One last thing, doctor," I say, now reluctant to continue, "Can I get a copy of those fact sheets—the ones you've been reading from? I'd like to learn all I can about my cancer."

He sits stone still for a moment, thinking. He reflects upon the assorted papers in his hands as if one more look will help decide the issue. "Actually, Mr.

Scribner, I'd rather not," he concludes finally. "Patients sometimes get confused . . . picking out the wrong information."

"But . . . since you've been referring to them and you got them for my cancer . . . I thought—"

He shakes his head as if to re-establish the firmness of his decision.

"Well, okay then," is all I can think of in response, in concession. "Also," I resume, feeling I have firm footing here, "I've been experiencing some painful rawness in my throat lately. Like a strep infection is coming on. Can you possibly take a look—or prescribe something?"

Aloofly, Dr. Drake taps, then aligns his cherished fact sheets on the desk top. "For that," he says with disdain, "you'll have to see your primary-care physician. I'm an oncologist. I take care of cancer issues; your primary takes care of things like that."

Driving home, Jane and I discuss the delusion that all doctors welcome a second opinion. It just isn't so. Drake's predictable irritation only served to reinforce my earlier beliefs. Jane, now a believer, at least for the moment, says, "Sure got upset, didn't he?"

"No kidding. Like I didn't predict it."

"He's even sort of a . . . jerk."

"Not sort of. And he's the doctor who's going to be treating my cancer."

Chinks are beginning to appear in the TDKB armor.

Each of us, in all we do, makes weighty choices. Most choices a cancer patient makes—if he is given choices—especially early in the diagnosis, are gut wrenching. Such was the case with the chemotherapy Drake recommended. All I knew about the horrors of chemo at that point I'd learned from Sunday night TV movies—but still, my first inclination, sitting in his office, was that I take an aggressive approach: jump at the opportunity to fight this cancer. A deeper sense of reason, however, said step back, look more closely at the long-term issues.

Six weeks after being off, I return to work. Since Jane's job allows her more time at home, she calls USC, arranges the second opinion. From Jane's first call, she's wowed by USC's professionalism and courtesy. She's even spoken with the endocrinologist who'll see us.

Secretly I held the belief—hope?—that USC, a major medical school and cancer center, would see to the bottom of this and say Drake's all wet, that nothing's seriously wrong with me. I don't have to do anything. No chemo, nothing. Being unfamiliar with this kind of cancer, Drake's overreacted. This isn't so much to be a second opinion, as an exoneration. This is my private dream. In retrospect, this fanciful thinking amounted to little more than outright denial.

The following week, without yet receiving the HMO's blessing on this second opinion, Jane and I drive to USC. The patient check-in area, carpeted and nicely furnished, is scattered with people like myself, sitting, fumbling nervously with arcane items—medical records, various papers, imposing x-ray, CT scan envelopes. Jane had requested a set of my pathology slides be mailed ahead for review.

After a few minutes' wait, we're escorted to Dr. Kyrouz' office—a small-boned woman, about forty, very precise. She, unlike Dr. Drake, stands as we enter, introducing herself with a gracious smile. Coming from behind her desk, she joins us in comfortable, padded wing chairs. Her office, a quiet shade of light brown, has unstained beige carpeting. On the walls are soothing watercolors of the Northern California coast ablaze in spring wild flowers. No carelessly displayed books on death.

Holding a kind smile, Dr. Kyrouz asks why—though she's spoken with Jane on the phone—we've come to USC. A standard and fair door opener, if you will.

Briefly I explain the exploratory surgery, my prior symptoms, the post-surgery pathology report—and Dr. Drake's recommended adjuvant therapy. To call upon her sympathies, I mention his displeasure in granting this second opinion. Dr. Kyrouz' dark, serious eyes remain on me as if she's picking up subtle details as we go.

"And what do you hope to accomplish . . . here?" she asks, with a noticeable accent. Her hands are now neatly folded in atop her crossed knees, on her smoothed-over ankle-length skirt.

I smile: my opportunity to really open up. This I hadn't covered with Jane. "Actually, doctor, I'm hoping you'll say these other people are all wet—that what they're calling cancer is not cancer at all but something else."

CHAPTER 10

BOY ON THE BEACH—
THE SECOND OPINION CONFIRMS THE FIRST

"How many times I have heard this," Dr. Kyrouz remarks sympathetically, nodding gently. "Many patients come here, wanting us to tell them something is not so."

The small office is quiet, save for the peaceful hum of air conditioning. The doctor deliberates a moment, looking to Jane. "And your feeling on this?"

"I want it not to be cancer, too," Jane replies pointedly.

Returning to me, Dr. Kyrouz: "This condition we are talking about—adrenal cortical carcinoma—is difficult to gather information on. I have not seen any cases of this myself."

Her words expand the forsakenness already overwhelming me. We're headed, I realize now, down a familiar pathway. Is this a never-ending nightmare?

"When I got your request," Dr. Kyrouz resumes, nodding toward a modest accumulation of papers on her desk, "I assigned several of my students to look into this."

Jane coughs reservedly, sitting forward in her chair.

"We have reviewed your slides," Dr. Kyrouz is saying, reaching for the papers on her desk, "and we concur with the original diagnosis. I am sorry. This is a malignancy of the adrenal cortex."

By this point, her words come as no surprise. "Is this cancer," I ask, feeling hope draining away, "as bad as my other doctor says?"

"There is so little data, Mr. Scribner, to go on," the doctor replies, appearing slightly ill at ease, as she reads silently from the papers in her lap. "This cancer, according to National Cancer Institute literature, only occurs once in every two million people."

"What causes it?" I ask, my mind grabbing at that incredible statistic, now meandering pointlessly "This mysterious cancer."

The naiveté of the question seems to catch the doctor unawares. "Adrenal carcinoma, you are asking?"

I nod yes.

"For this, as with most cancers, we have no answer."

"Well, how long would say I've had it?" I continue, figuring I might as well ask as many simpleminded questions as I can while this specialist's sitting before me. "How long was the . . . tumor there before it was discovered?"

"Again, no answers. Maybe for months . . . maybe for many years."

"—And now it must be treated? The cancer? Even though we think the surgeon got it all?"

"That would be our recommendation."

"And if I decide to do nothing?"

"Bad, Mr. Scribner, very bad," Dr. Kyrouz asserts gravely. "Very dangerous. This one likes to return."

"So . . . what's your advice?"

Dr. Kyrouz licks her thumb, rearranging the sheets in her lap. "A drug called Lysodren—or Mitotane," she offers.

"Same as Dr. Drake said," I say dejectedly. "It's a pretty bad drug, according to him. He called a doctor in Houston and they talked about it."

"Yes," Dr. Kyrouz says, "probably he spoke with the M. D. Anderson Cancer Center. That is where much of these data come from. If there is an institution with an experience base on this type of cancer, it is them."

Sunshine, flickering on the ocean spray in the large watercolor behind the doctor, catches my digressive eye. Flashing back, I relive for an instant the sense of innocence that dominated the carefree days I spent on the Chesapeake Bay in Maryland, as a kid, in the heavily humid air of summer, the fiery sun, never thinking of sinking toward death . . . . Now an indelible essence—the loving stench of my father's outboard, mixed with salty air—seizes me.

". . . Eight to ten grams a day, right?" I resume, blandly.

Dr. Kyrouz, scanning a sheet of paper. Her schooling on this disease is broadening as well. "That is the eventual dosage," she replies. "I would suggest starting much lower—at maybe one gram per day for a week or two. To see how the body tolerates. If tolerance is good, I would then increase the dosage until you reach eight to 10 grams a day. With this, I would also recommend taking replacement adrenal hormones as well."

"This is the first we've heard of this—" Jane puts in, "—these hormones."

"This drug, Mrs. Scribner, this Lysodren, will suppress—perhaps even destroy—your husband's remaining adrenal gland. Replacement hormones will prevent him from experiencing acute adrenal failure as the gland itself shuts down."

"That's a serious problem?"

"Oh, quite. It can result in death if not recognized and treated."

"But," I interject, "unlike Dr. Drake, you don't suggest starting at eight to ten grams a day?"

"Correct. It is best, I believe, to allow the body to adjust. We would start you slowly and build up, gradually. The literature suggests you achieve what is called 'MTD'—maximum tolerated dosage. Ideally, that would mean working up to 16 grams per day—or, the maximum dosage your body will tolerate: in other words, your own MTD."

Now realizing there's truly little known about this rare disease, I ask: "Then you really don't know how much to prescribe?"

"Not precisely," Dr. Kyrouz sighs, responding candidly. "This is not like, say, an antibiotic, where we know what a given amount will accomplish."

"So," Jane asks, "the more, the better?"

Dr. Kyrouz nods yes.

"How do we monitor the drug's success?" I want to know.

The doctor thumbs forward to yet another sheet of paper. "We would follow you with blood work and CT scans, every three months. Six months at the longest."

Having had training in industrial radiation and its exposure dangers early in my aerospace career, I ask: "There comes a time, doesn't there, when radiation exposure becomes a concern?"

"Some of our patients receive CT scans monthly. At this point," she continues, pausing thoughtfully, "radiation exposure is *not* your primary concern."

Again somewhat transfixed, I find myself looking beyond her, at the watercolor beach scene, seeing myself once again—a disease-free little boy, alone, roaming the sandy waterfront in search of other-world treasures that might've washed ashore during the night. "I see," I reply. "Would it be best, then, if I was treated here, at USC . . . instead of locally by the HMO's oncologist?"

Dr. Kyrouz deliberates a moment as doctors seem wont to do when asked questions involving other doctors. "We could treat you here, yes, but . . . in truth, the best location for treatment would the Anderson Cancer Center in Houston. It is *experience* you need."

As we stand to leave, I reluctantly ask Dr. Kyrouz if I can have a copy of the literature she's been quoting from. A smile, a warm, thin-fingered handshake, and she cheerfully agrees. No objections. "A patient," she volunteers, kindly touching my arm for emphasis, "should be educated in his disease. The more you understand, the better you will do."

"Classy lady," Jane laments as we drive home in the clutch of late-afternoon freeway traffic. "I was really impressed, weren't you? At least she didn't harp on those awful statistics. The ones Drake seems so proud of."

"I like her idea of starting the chemo at a lower dose. That makes a lot of sense to me."

Advice: Even if your doctor does as Dr. Drake and attempts to dissuade you from seeking a second opinion, insist on one anyway. A second opinion—and sometimes even a third—can prove extremely helpful in (1) precisely determining the type of cancer you're dealing with, and (2) possibly revealing a whole new slate of treatment options. This is especially true if your second opinion's performed at one of the many Comprehensive Cancer Centers throughout the U.S.

These centers see and treat all kinds of cancer each day—and perhaps most important, they will offer the most up-to-date, state-of-the-art treatment protocols. There is a great deal of satisfaction in knowing, via a second opinion, that you're correctly dealing with a particular cancer. There are numerous cases of patients having been treated for the wrong cancer—because they did not seek a second opinion. Even if you have to pay for it yourself, *get a second opinion.*

CHAPTER 11

THAT FIRST TASTE OF CHEMO

After driving in silence for a period, Jane observes, "They really don't like that word 'cure,' do they?" She's behind the wheel. I'm reading through the information Dr. Kyrouz gave me.

Ominous words like 'lethal' and 'dismal' leap at me like grotesque little parasites from the pages. "Looks like . . . I really have cancer," I confess hesitantly, without pretense, after a few minutes of reflective reading. "Much as I hate admitting it. I really . . . really have cancer." I detest the sound of the words, my own voice.

"Maybe, hon," she says buoyantly, reaching over, squeezing my kneecap, "this drug will do the trick. You'll be okay."

"It's hard understanding . . ." I reply, staring off at the endless sea of chrome and color hemming us in on the stagnant freeway, all the disinterested, glass-framed faces, "a disease that doesn't make you hurt or feel bad."

"You certainly look good," Jane confirms, "and feel good."

"I think now we're seeing the fallacy in that. What really counts is what the damn doctors see in their precious films."

"This means, then . . . you'll be telling Dr. Drake to go ahead? With the Mitotane?"

"Not a whole lot of choices out there. Besides, I'm not one to turn and run at the thought of a little nausea . . . or the possibility of the drug killing me."

"At least the endocrinologist, Dr. Kyrouz," Jane goes on, trying her best to elevate my spirits, "let us have copies of what her students put together. That was a pleasant switch."

"—Was it nice of her," I ask, looking across at Jane, who's intently watching a series of erratic lanes changes going on in front of her, "—or is Drake just a creep?"

"Don't call doctors creeps," she responds defensively, her instinctive protectiveness of physicians (TDKB again?) coming to the fore. "They're busy people."

"In my book, there comes a time when the things at hand become more important. I'm talking about dealing mercifully with the people who're unlucky enough to get cancer."

As we converse, I notice how we're both becoming more pacified with what had been an emotional catchword—cancer—though always before it had been used in relation to someone else, not me.

Several days later: We're sitting once again with my favorite oncologist, Dr. Drake. He's received word back from the tumor registry. Their findings are essentially the same as the original pathology report, though they seem even more vague in their conclusion, saying they'd like to see more of the tissue before committing fully to a diagnosis. Again, I'm unable to wrangle a copy of the tumor registry's report from Dr. Drake, despite telling him the doctor at USC had given me all she drew upon.

"Since we're on the subject," Dr. Drake says, thumbing through my file, "the UR group denied your request for a second opinion."

"What's that mean . . . in light of the fact that I've already gone to USC?"

"Two choices," Dr. Drake explains. "You can either pay for the USC visit yourself—or, you can go to the next level and appeal this decision with the HMO . . . . Let's see," he flips more pages, "here's your copy of the denial."

Attached to the denial form is Dr. Drake's request for the second opinion. Toward the bottom of his brief request, he's stated in no uncertain terms he opposes granting a USC visit. 'Needless,' is the word he's written and underlined. Reading this, I feel my insides, in an instant, grow branding-iron hot. Is this man—this doctor who took the Hippocratic Oath—on my side, or theirs? Strangely, I'm torn between disliking this man, my oncologist, and staying with him since he's all the HMO has to offer locally.

(I appealed this decision in writing. The good news: the HMO agreed to allow the second opinion. The bad news: The HMO's decision process took three months. Far, far too long to wait for a second opinion in the case of a deadly cancer.)

I tell Dr. Drake I've decided to begin taking the Mitotane. He directs his nurse to get the disclaimer he's prepared. This crudely done, hand-written sheet essentially spells out the reasons for which I will not sue him in the event some organ or gland or some such bodily thing ceases to function or has to be removed due to the Mitotane. There's also a statement to the effect that if I die my heirs will not sue either.

The whole exercise seems odd, unprofessional—overkill. With my signature on the disclaimer, Dr. Drake says he'll order the drug—and, he informs me, the HMO, mine, has agreed to cover the cost, expected to be somewhere in the neighborhood of $700 and $1100 a month . . . for the rest of my life. But, I am angrily thinking now, in light of this guy's outlook for me, how long did he tell the penny-pinching HMO that life would be?

Dr. Kyrouz' office had mailed each of us, Dr. Drake and myself, a copy of her second-opinion report. In it she recommends beginning the Mitotane at a low a dose—one gram per day—to check my tolerance. She also strongly advises concurrent replacement adrenal hormones. When I question Dr. Drake about the need for replacement drugs—what with his neglecting to mention them earlier—he adopts a blasé attitude, as though it's not a big issue, or an imperative, as far as he's concerned. When I ask what could happen if I don't take them, he mentions the possibility of acute adrenal failure.

I'd rather start taking the hormones now, I tell him—not wait till adrenal failure occurs, whatever that involves. When I ask about side effects, if any, of these replacement hormones, he indicates there may be some facial puffiness, stomach irritation, weight gain, mood swings, fat deposited on the midsection. Beyond that little would be noticeable to the naked eye. (In addition, other side effects of these replacement adrenal hormones [Prednisone and florinef] include: gastric or duodenal ulcers, weight gain or loss, potassium imbalance, muscle weakness, loss of muscle mass, slow wound healing, possible convulsions, and headaches to cite the major concerns.)

As suggested by the USC endocrinologist, Dr. Drake agrees to arrange a baseline CT and chest x-ray before beginning the Mitotane therapy. The Xeroxed sheet he'd given me at our previous meeting indicated Mitotane therapy should begin in a hospital setting so a patient's adverse reactions could be monitored closely. I remind Dr. Drake of this.

His irritated response: "You see, this is further evidence why patients should *not* be given printed matter. A little knowledge . . ."

But, he concedes, in this case, in that he's unfamiliar with the drug's side effects, he felt it necessary to give me the Mitotane printout. "You may want to take a few days off work. Once you start the Mitotane," he says, his hard little eyes looking dry behind his Freud-like glasses. "Just in case."

Hospitalization, he goes on condescendingly, is completely unnecessary. "We can deal with any issues that arise." This, to me, being new to this cancer business, seems an odd assumption—i.e., some of the recommendations in the literature on Mitotane are arbitrarily adhered to, while others, like the recommended hospitalization—something we all know costs the HMO money—are downplayed.

It's now late January, 1990, roughly two months since the surgery. Results of the baseline CT and x-ray are negative, meaning they're good. This negative-positive terminology's still confusing relative to CT, to x-ray results. When doctors say your CT's positive that means it's not good—they found something irregular. Negative means everything's okay— they found no irregularities. Then there are terms like 'false-positives' . . . and so on. Very confusing. At any rate, the baseline CT's clean—no new tumors.

Four days later: A call comes in from Dr. Drake's nurse—my drug is in. I pick it up at the small-scale pharmacy on the ground floor in the clinic where his office is. My co-pay's $7.00; actual cost of the drug for the first month: $870.00. Thank God for insurance—even if it is a begrudging, tight-fisted HMO.

At home, I cautiously open the intimidating soft-drink size pill container as one might a coffee can filled with those coiled snakes. The ghostly pills, a half-gram each, a bit thicker than Necco wafers and half the diameter, appear harmless. Bringing the pill container to my nose, no weird smells knock my head back. Nothing indicates the hazards or power of this pernicious medication. Sitting at the breakfast table am I. Jane's there also, watching this meeting of patient and medicine.

"What comes to mind?" she asks, blowing across a cup of hot tea.

"Fear, mostly, I guess," I respond truthfully. "What I'll do, I think, is have lunch," I go on procrastinating, "then pop one of these babies . . . and sit back and wait."

We've both taken a few days off work in case something arises requiring swift action. Like getting me to the emergency room quickly. After lunch—tuna sandwich and ice tea—I gulp down my first chemo pill, go in the den, flip on the TV and wait for the intestinal thunderstorms to commence. I fully expect to be hugging the commode within minutes. An hour passes: I'm still watching TV . . . without incident.

"Feel anything?" Jane asks, leaning forward, looking at me.

"Nada," I reply tentatively, running a quick mental analysis of my internal functions and feelings.

"Nothing? No upset stomach—nothing?"

I nod, quit pleased, actually, with my early reaction. The drug is in me, I know, being metabolized, but nothing's happening outwardly. The smiling tough guy in me says, So this is chemo?

That evening I take another half gram with dinner. Again, no backlash.

"See," Jane points out cheerfully, scratching my back playfully, "I said you were going to do okay."

I remind her I'm only at one gram . . . "A person could probably take one gram of anything—arsenic even—and not feel any ill effects."

She shakes her head in that special way wives do.

The following day I get really courageous and propose we go to our favorite outdoor café at the marina for a quiet lunch. After a lovely portion of grilled snapper and steamed vegetables, I down another pill, watching a series of sleek sailboats heading through the marina on their way out to sea. Again, nothing. This pattern goes on for a week. Then I up the dosage to two grams a day. Still nothing.

Seemingly, there aren't going to be any side effects—no stomach convulsions, no diarrhea, no nausea. Perhaps like many of the uninitiated, I'd been conditioned by dubious movie portrayals of patients 'on chemo,' and by the Xeroxed sheet stating that all cancer patients get inhumanely ill, always.

(Not to downplay this chemo business in any way, because many patients do become violently ill, but as cliché as it sounds, everyone is different; everyone reacts differently to chemo. Some will get ill taking low dosages, others not. Don't automatically assume you're going get sick with chemo. And if you do, there are wonderful drugs—like Zofran and Kytril—that can knock down most bouts of nausea.)

Shortly thereafter I bump the Mitotane dosage to three grams a day—one gram with breakfast, one with lunch, one with dinner. I remain at this dosage for approximately a month before advancing to four grams per day. Still, I notice little in the way of side effects. In fact, nothing I'd really ascribe to the drug itself. There are negligible bouts of indigestion and sporadic loose bowels, but that's no big deal. I was about to learn, though, the subtleness of this hefty white tablet.

FINDING HOPE WHEN DOCTORS SAY THERE IS NONE

CHAPTER 12

THE LONGEST JOURNEY— PHASE ONE OF MY RESEARCH

Still actively pursuing in-depth information on ACC, my first real break appears like a thin stream of light beneath a darkened doorway: The National Cancer Institute's 1-800-4-CANCER phone number for their Cancer Information Service. This free telephone service provides current, detailed information on almost every type of cancer imaginable. Two versions of the information are mailed out without charge: the Patient Version (less detailed) and a doctors' version, called Physicians Data Query, PDQ (much more detailed).

Asking for the Adrenocortical Carcinoma version of the PDQ, I fully expect the telephone volunteer to say, "Sorry, sir, that's a rare cancer—we don't have any information available. And, you're not a doctor so we can't send you the PDQ version anyway." This doesn't happen.

After I answer a few questions about my ACC and its staging, the volunteer encouragingly agrees to send the latest NCI fact sheets. Someone actually has information on ACC!

A timeless Buddhist passage declares with profound simplicity: The longest journey begins with the first step. This is mine. PDQ information from the NCI opens the door to a couple of things—not only does this provide germane information, but also empowers me, making me realize I can effectively research my own disease. Finally, I have a sense of moving ahead in this war.

Within seven days, free of charge, I receive a bulging manila envelope in my mailbox. Opening the material I'm a bit apprehensive—there may be things here I don't want to see. Statistics regarding my life expectancy, for example. Who knows what else.

Scanning the steps used in the staging procedure, I see how Drs. Drake and Kyrouz had placed my ACC between Stages II and III. (Stage IV being the most deadly.) Using the PDQ criteria, I subjectively place myself solidly within the tamer of the two—Stage II. As such, chances for my long-term survival—beyond five years—look good. In fact the only issue dragging me toward a Stage III designation is the actual size of the removed tumor.

To see an authoritative, an objective source, the PDQ, corroborating the use of Mitotane for ACC—in writing—is soothing. Yes, I'm a skeptic.

Since my days in college journalism I've researched topics to the nth degree. That, I find, is the surest route to a well-rounded, factual story. This time I have much more at stake—personally.

I dedicate myself to the pursuit of the undiscovered. Who's to say that I—Joe Layman—can't stumble upon the missing pieces . . . something that may prove pivotal to extending my life . . . something the doctors, because they're too close to the trees, have overlooked. (Later you'll see how this layman's search pays off in several ways, one of which is a self-devised chemo plan.)

Also about this time, fall of 1990, Jane begins to grossly misinterpret my hunger for cancer information. To her I'm dwelling unhealthily on the subject. 'We've done all we can up to this point,' she reasons, 'so let's move on.' She sees this quest of mine, apparently, as a freakish form of hypochondria.

In frustration, I disagree, explaining I'm justifiably searching out any bit of information that'll benefit me . . . in any way. Nonetheless, she grows quite rattled when she finds me 'dwelling on something' I've found. I am not, to my way of thinking, dwelling unhealthily on anything. If answers are out there, by God, I'm going to unearth them.

In books and articles I keep coming upon writers—one author seems to lead to another—who've totally recovered, or at least greatly improved their odds in the cancer trenches, with major modifications to their diets. Some greatly increased their fruit and vegetable intake, some became strict vegetarians . . . some even advise of something called the macrobiotic diet.

All this seems too severe for my liking, at this point, anyway.

In my heart, however, as I read these accounts, these testimonials, there's a growing and obvious truth in what these authors are saying about the cancer vs. diet connection. Every cell in our body's created from the food we put in our mouths. It's that simple. To say what we eat does not effect our cancer is absolute nonsense.

Early on, though, I don't want to surrender my high-fat, meat-oriented diet to this demoralizing disease. Go even a week without an oozing grilled cheeseburger, a barbecued steak, a plateful of greasy bacon and eggs—no way!

Eventually, though, I come to watch my diet closely, very closely. (After being found to have inoperable Stage IV metastatic ACC in 1993 by surgeons at M. D. Anderson, I jump in and become a full-on vegetarian. With this final doctors' diagnosis, I'm adrift, on my own, so to speak—no more radiation, no more surgery. Only questionable chemo remains. I have to do everything I can—within my power—do to rescue myself. Details on this in later chapters.)

Over a period of eight months, I work my way up to 8 grams of Mitotane per day—16 very large pills a day. I'm consuming five pills after breakfast, five after lunch, six after dinner. Also included are replacement adrenal hormones: another five small pills with breakfast, another five with dinner.

Mitotane's strange side effects have finally emerged . . . and are indeed troubling, even if somewhat subtle.

A deep-down sense of weariness—unlike an ordinary feeling of being tired, almost a sense of forlorness at times—eventually overtakes me. There are also extended periods of cramping indigestion. Also I find it near impossible to rise in the morning—to physically awaken—and go to work. When the alarm sounds, my sense of consciousness just doesn't react like it used to: I have to force myself out of bed as a mental, not physical process. (Not until much later do I learn to intelligently manipulate—adjust up and down—my daily adrenal hormones to garner their best energy and stamina advantage to minimize Mitotane's hangover effect.)

Some of Mitotane's side effects are so unusual so as to not be immediately recognized. There is, for example, a gradual loss of libido, and my breasts are becoming slightly enlarged, quite sensitive. Dr. Drake checks my serum testosterone and finds it running low. Recommended solution? Add bi-weekly injections of testosterone to all I'm already doing.

The day after the first testosterone injection, a brutal headache sets in, lasting four full days. The almost intolerable pain's enough to force me to pack my head in ice for hours. Just for some minor relief. Aspirin, even prescription pain medications are about as effective as a water pistol against a raging forest fire.

When the same pattern emerges following the next testosterone injection two weeks later, I discuss this agonizing problem with Dr. Drake. Making light of the issue, as though headaches are frivolous, he says something to the effect that this is the price one has to pay for a passable sex life, a reduction in breast tissue.

Recurrent testosterone headaches become so oppressive that I seriously consider halting the injections. Dr. Drake advises that not only do I need the injections for libido and breast-size reduction, but the male body requires appreciable amounts of testosterone in the blood for other normal bodily functions. He suggests I'm allergic to the injected testosterone.

In light of my family's prostate cancer history, I ask about the wisdom of these injections, about the possible correlation between testosterone injections and the inducement of testicular or prostate malignancies. Offering little by way of explanation, Dr. Drake seems to scoff at this notion.

One day at work, while enduring an especially torturous testosterone headache, I take matters in my own hands: I call the M. D. Anderson Cancer Center in Houston. Once connected with MDA and explaining my purpose, a sweet-natured young woman puts me through—much to my amazement—to an Anderson endocrinologist.

Dr. Frank's inordinately patient with my questions, almost seeming too considerate in giving an ear to my story. They (MDA) have observed this breast tenderness condition—'gynecomastia,' he calls it—in men taking Mitotane. This can be countered, he says, with yet another chemotherapeutic agent. A drug that's most often associated with women's breast cancer: Tamoxifen.

Tamoxifen, he explains, reduces gynecomastia (breast enlargement in men) by suppressing the production or conversion of testosterone to estrogen. I hadn't realized men also manufacture estrogen until Dr. Frank explains this. He recommends an adequate dose of Tamoxifen: 20mgs, taken twice daily.

I ask about other patients and testosterone headaches. While sympathizing, he can offer no explanation. Folks respond differently to different hormones, is all he can offer. (Two painful years later, I discover the actual reason for my tormenting response to testosterone by way of an unrelated urological visit—a very good reason to ask old questions of new doctors. More on this later, also.)

My next visit with Dr. Drake: He studies me rather strangely over his round glasses as I tell him of calling M. D. Anderson. He seems more dumbstruck than offended. Another interesting phenomenon relative to doctors in general, one I've experienced numerous times, is that if you tell a doctor something you've discovered, he probably won't pay much attention. But, if you pass along something another doctor's told you—not written out and sent along, mind you—your doctor will probably not only listen, but will agree to whatever that other doctor's suggested, without evidence. Thus it is with Dr. Drake.

When I relay what Dr. Frank had said, he, Dr. Drake, without batting an eye, without calling Dr. Frank for verification, removes a small prescription pad from his coat pocket and writes the order for Tamoxifen.

"They've used this before, I presume," he asks, scribbling, "—in the past?"

I answer in the affirmative.

"What can I expect . . . by way of side effects from this new drug, doctor?"

"I wouldn't look for much," Dr. Drake replies offhandedly. "It's a pretty innocuous, for the most part."

Next day I'm taking yet another chemo drug—two more pills a day. After about a month, I notice a slight reduction in gynecomastia. The breast sensitivity's all but gone. Dr. Frank guessed it'd take three to four months to see meaningful results.

Resolution of the issues involved here was the outcome of my work, my calling MDA. In today's often-confusing and disheartening maze of HMO medicine, if you want answers, you best seek them yourself. Sadly, you are your own health advocate.

Advice: Learn as much as much as possible about your disease. Most people, when they make a significant acquisition—an automobile or a home—research all options. Do the same with your disease. This illness *will* alter your life, the way you view life. Take every opportunity to learn: knowledge in the battle against cancer is definitely power. And continue to learn, learn, learn, don't stop just because 'you think that's all there is.' Arm yourself! You can never know too much. New treatments are popping up everyday. Keep that in mind.

Read, ask question after question, listen to anything anyone has to say, be open to sensible suggestions . . . Start by calling 1-800-4-CANCER and getting current NCI information on your cancer. Because, only with knowledge can you be a wise consumer of medical information, a wise decision-maker when it comes to treatments and options you'll be offered.

Other numbers to call: The M. D. Anderson Patient Network—800-345-6324—and the Block Cancer Foundation—800-433-0464. Both organizations will connect you, via telephone, without cost to you, with someone with a like cancer diagnosis. You can then talk at length to that person about his or her real-life experiences with 'your type of cancer.'

These are among the best patient resources in America today. By calling these organizations, by being linked with another patient, you can find out immediately first-hand information about most cancers—what treatments various people have undergone, where they had those treatments, how those treatments work, the side effects, the success rates.

Make it your policy to sift through whatever everyone has to say about cancer—no matter how off the wall it seems. Who knows where your answers will come from? When people tell me they saw an interesting cancer article in the *Enquirer*, I look it up. When someone mentions *Newsweek* as source, I track it down. I'll go anywhere for the truth. Frequently the wisdom you gather is all you have to go on. Later we'll see how the knowledge I gained saved my life.

FINDING HOPE WHEN DOCTORS SAY THERE IS NONE

CHAPTER 13

NOT SO CLEAR AND PRESENT DANGER—
A SHADOW APPEARS ON THE CT FILM

Mid-1991... Admittedly, with the surgery now a distant memory, I've become a bit smug. For over a year now I've been taking Mitotane without encountering any unsolvable medical mysteries—side effects or otherwise—that severely restrict or alter my everyday lifestyle. Eight grams a day, 16 pills, is the dosage I top off at. That's my MTD. My body seems to have adapted as best it can to this alien chemical regimen. Above 16 pills a day and I find myself very light-headed, almost drunk—unable to think coherently, often losing my train of thought mid-sentence. Tamoxifen's done its job. My breasts have shrunken to as near normal as they're going to get, according to Dr. Drake.

Going to work each day now, I'm back to putting in eight hours a day in a ragged, windowless office and driving 45 grueling miles each way on the bumper-to-bumper, nerve-racking 101 freeway. But I'm doing okay. I've survived to this point—and the company's singled me out to receive a prestigious NASA Astronauts Award for exemplary achievements over the years. Jane and I will be VIPs at an upcoming shuttle launch, following a cocktail reception with a group of astronauts. Quite an honor.

The only tangible ongoing problems I'm confronted with—in my own self-indulgent tunnel vision—are the thunderous headaches that roar in following each testosterone injection. As a partial solution, I decide, on my own, to have the shots every four weeks—instead of every two as originally planned. This partial solution extends the headache-free period between each of the injections. No one seems to object to or notice this change—not Dr. Drake, not his nurse.

After being cancer-free for almost a year and a half, I've become shortsightedly complacent, feeling, at times, like it's all behind me now— believing my only serious problems now or in the future will arise from the drugs I'll be taking the rest of my life: Mitotane and replacement adrenal hormones.

That my cancer can recur is a distant fear at best. The farther one is removed from a source of fear, the more that fear loses its sting. Even the usually stoic and hard-to-impress Dr. Drake admits, when I pass the one-year, cancer-free mark, the future looks considerably brighter. (Politely, I don't mention the death sentence he'd so arrogantly advanced at our introductory meeting.) "That first year," he offers ungenerously, "is the most critical."

Well, not exactly, as I'm soon to learn.

I'd recently had a routine follow-up CT scan-chest, abdomen, pelvis. This relatively painless test, as any cancer patient can attest, is accompanied by tremendous emotional and physical apprehension. Negative CT results—*mere words on paper*, mind you—can instantly turn your otherwise contented world upside-down. Truly it's astonishing how we, as human beings, can feel so triumphant one day, then undergo a CT, get subverting report results three days later and abruptly our beautiful world flip-flops to one of utter despair. It's ink on paper—not the actual onset of physical symptoms—that accomplishes this feat.

You may not physically feel any different, but the simple fact that a doctor—that supreme authority figure—has told you your CT results are negative, makes you instantly feel befouled, tainted. This prime example of the negative placebo effect (when your doctor gives you the bad news and, because you believe in him, it comes true) is what authors like Deepak Chopra and Bernie Siegel mean when they talk about the mind-body connection: the body feels fat and happy till the ever-powerful mind registers bad news, then all mental and physical positiveness vanishes, replaced by a pervasive negativity.

At any rate, this routine, follow-up CT reveals something—a shadow—an abnormality of some sort in the exact area of the original tumor. My initial response is one of escape, disbelief. Deep down, I'm convinced I'll never have to deal with active cancer again. This interpretation is, perhaps, one of Nature's warm-blanket defense mechanisms. Without it I'd probably go bonkers with fear, with worry.

Dr. Drake takes this auspicious occasion to launch into his This-Is-The-Reason-I-Don't-Like-Frequent-CT speeches. "These kinds of things," he notes, pausing while reading aloud about the abnormality vaguely described in the radiologist's report, "cause patients a good deal of consternation. This shadow that the radiologist is talking about." (I never knew the usually unoffending word *shadow* could impart such foreboding till I hear it used in reference to me—my insides, my future.)

"Does he say at all . . ." I ask, recoiling, sensing this to be at least a wake-up call, "what it is?"

"No. Only that it's in the same location as your surgery. Regrowth is always a possibility."

"Of the tumor, you're saying?" I persist, unconsciously fingering a jagged tear in the vinyl covering the exam table.

"Well, naturally," Dr. Drake responds nonchalantly. (Again, I think some people derive a perverted sense of authority or pleasure in delivering jarring news to others—be they doctors or not.)

"What . . . do we do now?" I use the plural on purpose: I feel the need to make him feel he's involved, too.

"We wait," he responds with a strange grin, looking a bit too all-knowing. "Till next time. Then we compare."

"—And," I ask, feeling again very much cut adrift in the murky sea of cancer treatment and diagnostics, "what do I do in the meantime? How do I sleep?"

"As I said moments ago, Mr. Scribner, this is the primary reason I'm opposed to giving patients CTs too often."

"Well . . ." I begin, feeling my insides infused with a new sense of fear, a depthless unknown, "how soon can we look to do the next CT?"

"Maybe four months. We'll think about it."

"I've got to live with this for *four* months?" I continue, thrust once again up against the finality of this disease. "What about . . . if something *is* going on?"

"Your HMO won't authorize another CT any sooner. I wouldn't be really too troubled," he concludes in his ever-blasé manner. "Not much can be done. Four months isn't long."

Easy for him to say—it's not his damn cancer we're watching grow. "To me, it will be."

Over the next four months, while trying to cope with an uninterrupted flood of 'constermation'—minute-to-minute fear the cancer's coming back and is consuming me—and logging many a sleepless night, I take Dr. Drake's word (that my HMO won't authorize another CT so soon—TDKB, remember?), and wait. This isn't easy, by any means. But again, the weak but lingering belief the cancer's behind me helps bolster my outlook.

The four-month scan: Clearly, I remember slipping on a loose-fitting hospital gown, lying nervously on the icy CT table. An obliging and diplomatic female technician, properly detecting my harried state, tries her smiling best to comfort me. Though feeling and looking quite healthy, I know that, within a couple of days, with the reading of these test results, all that can do a one-eighty depending upon what 'they' find.

When I say I feel good that should be qualified. Almost always prior to a CT exam all parts of my body, especially my left side where Dr. Lutes sliced me open, begins to deliver odd, uncomfortable sensations. Things hurt in odd places. There are all sorts of weird stabbing pains. Again, the mind-body connection's flexing its muscle.

These CTs usually take about an hour to an hour and a half, depending on whether they scan all three areas, abdomen, chest, pelvis. This time, with the contrast needle jabbed painfully into a vein at my right wrist, each time I sense the technician pausing unnaturally at her console, I'm sure she's noticed some abnormality inside me and has stopped to report this unportentious 'thing' to the radiologist.

Finishing, she offers nothing more than a polite "Best of luck." A good-bye. For most professional technicians, this is customary. They won't offer any unfounded opinions, good or otherwise, unlike my first CT technician and radiologist who offered at first glance, as you'll recall, that I only had an enlarged spleen. Yeah, sure. Human nature being what it is, the tendency's to ask technicians how things went, how the scans look—or, to at least try to decipher the tech's poker face. But as a patient, you soon get over this curiosity . . . a few more days in the dark's often welcomed.

In Dr. Drake's office, five days later, he reads Jane and me the test results (I've always hoped he—and other doctors I've seen—would've read the report beforehand and digested its results, but sadly they never do: they're always too busy and thus read it for the first time in your presence.)

"Apparently," Dr. Drake begins, almost disinterestedly, "what they detected last go-round, from what's reported here, was the tail of the pancreas. That was the shadowy thing. Everything appears fine this time."

As Jane and I drive home there's no real sense of cheerfulness, of triumph, like you might expect. Instead, Dr. Drake's somberness seems to stay with us, coloring our moods.

As we go along here I'm sure it becomes apparent that the typical cancer patient lives in the front seat of a blinding roller-coaster ride, never sure what the next day, the next peek or valley, will bring. Or if some minor ache or pain (that earlier in life wouldn't have been noticed) is actually a physical prologue of the cancer renewing its attack.

CHAPTER 14

A STEP BACKWARD—
IN THE HOSPITAL AGAIN

Somewhere around month seven, 1991, I'm in bed one night, a Friday night around ten o'clock, sound asleep. About three hours later, I'm explosively awake. One of the most inexplicable and disquieting sensations of my life's swarming over me like quick-tempered yellow jackets: I'm shaking so violently, so uncontrollably, that I can't see. I feel as if I'm freezing to death despite the bedroom being at least 65 degrees.

Jane, standing over me, is all but shouting in my face.

"Eric! Eric! What is going on!" she's crying, shaking my shoulder, her face near mine. "You're bouncing around like you're having a seizure!"

Strange as it seems, I don't really realize anything's amiss till I'm fully awake. I'd literally slept through the early portion of this. Convulsing as I am, it's like I've awakened within someone else's bizarre, deranged body. Nothing I do deters these tremors.

"Pile on . . . some more . . . blankets!" I manage to say through chattering teeth. Jane hastily flings on at least four more weighty blankets. This solves nothing.

"We have to get you over to emergency!" Jane decides, frantically yanking on her clothes, then helping me into sweat pants and shirt. Still, I can't stop shaking. I've never experienced this out-of-control feeling. I'm trembling so aggressively, in fact, I can hardly stand upright, or walk.

Neither of us verbalize the word we know is on our minds—*cancer*. We both know the word's perched in the darkness of our thoughts, like a resting vulture. I hadn't been sick with a cold or the flu, nothing. This is out of the blue.

In five minutes, we're dressed, downstairs in the car. The demonic shaking persists in defiance of me being up and dressed in thick sweat clothes and coiled in several hefty blankets. Within minutes the car heater has the interior warmed considerably—but that does little good.

The hospital emergency room's roughly eight miles away. Approximately halfway, the shaking disappears altogether, abruptly, as if being lifted by the hand of some fiendish magician. Taking a discerning breath, I feel at once, remarkably, near normal. The calm within reminds me of the edgy peacefulness that hangs in the air following an earthquake. I do, however, feel war weary. My scalp's searing like a stove top.

At that point, I suggest we turn around, go home—all this is for naught. Jane will hear nothing of it. The condition, she insists, warrants the competent eye of a physician. "Especially in light of your history."

She's right, but desperately I don't want to return to the hospital: this symbolizes a significant step rearward in my fight to put cancer forever behind me. Going to ER's a defeat—albeit a minor one.

Still wrapped in a cumbersome blanket, I'm promptly escorted to an emergency exam table. ER's peaceful, all but uninhabited at this hour. Jane explains briefly the highs, the lows of my medical history to the young, tan-faced attending physician. He and the duty nurse begin giving me the once over.

"He's running a pretty good fever," the fast-moving RN notes. "Pulse's way up, too."

"Severe chills, I believe," the doctor says, as if tutoring me, moving a tiny flashlight from eye to eye, "are indicative of that. People sometimes experience severe shaking just prior to their temperatures zooming."

I watch them in conversation, hearing nothing, as though they're behind soundproof glass. Groggily viewing Jane I recollect an afternoon—before all this cancer crap—when we stood on the high rocks at Morro Bay, the sea gusts shifting her flaxen hair, making it lie in uneven patterns the way towering grass does in a wind-swept meadow, exposing her scalp in unsymmetrical parts . . . The-World-is-a-Beautiful-Place, I-Love-You expression on her face.

"With his medical background," the doctor's saying to Jane, as if I weren't there or mindful, "I'd like to keep him a day or two, put him on antibiotics, watch him."

Back in the present, I disagree. But Jane, the doctor, the nurse prevail.

So here I am: stuck in the same damn hospital where I'd had my original operation, now almost two years ago. A harsh sense of defeat drags me rearward. Once in a room, a private room, a bright-eyed nurse, looking as if she's just come on duty, comes in and starts an IV. Then, for fifteen minutes or so, she sits with me, making notes on my medical history within my chart. (Private rooms are always preferable to semi-private rooms for self-evident reasons—quiet, personal bathroom, solitude. The added expense, just a few dollars a day over what an insurance company will pay for a semi-private room, is well worth the expedience, the peace of mind.)

"You certainly don't look like you're on any sort of chemotherapy, Mr. Scribner," she says, clicking her ballpoint. "If that's any consolation." (Amazing how even trained members of the medical profession are driven by basic, and often false, everyday human assumptions: if you look good, you must feel good. This rationalism's even in effect when you visit a doctor—you will get more attentive treatment if you *look* sick. On occasion I've purposely looked worse than I feel—unshowered, unshaved, for example—to better capture a doctor's attention.)

Away from the tumult of the closing bar on the street below, I'm on the other wing of the hospital. Within ten minutes after the nurse's started the IV, the on-duty HMO doctor shows up. Not the same doctor I'd seen minutes before in ER. This is Dr. Inouye, a thickset fortyish internist. He comes off as wonderfully dedicated, actually interested in my general physical state and medical history. He makes notes in the margins next to the information the nurse's gathered. I'm impressed.

Dr. Inouye gives me the once-over with stethoscope, flashlight, and poking fingers. Right away I like this guy, his country-doctor manner. He seems sincerely caught up in patient care.

"Any idea what we're dealing with?" I ask.

"Very hard to say, quite frankly," he offers, smiling. "We're seeing a lot of strange bugs lately. So what we'll do is keep you on a series of antibiotics for a few days . . . as a precaution. You present a very unique situation, Mr. Scribner."

Defeat—and the uniqueness of my disease—races bitterly through me.

"You don't think this is . . . a reaction to Mitotane? The chemo?" I ask knowing, though, that this doctor probably knows little or nothing about the drug.

"Chemotherapy, I'm afraid that's not my bailiwick. We'll run your question by Dr. Drake on Monday. I'm certain he'll want to be brought on-board."

At once I'm struck with the knowledge that I'm in the hospital and my No. 1 doctor, my oncologist, isn't being apprised till Monday, two days hence. I hold my tongue: I don't want to alienate Dr. Inouye. Besides, this postponement in involving Dr. Drake's probably some HMO regulation anyway.

"What did Dr. Inouye tell you I have?" I ask the nurse, when she reappears following the doctor's departure.

"Probably what he told you. He only told me what antibiotics to start." Dangling several more bags of transparent solution on the chrome IV pole, she continues, almost whispering: "But I can tell you this—you're in good hands. He's one of the good ones . . . . He's your regular doctor?"

"No. Actually Dr. Zindler's my regular doctor." Catching a quick look of disapproval in the nurse's eye, I hesitate, feeling curiously laid bare or shamed at having to announce this—though I don't know why. A bit intimidated, I offer feebly: "He's got the office right next to my oncologist. What do you make of him—Zindler?"

Reading her eyes, listening to the pitch of her voice, I get a obvious picture of her opinion. "Oh, Dr. Zindler, he's . . . pretty good, yeah. But us nurses, we're kind of partial to Dr. Inouye."

She's not referring to anything as crude as his looks or sexual prowess or something of that nature—she referring to Dr. Inouye's medical know-how. In that

I wasn't enamored with Dr. Zindler, I make a mental memo to switch primary physicians at my next opportunity.

'He's one of the good ones.' With the nurse's observation soothing my sense of misfortune at being in the hospital again, I doze off to the resonance of a forlorn jetliner high in the night sky. It's now well after 2:00 a.m.

Advice: Your most reliable source of medical information is an honest nurse. One thing I've learned over the course of this illness—get on a nurse's good side and then ask penetrating questions. Listen closely to what she says, particularly when she's discussing your doctor or the treatment strategies he's proposing. Often your most rewarding insight will come from nurses. No one knows a physician's overall skill better than a nurse. Surgical nurses are eminently beneficial in revealing who's trustworthy with scalpel and . . . who's not.

Chapter 15

More Questions Than Answers—
Many Antibiotics, Few Reasons

When I awaken in the morning to the predictable hospital pandemonium, it's around six-thirty. A lithesome, refined-looking ebony nurse's standing as quietly as possible beside my bed modifying the IV drip rate. She grins sensing my open eyes.

"What do you have, mon?" she asks softly, in a pithy Jamaican accent. Is this an illusion, I wonder . . . or some weird prank?

"I was hoping you could fill me in," I answer, gaining my whereabouts. "You my new nurse? What's your name?"

She displays a pinned-on ID with her likeness. "Gloria's the name and I cannot tell you what you have, mon. But this I can tell you, I have never seen so many antibiotics poured into one body before. Are you famous?"

Only for the scarcity of my disease, I think begrudgingly. "Not yet, anyway," I reply. "Came in last night with bad chills—really bad chills, and a temperature. Otherwise, I feel okay."

Nurse Gloria, hands on her hips, is looking at the assorted bottles and bags of liquids dripping into a solitary tube that ultimately winds its way to a vein in my forearm. "Um-um-um," she mutters to herself in obvious wonder, shaking her head.

"I take it this is unusual—having so many bottles?"

"Oh, yes, mon. I have never seen anyone treated with so many drugs at one time. I will have to look and see why."

"I'm . . . also a cancer patient," I volunteer, not considering my words, perhaps looking for condolence, perhaps thinking this may explain matters.

(I always refer to myself in the neutral, as a cancer patient, rather than using a self-condemning term like, 'I have cancer.' Since no one knows for sure whether you do or do not have cancer by your appearance, when you look and feel good, why not refer to yourself simply as 'a cancer patient?' Without visible signs to the contrary, I favor the term 'cancer-free.' This isn't a form of negation; the words simply state that at this moment, to my knowledge, the knowledge of my doctors, I'm without any sign of cancer. Also, early on, I took a vehement dislike to the term 'remission.' This over-wrought designation signifies that doctors and others feel that, yes, the disease's still present, but is being held at bay—is hiding in the wings, so to speak, awaiting its next occasion to strike.)

Gloria nods in a calculated way. In her eyes, I can see this answers some of her doubts. "I take special care of you, mon," she promises, winking as she leaves the room.

Shortly thereafter Jane arrives. She too looks at the five bottles suspended over the bed. "What're they doing to you?" Jane remarks, preoccupied. "Looks like some kind of dangling aquarium."

"Apparently they're giving me everything in the book. I'll have to wait till Dr. Zindler gets here. Should be any time. He supposedly makes his morning rounds around eight. Strange . . .how you don't stay with the doctor who admits you. Aren't HMOs wonderful?"

"It's Saturday, you realize," Jane offers as if this answers something, setting her small deerskin purse on the lower part of the bed. "How do you feel this morning? Anymore shaking?"

"I was thinking—I bet the Mitotane has thrown off my sense of balance. Internally, you know."

"The ER doc last night sure didn't know what to make of you."

"There aren't many, it seems, who've heard of adrenal cortical carcinoma," I say, feeling disagreeably singular, distressed.

"Funny," Jane remarks, scooting her chair nearer the bed, "how we come to think of doctors as knowing everything, isn't it?"

My breakfast arrives—two eggs, sausage, toast, orange juice, and coffee—looking like it came from a Las Vegas buffet table. Well, at least I get to eat. "Should of thought to bring you something," Jane laments as the volunteer takes the lid from my meal.

Sitting quietly for a minute, looking about, Jane says: "See any nurses you recognize—from last time?"

"Thank God, no. You know, it's funny how the nurses here, on this floor, are more attentive than the ones on the post-surgery floor. Seems like it'd be just the opposite."

The hospital is in full swing now. Humankind of all sorts zooming by the doorway: nurses, doctors, technicians, candy-stripers, and white-clad janitors. The morning TV news is on when Dr. Zindler strides in—faded jeans, striped polo shirt, no spit, no polish.

Dr. Zindler is a compressed fellow of about thirty-five, maybe older. (Younger than me, at any rate.) I chose him as my primary-care physician because I thought he'd be unique for two reasons: (1) he's an intimate crony of Dr. Drake—I saw this as a plus: they could knowingly share the overlapping issues of my case; and (2) his office's located conveniently across the hallway from Dr. Drake's.

In the three or four times I've seen Dr. Zindler, he and I haven't reached a great sense of compatibility. His stock greeting, as he breezes into the exam room, is, "Well, Mr. Scribner, you're not dead yet, so let's have a look at you." This isn't accompanied by a laugh or even a smile—not that that would make it appropriate. This disturbing opening observation, I gather, summarizes the discussions he's had with Dr. Drake relative to my fate.

So outraged have I become at this mockery, I decide to go to the HMO's resident patient advocate to complain. She, the advocate, seems righteously concerned, appearing as though she'll take suitable action, till I realize (some time later) that she and the doctors are paid by the same source. Shining example of the fox and the hen house.

Needless to say the HMO patient advocate position is in name only. As such, she does little beside lend a commiserating ear to patient complaints. She takes no action on my behalf. Thus it was that Dr. Inouye, the on-duty physician who'd seen me last night with such professionalism—and had won the recognition of the floor nurses—interested me instantly as a potential new primary-care physician.

Stone-faced, Dr. Zindler nods a vague, nonverbal 'Hello,' as he helps himself to my TV control and hits the Off button. I'm not ill-mannered. I'd fully planned to do the same—before he began speaking. Next he reaches out, fingering the clear tubing leading from the IV bottles to my arm, as if this educated handling communicates something. Whipping his stethoscope from around his neck and, with its business end headed my way, he asks mechanically how I am. Never does he say: "Good morning," to either Jane or myself. I might as well have been a mute animal lying there for all he cared.

After bringing him up to speed, I summarize by saying: "The whole thing had me pretty scared, actually. I didn't know your body could do something like that—on its own, I mean, without me telling it to."

Lightly digesting my words in his own I-Could-Care-Less manner, Dr. Zindler, dark hair parted in the center, says, "The body is quite capable of extraordinary reflexive behavior. Convulsive chills being just one of them. How do you feel now—this minute?"

"Like I want to go home."

"Well, you'll have to adjust those feelings. I want to get some more of these antibiotics in you. And run a test or two."

"What am I being treated for?" I ask, idly trying to conceive of what species of music this character listens to . . . what his wife and children look like.

"Couldn't say at this point. That's why I'm opting to be cautious, considering," he says, making a ceremony of re-draping his stethoscope around his neck, standing to leave. "I'll have somebody check on you later. I'll be back tomorrow. We'll look at sending you home then."

As he gets to the door, he stops. "I have to remind you of something . . . . Were you aware you were supposed to call the HMO urgent care unit to get permission to come here last night? Patients don't just *decide* to go to ER themselves."

"But," Jane offers, "this was an emergency. Eric's a cancer patient. We didn't know."

"The on-duty HMO doctor has to approve your coming here."

"It was after midnight."

"That matters little. Call urgent care and the operator will contact the duty physician and he'll then contact you with instructions as to how to proceed."

"All that takes time," Jane resumes angrily. "We had to act."

"Be that as it may, Mrs. Scribner."

"Well," I say as he walks out, "let's hope there isn't a next time."

"Pleasant soul," Jane observes, having now met the ignoble Dr. Zindler for the first time. "He's the one you talked to the HMO about, right?"

"In the flesh."

"Does seem a bit of a cold fish."

"To put it mildly. You wonder, don't you, how some of these people get to be MDs?"

"Doesn't seem like a whole lot of them are in it for love of the patient. He did, however, indicate he's doing all this because of your condition. When he talked about being cautious."

"Yeah. I wonder what he would've done if he'd admitted me last night, instead of Dr. Inouye? Would I have all these antibiotics? Would I even be here?"

"Every profession has its good and bad."

Later in the day a Respiratory Therapist comes in and attempts to get me to hack up something—sputum, I believe she called it—that can be examined in the lab. This apparently is what Dr. Zindler was referring to when he referred to testing.

Dr. Inouye, a welcomed faced, comes by once in the evening to check on me. He's on his usual rounds.

The next morning while Dr. Zindler's listening to my lungs, I ask him, "Anything come of the tests you ran?"

"Nothing conclusive," he says, re-draping his stethoscope around his neck. Contemplating the five bottles dangling on the IV pole, he decides, "So what we'll do is keep you for at least another day."

"Has Dr. Drake been called or anything?" I ask, thinking this a sensible query.

"He'll get my report later this week."

"He . . . doesn't get involved . . . in some way . . . in this hospital stay? I mean, I am his patient," I say, wondering to myself what would happen if I were there for a recognized cancer issue. Would Drake deign to show up?

"His focus is the oncology portion of your case."

Not really wanting to link this current mystery condition and cancer, I say: "How do we know this isn't related? Or that it isn't a result of the drug he's got me taking. Mitotane."

"Because, Mr. Scribner, that's not the way our system works," Dr. Zindler says as if speaking to an offending adolescent. "You worry about getting well. Leave the doctoring to us—okay?"

FINDING HOPE WHEN DOCTORS SAY THERE IS NONE

CHAPTER 16

PSYCHOLOGY AS VOODOO—
DR. DRAKE'S LABEL FOR PSYCHOTHERAPY

Soon as I'm released from the hospital (without ever learning what I had), I go to the HMO clinic to request—no, demand—a different primary physician. This is well within my advertised rights as an HMO patient. Again, I have to bargain with the same impotent clerk who 'helped' me previously, the patient coordinator. I want to become Dr. Inouye's patient, but the coordinator says he isn't accepting new patients. Understandably, his practice is full. Ultimately, the clerk does cooperate, albeit unknowingly.

She reveals that a unique doctor's joining the staff in a week or two. She'll see that my name gets on this doctor's new-patient list. The new doctor's an internist and a nephrologist, a kidney specialist. Kidneys aren't exactly adrenals, but they're close. The adrenal glands, each roughly the size of a grape, sit atop each kidney.

The patient coordinator is presumably inspired to volunteer this settlement when I tell her if Dr. Zindler one more time greets me with, "Well, I see you're not dead yet, Mr. Scribner, so let's have a look at you," I'm going to come off the table and loosen his teeth, doctor or no doctor. How dare this man be so openly insensitive!

From all I'd read—I was still researching profusely—your faith and confidence in your medical team, as many books put it, is of paramount consequence to your eventual recovery. This line of thinking, of course, presupposes you have the right doctors—the right medical team in the sense that they truly know what they're talking about—and actually care about you.

Intuitively, this trust/mistrust issue's been eating at me: I don't have enormous faith or trust in either Dr. Drake or Zindler. My team. How can I hope to enrich my survival chances unless I believe that they believe—or care about—what they're saying?

Example: After reading time and again that a psychologist should be part of a cancer patient's 'medical team' (medical team in quotes because I believe I had anything but a team working for me), I bring this notion up with Dr. Drake. I assume (yes, I know about assume: it makes an ass out of you and me), that he'll know of various psychologists and will gladly suggest a seasoned soul. Instead, in his characteristic off-base fashion, he simply nods, saying he knows of none. Not a one. He's also unaware of any local support groups for cancer patients.

"There's *no one* you can refer me too?" I ask, in disbelief. "We've got local groups to help people quit smoking, loose weight, and stop gambling—but nothing for cancer patients?"

"Mr. Scribner," he begins in his droll fashion, "the practice of psychotherapy is little more than prevailing voodoo. There's no evidence that this sort of therapy in any way aids cancer patients. Cancer, plain and simple, is a disease of the body."

Again, is this the doctor talking or the Penny-Pinching, You-Don't-Need-Another-Referral-To-A-Specialist HMO speaking through him?

Okay. I figured if I want to see a shrink (I lump all therapists, psychiatrists and psychologists, in this category), I have to uncover one myself. Which is exactly what I did, albeit not scientifically: Using the yellow pages, I call several therapists till I hit upon one I think has some expertise assisting people with chronic and life-threatening afflictions.

Dr. Reginald Holt, my first therapist, is, more than anything, a troubled-youth and marriage counselor, but for me, he's a satisfactory start; a perceptive ear. He says he can help. His doctorate is from a school of divinity. This makes no difference, I decide, in that I'm sure he's been well-grounded in human relations in general. Life and death, obviously, being an indivisible part of that.

At our initial meeting, he seems entirely untroubled talking about cancer's ugly side. His wife, it seems, had a touch-and-go bout with breast cancer approximately ten years earlier. She's now doing well. Propitious news, indeed. We cancer patients are always up for an honest survival story—nothing's quite as enriching.

Dr. Holt wears loafers, casual pants, open-necked shirts. (This doesn't sit too well with me: Doctors and other professionals should be seen in the appropriate uniform—shirt and tie and suitable dress shoes. No clogs, no contemptible tennis sneakers.)

At our opening session we sit one-on-one in a restful den-like setting, in a one-story stucco office building, called The Counseling Center. Cars zoom noisily by in the late-afternoon sun as we talk. I open by saying that I want to discuss only my prevalent medical situation. I'm not here for a Freudian analysis of my adolescence or my dependence on my parents or their traumas.

Dr. Holt seems somewhat pained at this announcement. I'm convinced—later I formed this opinion—he was educated in a mold, or system, much like a hairdresser or barber who learns to perform tasks only a certain way and, when I asked to go outside that mold, outside his habitual methodology, he'd follow only involuntarily.

Initially, Dr. Holt does agree: no delving into my childhood—for any reason. We're to stick with the here, the now: cancer.

These hour-long sessions are valuable. If nothing else, they allow me to completely bare myself, to reveal the dread I'd kept hidden, to get educated feedback. Right away, I voice the concerns I have with my medical team—Drs. Drake and Zindler. As I itemize my fears, it's soothing to hear another mortal, a professional, agree that these doctors are not necessarily worthy of my trust.

I advise the shrink how Dr. Drake referred to psychotherapy as voodoo. And I describe Dr. Zindler's belittling salutations. I also tell Dr. Holt that, since Dr. Drake won't sanction these visits, he has to get in touch with Dr. Drake directly and persuade him these consultations are worthwhile in order to get an HMO authorization.

Dr. Holt knows distantly of Dr. Drake. He's heard of Dr. Drake's less-than-appealing nature. After seeing me a few times, however, he is able to win over Dr. Drake that these sessions are rewarding. Dr. Drake concedes to submitting the requisite paperwork for the HMO's consent.

Advice: I highly advocate that every cancer patient regularly consult and abide by the admonitions of a discerning psychotherapist or psychiatrist. He/she is the consummate non-partisan third-party listener, one who'll offer incisive and well-informed guidance relative to your concerns, your questions.

I, by the way, had hitherto been wholly averse to the notion of anyone needing the services of psychologist. I theorized all shrinks should be hauled out to sea and drowned. Mankind would be better served. (Perhaps I was like Dr. Drake . . . till I actually needed guidance myself.)

A conscientious shrink's a vital element—at times the centermost—of your recovery team. He/she will commonly be the only one interjecting enlightened, unbiased convictions into the chaotic process of cancer healing. Your friends and kindred, while well-meaning, are too devoted to discern the trees. . . .

FINDING HOPE WHEN DOCTORS SAY THERE IS NONE

Chapter 17

An Old Foe Rears Its Head—
The Shrink Turns Traitor

Now I'm back working full time—still experiencing killer testosterone headaches and a near impossible time waking up in the morning—and seeing the shrink once a week after work. I've been following this routine for a couple of months. Jane thinks this a capital plan. I emerge from these shrink sessions, she observes, a more mellow human being.

I do feel comfortably unraveled, freshened after each session. Perhaps it's just being able to commune with someone possessing the title doctor, to spew openly about the eventual conclusions preying upon me, to have someone give an ear and respond civilly. As much as I don't want to face it, way, way, way down inside I'm still scared shitless of dying an abject cancer death.

Dr. Drake had assured me in his ever-polite manner it would happen . . . most NCI literature indicates it will . . . and, unlike other cancers, ACC offers no five-year cure rate to work toward. I'll be taking Mitotane forever. At a minimum, the drug's guaranteed to extinguish my one remaining adrenal gland. Then I'll have to deal with whatever repercussions that spawns. And there are other issues: the PDQ indicates that patients on long-term Mitotane are subject to 'brain damage and impairment of function.' These and other concerns I reveal openly with Dr. Holt.

Despite my earlier admonitions (that we not delve into my childhood or areas other than cancer treatment and recovery), Dr. Holt feels it necessary to resolve the relationship I have—or didn't have, actually—with my youngest son, Gregory. For about five years, since his mother and I'd divorced, he and I hadn't exchanged a word.

Dr. Holt feels it's up to me, the adult in this situation (despite my son being 24), to take the initiative. This unappreciative kid hadn't bothered to come to the hospital or even call following my cancer surgery. But I agree to make a real effort to talk with him, to see if we can arrange at least one dinner meeting to iron-out our unclear differences.

After two face-to-face exchanges with Greg to set up this dinner (he's very mannerly, very agreeable), he comes up with last-minute reasons for not showing up—his way of saying, 'Thanks, but no thanks.' His position, I believe, was one of convenience—he found it less burdensome to avoid seeing me, speaking with me: He could remove himself from the tangle of his father's uncertain fate. It was too early in my counseling to fathom the real value of unqualified forgiveness in your total healing (that'll come later when I return to my religious roots).

After few sessions with Dr. Holt, I decide that, despite his overly casual attire and his offhand manner, he's an okay guy—that it'd be a good idea to have Jane see him a time or two. Cancer, we patients soon learn, reaches its malignant tentacles just as mysteriously into the hearts and minds of otherwise healthy family members. Dr. Holt agrees.

This arrangement, however, proves to be our undoing.

In going over things with Jane, I hoped Holt would positively reshape some of the ill-defined notions she held, bringing her on-board relative to the inner fears of your everyday cancer patient. She could voice her deep-seated concerns—those life-and-death issues she kindly withheld from me—and have a doctor shepherd her.

Midway through dinner on the evening she'd seen Dr. Holt, I'm eager to hear what she thinks of this guy as a mentor.

"Oh," Jane comments impassively, curiously distant, spooning some dressing on her salad, "he seems a likable person."

"Well," I persist, "what did you come away with?"

Jane, cocking her head, makes an odd face. For some reason she doesn't want to go on. I persist.

"Okay," she begins warily, pondering for a moment a forkful of mashed potatoes, "he said, he thought you were . . . well . . . wallowing in self-pity. Acting like a child . . . about this whole thing."

"All right, hon, enough kidding," I say, chuckling. "What did you guys *really* talk about?"

"What I just said. That my husband's over-reacting." After a moment she adds: "Like I've been saying all along."

My stomach, discerning with this off-the-wall account, contracts instantly into a tense, angry lump. I've been . . . betrayed? No, this can't be. Their meeting was supposed to result in an enlightenment of sorts. "You're . . . putting me on," I say, poking at the half-uneaten pork chop on my plate, hoping desperately she is toying with me—but again, feeling as if I've lost another round to this merciless foe, this cancer.

"He said," Jane resumes discreetly, again almost unwillingly, "he thought you were well over the crisis point. That you're dwelling too heavily on this whole business."

"Why would he say something to you . . . he never said to me?"

Chewing quietly, Jane shrugs blamelessly.

"I cannot believe this. Here I've been trying intelligently to come to grips with this whole situation—this friggin' cancer-in-me thing . . . this disease Drake says is going to do me in—and this jerk tells you I'm a baby. That I'm overreacting . . . Shit!" Shoving my plate away, I go on, "In my own way, I thought I was doing right. This just rips me up."

"—According to him," Jane goes on, now oddly infused, adopting more of an I-Told-You-So attitude, "you can only go so far. This research business then becomes an obsession."

"That complete asshole!" I blurt out, furious, hearing these words coming, not from my wife, but some double-dealing psychologist. "The reading I do's a precautionary measure . . . a preemptive strike—I feel—in the battle to beat this disease. I don't want this shit sneaking up on me, when I know I could've done something. It's cliché, I know, but to defeat one's enemy, one must understand that enemy . . ." Pausing, I quickly sift these disturbing thoughts, trying to understand why my wife finds harm in researching a disease. "That rotten bastard, one meeting, and he's set us—you and me—back a hundred years."

"He's right, though, Eric. I've said this all along."

"All right, I'll say it: I'm scared as hell this cancer's going to eat me up when I'm not looking. Are you friggin' satisfied? I'm a man and I'm scared. Okay?"

"You don't have to tell me that."

"I thought finally you understood."

"I'm living with a lot too."

"That was the whole purpose of this Holt thing."

"Only, I don't need a shrink."

"We were well past this He's-Dwelling-On-His-Disease crap, I thought . . . . Reading, Jane, is my way of coping. My armament. Tell me: Do you see me wallowing? Ever? Moping about, crying in my friggin' beer? You really want to know why I'm always searching? (Raising her eyebrows, Jane sips her ice tea.) I'm hoping to stumble on something that says all these doctors are wacko—that there's not a damn thing wrong with me. I know, I know, it's stupid. But it's my hope. I'm doing what makes me comfortable. I want to understand everything about this cancer. I want to be standing and ready . . . if ever the day comes. Knowledge is like insurance to me."

"It's never coming back, I told you," Jane asserts, now reaching lovingly across the table to squeeze my hand. "You just need more confidence."

"Jane, if anything, I'm a realist."

Later that evening, trekking unaccompanied on our breezy, moonless beach, I try picturing how the dialogue must've gone . . . Holt holding court, wiggling his sandaled foot, maybe pretending to read from his notes. Why would he offer such a malicious, destructive critique? If he's truly a professional, why didn't he have enough prudence *not* to dredge up an injurious assumption—even if he believed it.

With the October wind whipping my thin nylon jacket, the mist of the pounding surf pelting my face, I momentarily let go of my resentment and resolve to call and lock horns with this double-dealing character in the morning.

Mostly, I feel emotionally violated—as when someone rummages through your personal belongings, then laughingly tells everyone your secrets. As I try sleeping that night, Holt's rending words take on a life of their own—Is he, I wonder, somehow, correct? Am I oblivious to this side of myself?

In a cramped phone booth down the hall from my office (for privacy's sake), I dial Dr. Holt's office the next morning. "Hey, Eric," he says affably. "Calling about our next session, are you?"

"Not exactly, Dr. Holt," I reply, baiting him, I suppose. "There isn't going to *be* a next session."

Following an unexpected, drawn-out pause: "Why the uncertainty, Mr. Scribner?" Holt changes gears, a new tone entering his words. At least he's incisive enough to perceive there is something eating me.

"Jane and I . . . had a little talk last night. About what you guys went over."

"Okay . . .?"

"Frankly, I feel laughed-at, for lack of a better term. You *really* told Jane I was over-reacting? That I was being a baby?"

No comeback from the shrink. A faint buzzing silence on the line. A vice president's secretary walks hurriedly by the phone booth, smiling at me awkwardly as if to discern the content of this conversation.

"Want me to tell you what you accomplished, doctor?" I volunteer, resuming. "Single-handedly you punched a major hole in our relationship—mine and my wife's. She's now back where she was eight months ago—on this kick that I'm over-researching the cancer, that I'm dwelling on it like some hypochondriac."

"Mr. Scribner, I seriously doubt that, in one session, I could accomplish a reversal of that sort," Dr. Holt says protectively. "If that's in fact what happened, then we must assume your wife's a relatively superficial individual. We discussed you, certainly, but I don't think that was the conclusion we came to. It's possible your wife misinterpreted what I said. Again, I don't think anyone can change other's opinion in a single hour."

"Isn't that fairly naive of you?" I ask, a biting acid now flowing across my stomach walls. "You're the one carrying the title doctor. That makes you, in case you forgot, an authority figure. We commoners tend to believe things you spew. Educated opinions do carry weight with most plain folk—especially when they reinforce distant, already held beliefs. You and I've talked about this very thing."

"Well, if that's what materialized, it wasn't my intention."

"Why were you never honest with me about this?"

"I thought we'd said as much, in so many words."

"Communication is supposed to be one of your strong suits, doctor."

"Certain listening skills are likewise required of the patient."

"So, anyway, I have to live with the consequences now. Re-fight this battle, as it were. Whether that was your intention or not, that's how things were perceived. To repeat: I won't be coming back to see you. If this is a sample of the back-handed family counseling you dish up, maybe you should also consider selling a variety of ammunition—"

"Mr. Scribner, I'm afraid I don't need this. *Good*-bye," Dr. Holt mutters, hanging up.

"I thought you were on my side, doctor," I whisper into the dead phone.

Notwithstanding this encounter, I didn't stop reading nor did I lose faith in making a shrink a part of my recovery team. Soon after this, with a little help from my new primary-care physician, I locate my next psychologist. He, unlike Dr. Holt, is a legitimate, licensed clinical psychologist. Come to find out, he and Holt are distant acquaintances. This new shrink's opinion of my former therapist? "A third-rate social worker, at best. In way over his head if he's seeing cancer patients."

CHAPTER 18

A BREAK IN THE CLOUDS—
NEW DOCTORS TAKE CONTROL

Long about this time, a call comes from Dr. Drake's nurse, April. Dr. Drake's been in a minor car accident, she tells me. It looks like he'll be out for six weeks or so while his doctors decide what to do. How serious is the injury, I ask. Well, it appears it's just a minor case of whiplash, I believe, April confides. Interesting turn of events, I'm thinking, vindictively amused inside. So . . . now the tough guy, Drake, will be dealing with *his* doctors. How interesting.

I'm not scheduled to see him for a couple of weeks. So this doesn't prove any great inconvenience. Give the doctor my best, I tell April. I really want to say: Tell the good doctor to quit being such a wimp! Tell him most people continue working with a minor whiplash. Tell him he inflicts far greater harm on his patients than any silly whiplash by telling them they're going to die soon! But I bite my tongue.

For the last couple of weeks I'd been noticing a worrisome pattern in my breathing. At times I'd suck in quick, short breaths, involuntarily, for no apparent reason. And my lungs, my breathing in general, seemed unusually constricted. This condition has me concerned, as do all little glitches or unexplained physical changes, be they painful or not. Am I becoming a hypochondriac? Fortunately, my new primary-care physician, Dr. Margaret Bristol, a distinguished-looking, silver-haired lady in her early sixties comes on the scene.

Our initial meeting goes well, considering my recent luck with doctors. Realizing it probably doesn't matter one way or the other, I tell her of my encounters with Dr. Zindler, of his unrefined bedside manner. Dr. Bristol, being duly indoctrinated in the 'brotherhood of the AMA,' offers little more than, "Hm . . . I see." This I don't hold against her. I didn't anticipate she'd say much, if anything, about a colleague. I just had to get the words off my chest.

Dr. Bristol has a take-charge, but gracious, sincere, respectful, bigger-than-life, matronly air about her. Quite refreshing is she after all the detached male doctors I've dealt with of late. Not only is she a nephrologist, but she'd apparently retired as chief administrator of a prestigious medical facility in Los Angeles prior to joining this local HMO clinic. In conversation she mentions she tried to retire, but found it vexatious (her word). She and I seem to hit it off pretty well from the get-go. She, I believe, has heard of some of the indelicate treatment I'd received at the hands of Dr. Zindler and is accordingly supportive.

Taking time to read over my medical records—actually read them!—she listens attentively as I describe this newly noted condition in my lungs and breathing. I explain how I'd been led to believe, via Dr. Drake and various literature, that ACC is most likely to metastasize to the lungs. Knowing this, I'm concerned. She's actually listening to me—something I find very unusual for a doctor. Everything about her says she's involved: her unaffected and keen questions, and the relaxed manner in which she examines me, listening especially to my lungs and feeling for enlarged lymph nodes in my neck.

"You know, doctor, I've been considering something for some time now," I begin hesitantly, as she examines me, knowing I'm venturing out on a limb. "I'd really like to go to M.D. Anderson, in Houston, to talk to those doctors. Being that this is a such a rare condition I'd really like to sit face to face with someone who's actually been in the trenches." This bit of boldness, I hope, will not short-circuit or offend her sense of professionalism, of expertise, a la Drake.

"I take it from your records," she asks rationally, looking up from my ever-thickening medical file, "that they're the authorities—in this type of cancer?"

"From all I've read, yes," I respond, immediately appreciating that she isn't referring to this as 'my cancer.' "And from what Dr. Drake and the doctor at USC said."

With her now looking me dead in the eye, I'm thinking, Uh-oh, here comes that venomous HMO spiel. "I wholeheartedly agree," she says, scratching some sort of note in my file. "I know if I had some rare cancer I'd certainly want to sit down with the experts."

What? Are my ears deceiving me? I'd been conditioned of late to expect only negative responses. Indirectly she's admitted she isn't an authority on this disease. To have any doctor admit this is remarkably refreshing. "You . . . *agree?*" I say, smiling incredulously.

She seems amused. "You're finding this peculiar?"

"Long, tangled story. I'm just impressed that you said yes."

"You make the travel arrangements. I'll take care of the paperwork," she continues. "I'd like us to do some testing here before you go. Check those lungs—pulmonary tests and possibly another CT. And I guess you heard Dr. Drake's out for a while, so Dr. Malone, a private-practice oncologist, will be filling in for him. She probably should be onboard with this trip thing, too."

Another stroke of good luck! Other cancer patients had said nice things about my new, but temporary oncologist, Dr. Anne Malone. But—two women doctors? While I am going to a far-off, unfamiliar city on rather esoteric medical business—kind of a good-news/bad-news sort of thing—I'm quite elated at this fortuitous turn of events. Finally I'll get to meet the ACC authorities. Maybe, just maybe, they'll offer new treatment options—or, who knows, new hope.

The following week Jane and I make arrangements for the flight to Houston. Calling Dr. Frank at M.D. Anderson, I remind him who I am—the ACC patient in California who took Tamoxifen for male breast enlargement. "Oh, yes!" he says heartily. In minutes, he explains the procedure for setting up a consultation at MDA. (A medical practitioner of some sort usually makes the referral. Dr. Bristol readily agreed to call MDA and arrange things. She seems too good to be true—an old-style doctor who doesn't cow-tow to HMO dictates.)

So now, locally, I have a new oncologist, a series of pulmonary tests and a CT of the chest to go through. I also have to gather all the necessary medical records, slides and previous CT results and data from these tests, then head off to the great unknown—Houston.

Despite this happy turn of events—two new doctors, a trip to Houston—a deep-seated sense of dread's nagging at me: Could this new breathing problem in fact be a recurrence?

FINDING HOPE WHEN DOCTORS SAY THERE IS NONE

CHAPTER 19

THE FIRST OF THREE TRIPS TO HOUSTON

Dr. Anne Malone, a demure, mousy little person, seems disappointingly withdrawn even in her physical demeanor, as she listens with a questioning curiosity as I recount my initial symptoms, the surgery and my present chemo regimen. Naively, I assume she's at least heard of Mitotane. I can't, however, ascertain whether she has from her unresponsive stare. And I'm afraid to ask—for fear her negative answer will undermine my belief in her. As we talk, she, like a cowering sparrow, maintains a clear distance—leaning as she is on the narrow writing ledge at the far side of the exam room.

When I finish she comes forward, asking me to lie back so she can feel (palpate) my abdomen. Her technique's disappointing—too delicate, too inhibited, in light of the weighty pawing other doctors had used. But who am I to pass judgment, I wonder quickly, maybe a light touch is all one needs to identify internal malformations. One positive outcome of this meeting, though: Dr. Malone agrees to endorse my trek to Houston to see the ACC experts. But she does so with a bit of misgiving, it seems, as though she's somehow leery of a patient who's brassy enough, on his initial visit, to make such a grandiose request.

Later I'm struck with three quick deductions: (1) either Dr. Malone feels uncomfortable with men in general, or (2) she is, for some reason, intimidated by me, which I doubt, or (3) she's just timorous by nature, which I also doubt. I don't quite know what to make of her . . . is she in fact a step up from Dr. Drake? Am I being too judgmental? Am I becoming gun shy of doctors in general?

At any rate, almost anything's better than the ever-sour Drake. I do, after all, want to get rid of him, if for no other reason than to sample another oncologist's approach. Drake's accident appears to be my only immediate hope of changing oncologists in this era of HMO-dominated medicine. At least Dr. Malone doesn't talk of my imminent death.

(My local HMO clinic had only one oncologist on staff—Dr. Drake. To get a referral to a private-practice oncologist would've been near impossible in that Dr. Drake was available and providing 'adequate care' in the eyes of HMO authorities. To further pursue a change, I would've had to [1] appeal my case in writing to the HMO higher-ups, or [2] wait for the once-at-year 'open enrollment' period with my employer, then change HMOs, or [3] convince my employer that my current HMO was not serving me well and request a change of HMOs via that route. Any of these approaches could take months . . . or longer.)

With the trip to Houston coming up quickly, completing the tests Dr. Bristol wants and the gathering the results becomes quite hectic. I'm running breathlessly everywhere, it seems. Finally, all's done and Jane and I can relax. My unoccupied mind now can settle in on the business of worrying about test results. This concern *isn't* unjustified. For example, while the pulmonary tests results proved normal, the chest CT results aren't so clear-cut.

Though there isn't outright evidence of recurrent cancer, in the chest (lungs), the radiologist notes something called 'multifocal alveolar infiltrates.' While this notation sounds medically precise, no one (various doctors) can tell me exactly what infiltrates are, nor can they say whether the condition's deadly. Apparently there'd been at least some discussion among local radiologists—yes, those doctors again—about these infiltrates representing a metastasis, a new cancer. These doctors though, admit, they haven't seen enough recurring ACC (can we say none?) to offer a conclusive opinion.

Needless to say, from the time I learned of this finding until we get off the plane in Houston, I'm more than distressed. Again, there are nights of tossing, turning, dwelling on this and that, watching the empty window as the moon slides soulessly across the dawdling night sky.

May 1, 1991: As the landing gear retracts, thudding in place beneath the plane, I lay my head back watching Los Angeles, a city of mustard-colored air, of uncountable criss-crossing asphalt stripes, dissolve below. Finally, we're on our way. It's mid-afternoon. We're to arrive shortly after dark, go to our hotel, and in the morning meet Dr. Frank. I'd attempted to arrange a consultation with the chief endocrinologist, author of many medical journal articles on ACC, but sadly was informed he was too ill—he'd suffered a severe stroke.

"So," Jane says, accepting a Coke from a smiling flight attendant, "now that we're in the air, what're you thinking?"

"Like . . . I'm going home. After all the reading I've done."

"That again?"

"This business with my lungs has me concerned. Why can't you be wifely about this and support me, damn it? I don't understand."

"You worry too much, I'm telling you."

"Now's probably not the time for this . . . again."

Dying for a beer or glass of wine, I am, something to relax the soul. But the Mitotane in my system won't permit drinking even a small amount of alcohol without severe lightheadedness, and a very weird kind of prolonged muscle weakness.

"I'll just be glad to see someone who understands this disease," I continue, now watching the fawn-colored, barren California desert slide beneath the wing.

"We certainly brought enough stuff," Jane comments lightly, referring to the items safely stowed overhead—the package of CT films, pathology slides, written test results, a steno pad brimming with questions for Dr. Frank.

"They said I'd need it all," I say, hoping still, as I gaze at checkerboard fields of emerald alfalfa below, that Anderson doctors will notice some loophole . . . saying something like 'Mr. Scribner, since you've done so well for so long we're going to give you a clean bill of health' . . . . Or maybe they'll throw up their hands, saying it's been a momentous mistake, made by people unfamiliar with this disease. Wild ideas, yes.

"If nothing else," Jane goes on opening a *Time* magazine, "we get to experience a new city."

"Sure. Like . . . this is how I want to see a new city."

"Eric, we ought to try, really try, to make this more than just another doctor visit." Jan is grinning subtlely. She loves traveling—and antagonizing me at odd times. "I'm sure your question will be answered. Finally we'll be able to put this . . . . Well, I don't need to say anymore."

Still Jane entertained the hypothesis—reinforced a while back by good old Dr. Holt—that my anxieties are a form of over-reaction, if not outright neurosis. Having been nurtured (as most of us were) in the sheltered environment of TDKB, Jane had recently come to the conclusion I'm getting adequate and reasonable guardianship at the HMO clinic—so, why continually rock the boat?

I'd given up trying to influence her otherwise. This had become a subject verboten—a topic no longer openly discussed. No matter what, it was my life—my fight. So I went on with my hunt for cancer understanding—patient power, as I'd taken to calling it in my mind.

An 8:00 a.m. appointment. Getting up the next morning in a unfamiliar hotel in an unfamiliar city, breathing unfamiliar air, I feel inexplicably separated, alone. Many if not all the hotels in the area cater to visitors and patients of the M.D. Anderson Cancer Center or other specialized hospitals in the area, all part of the sprawling complex known as the Texas Medical Center. Our hotel, for example, provided free transportation to and from the hospital—though the hospital, as we learned, was only blocks away.

The 10-story, rose-hued Anderson complex is imposing, to say the least. The structure looks like what a influential cancer facility should look like—impressive, stately. Standing before it, looking up, makes you feel good . . . just knowing a facility of this magnitude's devoted solely to the care and treatment of you—the cancer patient. Off to the left and right, down the street, multi-storied structures surge skyward all around, making MDA appear as though its facilities are a city within a city.

No sooner do your feet hit the pavement, stepping from the hotel van, when you get your first taste of Southern hospitality: a member of the Anderson staff greets you, attentively guiding you in the appropriate direction. This may seem trivial, but when you consider this facility sees over 16,000 new cancer patients a year, this well-mannered approach is noteworthy, and comforting. I soon feel that I'm in—if nothing else—indulgent hands.

Within a half hour, during which I complete the unavoidable sign-in and insurance papers, we're on our way up an elevator to Dr. Frank's station on the 7th floor. At the Endocrinology desk, a nurse leads Jane and me to an area where she records my physical particulars: height, weight, blood pressure and so forth. From there we convene with Dr. Frank. I don't recall waiting at all. It's as though they were catering only to me. Corny, I know.

MDA examination rooms are sparklingly tidy and spacious enough to move about with ease. Self-contained, they have a curtained-off disrobing area, a patient exam table, and a modest built-in desk, a chair for doctors' use. Again, things seem impressively suitable.

Dr. Frank, about six foot, a native of Belize, is much more youthful than I'd imagined, looking to be in his late thirties. Young or not, I find myself saying, if he's here, at Anderson, he's got to be a top-notch physician . . . and I'm really looking forward to what he has to say.

Advice: One of the primary—though at all not self-evident—liabilities in belonging to an HMO is this: If your regional HMO medical group has but one specialist—say a single oncologist—on its staff, and you and he/she don't hit it off . . . you're in a tough spot, probably stuck with him or her unless you change HMOs entirely or some external force intervenes.

While this issue isn't an *obvious* up-front liability in joining an HMO, it definitely should be: As a cancer patient, in the dubious hands of a profit-motivated HMO, you must believe in your doctors. In an HMO framework, sadly, you may have to jeopardize your welling-being by accepting a doctor who you don't really care for and in whom you have little confidence—because the HMO has no others to offer.

Unfortunately, you seldom know the kinds of specialists you're going to need in advance of joining an insurance plan, be it an HMO or otherwise. However, this should be taken into consideration when deciding on whether to join an HMO.

CHAPTER 20

AT HOME IN HOUSTON— SITTING WITH THE *REAL* SPECIALISTS

Prior to the trip, I purchased a pocket-sized tape recorder and a handful of blank tapes. Through reading and talking with other patients I learned it's a good idea to keep accurate records—tape recordings and such—of important meetings with specialists for later reference.

When I ask Dr. Frank—a man with lively, remarkably boyish eyes—if he minds my taping our dialogue, he says not in the least, in fact he invites it. With the three of us sitting around the small informal desk in the exam room, he takes a few minutes digesting my half-inch-thick medical records. Not a superficial reading, either—he many times stops, questioning a specific procedure or test as it catches his eye.

Sticking a series of CT films up on a light board to study the infiltrates, Dr. Frank points out the suspect areas. He says 'infiltrate' is sort of a catch-all term, meaning many things. Because of the term's vagueness, he wants an Anderson radiologist—one acquainted with recurrent ACC—to study the films.

"I must tell you, Mr. Scribner," Dr. Frank goes on, being unmistakably direct, "what is called an infiltrate is often new tumor growth."

"I figured that," I admit fearfully. In some curious fashion this dire language, coming from a recognized authority, seems less confrontational. "But I'm hoping."

"We'll know soon enough," he says assertively, calling someone on the phone to pick up the pathology slides and CT films for review. Like Dr. Kyrouz at USC, Dr. Frank asks what brings me to Anderson, what's happened to this point in my treatment.

Flipping the steno pad open, in which I'd jotted nearly a hundred questions, I begin.

These are questions/issues I'd begun putting on paper as they occurred to me, over a period of many months. Because there are so many overlapping problems for a cancer patient to contemplate, whenever an area of concern arose, I wrote it down so as not to overlook it when the time came. Every minute here's going to count: no fumbling for what to ask next.

(This approach is one I recommend to anyone facing a strategic discussion with an authority on their disease. Get *all* of your questions on paper and organize them in order of importance *beforehand* so you don't find yourself getting lost, later saying, 'Gee, I wish would've asked this or that.')

One of Dr. Frank's initial questions, after listening to my story, has to do with my thyroid condition. He wants to know if the gland's performance is sound. "I didn't see any indication of a workup in your tests," he notes. He's relaxed, patient—and engaging.

Looking to Jane as if to say, 'See, he's already digging in new areas,' I tell him no one's mentioned or checked my thyroid for anything.

"Frequently," he goes on, his eyes little-boyish in their simplicity, "patients on Mitotane experience some thyroid dysfunction, sometimes permanently. You're on . . . let's see . . . seven grams a day. I strongly recommend you have your TSH—your thyroid function—checked when you get home. It's a simple blood test. Any GI problems at that dose?"

"Like upset stomachs, you mean?"

"That, nausea, anything else."

"Well, some rather weird stuff does happen: first, when I eat something containing sugar, I get lightheaded—for lack of a better word—like I've gulped a strong drink or two. Second, cheeses sometimes cause the same problem. And third, even a small amount of alcohol—say, half a beer—will make me very unsteady and weak." I want to say I'm a cheap drunk but it doesn't seem apropos, considering Dr. Frank's professionalism.

The doctor, explaining that for undiscovered reasons certain foods bring about adverse reactions in many patients on Mitotane, offers two thoughts: (1) be conscious of the irritabilities and note the contents in what I eat, or (2) consider reducing my Mitotane dosage. "So you feel more human," as he puts it.

We examine the pluses and minuses of both alternatives, with me telling him I'm least untroubled psychologically—as a hawkish cancer patient—taking the maximum quantity of Mitotane. He grins discerningly, saying he thought I'd go that direction. "For whatever reason," he says, "I've seen artificial cheeses cause conditions like you describe. You might try eating only real cheese."

"Sounds like we got some kind of pizza commercial going here."

"I'm truly surprised you can handle seven grams a day, Mr. Scribner," he continues with a degree of astonishment. "And, for that long. Most patients can tolerate only half that. How long have you been at seven grams?"

"Maybe a year now," I answer, checking my tape recorder to be sure it's still working. (Always use fresh batteries and regularly look to make sure your recorder's indeed active.)

Jane nods in agreement.

Despite the potential for regretful news at Anderson, I'm thrilled to be here, talking with another human being—a noted medical authority—who actually understands the cryptic vernacular of cancer, of endocrinology, of Mitotane, of ACC.

As we talk, Dr. Frank scratches notes on a tablet he's pulled from the desk drawer. He asks more about my present symptoms—the chest tightness and so forth. He also notes, thumbing through various pages of my medical record, that I'd lost a few a pounds over the last few months. This, he says, could be the result of many things, one of them being faulty thyroid function. "But recurrent disease can't be ruled out."

While appearing as though he's uneasy doing so, Dr. Frank spells out how this disease—just as I'd previously had drilled into me—has a unmistakable propensity to scatter, to metastasize, to the lungs, liver, bones, and sometimes, brain. He seems troubled offering this, but plainly feels it's imperative—I may not have been told previously.

"That brings up a question, doctor. What other treatments are available for ACC? Do you ever use radiation, for example?"

"Because ACC is so rare, there's not much incentive for drug manufacturers to research treatments. Currently Mitotane is about all we have." Pausing, Dr. Frank's smiling oddly. "Are you aware of the story of Mitotane, Mr. Scribner?"

"Who . . . discovered it, you mean?"

"It was originally," he resumes, "a type of widely used pesticide. Over time, more and more field workers began coming down with adrenal insufficiency—a very serious matter. After investigating, authorities found a pesticide was causing the problem. Not long after that a pharmaceutical company created Mitotane. Its chemical make up, in case you hadn't noticed, is quite close to DDT."

"So . . . I'm being treated with a chemical designed to kill bugs?"

"A refined version, I assure you. But to answer your original question: the first line of defense against ACC is surgery. Next we look to Mitotane. There are other chemotherapies —such as Suramin—that we're looking into. None of them, as yet, seems to hold much promise."

"And radiation?"

"We have not found radiation to be of any positive effect. In fact, it may be just the opposite."

"How can that be?"

"Well, it's a convoluted process, but radiation seems to kill off only the most inferior cells—leaving the aggressive cells, the virulent ones, behind to stir up real problems."

"But, doctor, look at my husband," Jane interjects, "he looks like a million bucks."

As others had before him, Dr. Frank politely asserts it's by tests alone that he and others base their cancer opinions.

As I continue with my questions, Dr. Frank remains thoroughgoing, untiring. He does, at one point, nod toward the tablet and in jest refer to me as 'The Man of a Thousand Questions.' This is good, though, because I know he'll forever connect me with that title. Years later, he'll recall Eric Scribner—The Man of a Thousand Questions.

Following a lunch break in the ground-floor cafeteria—and my initial heart-rending encounter with bone-thin children, a pint-sized generation of unsmiling and baldheaded cancer patients being conveyed about in wheelchairs—we resume our discussion.

Shortly after we—Dr. Frank, Jane and I—begin talking, another white-coated physician, a rather stern black-haired woman, breezes in, introducing herself. Clutching a clipboard, she seems at once a no-nonsense individual. With her unmistakable demeanor, she lets it be known she's Dr. Frank's superior and that he answers to her.

"Yes," she says matter-of-factly, sans a smile, extending a gaunt hand my way, "I'm Dr. Saltz. You're from California, I understand, and Dr. Frank's been going over adrenocortical carcinoma treatment with you."

Glancing in the vicinity of Dr. Frank, but speaking to me, she goes on. "I hope he's made it clear this can be a very troublesome disease—that it has many ways of reappearing . . . causing real trouble."

I nod yes.

"Good. This is a particularly lethal and aggressive form of cancer. I want to be sure you understand that, Mr. Scribner."

Her emphasis on the word lethal makes the situation seem grimmer, far less hopeful. In fact, I remember her using the word 'grim' in her lead sentence in a journal article on ACC and its 'dismal' prognosis, written the preceding year. From the moment she surfaced, I didn't care for this lady, her brusque manner: her words reeking of negativity.

"He did cover all that," I confirm. "He also mentioned getting my thyroid checked; said a lot of Mitotane patients have problems with theirs."

Dr. Saltz casts an impatient, hostile glance Dr. Frank's way. "No. I won't agree that's true. In the literature very few patients have experienced thyroid dysfunction due to Mitotane," she says, as if reprimanding and informing Dr. Frank at the same time.

"I should get mine checked, he said."

"Okay," she says stiffly, making her disapproval known, "that's between you and your local physician." No friendliness about this woman. You wonder, even, if she smiles at her own children. Her vacuous nut-brown eyes seem fashioned of glass in their tepidness. Perhaps it's her vocation—doctor of cancer—that's hardened her. Whatever. At any rate, she has the heart of a rock.

With a definite brittleness in the air, fostered by her presence, the next five or ten minutes' worth of questioning on her part seems mechanical—compared to Dr. Frank's good-natured approach—and many times intended to refute what he's said. Once she's wrapped things up, she stands, excusing herself with same aloofness she exhibited upon entry. With her departure, Dr. Frank seems revived and at once returns to his down-to-earth self.

In the sticky afternoon Texas sunshine, Jane and I take leisurely walk back to the hotel. A short hike, maybe two blocks from the hospital to hotel. In our room, we cat nap for an hour or so. Dr. Frank said he'd have the interpretation of my CT films in the morning.

"Duly impressed, you are, right?" Jane asks, buttering a roll later at dinner.

"Him, I liked. Her, no."

"Now how did I know that?" Jane goes on. "What else?"

"I feel really at home here," I reply, thinking. "Like finally I'm in the right place."

"You think this'll end your search?"

"They know their stuff and they're sure geared to catering to the patient. Cancer's all they do, but I can't say whether I'll stop looking."

As we devour a crisp dinner salad, followed by tasty baked chicken and potatoes in the hotel's tasteful wood-finished dining room, I resume: "But that's not my real concern. I'm wondering about those damn films. What they'll show. And that other doctor, shit. . . ."

"Dr. Frank said in the morning, right?"

"He seems like an unusual guy. Answering all those questions."

Jane reaches over, squeezing my fingers. "It's going to be okay, sweetie, I know. I dreamed it last night. I love you, you know."

"I appreciate that, but it'd really help if you got involved—started asking a few questions."

"You're doing such a good job. And you know me."

"You are truly one weird person," I remark as we get on the elevator to our room. "Wedded wife or not."

"Now, now."

CHAPTER 21

BAD NEWS IS GOOD NEWS—
TRADING ONE DISEASE FOR ANOTHER

In the morning, I awaken early, a bit fearful, but feeling richly confident Anderson radiologists haven't found anything evil in my CT films. Maybe Jane's saying so—that she'd dreamed it—reinforces this. We eat our fill of sausage, eggs and toast at the hotel's buffet before heading for the hospital.

After waiting a few minutes on the 7th floor, Endocrinology, Dr. Frank himself appears, greeting us. "Your report's back," he begins without ado, studying a single sheet of paper. He seems from all appearances to be phrasing precisely his words. "They're saying . . . your infiltrates—" in this one split second, where he pauses, my mind rockets ahead, pelting me with morbid images . . . "are a form of pneumonia. And the pathology review confirms your condition as adrenocortical carcinoma."

Exhaling audibly, I say, "*Pneumonia? Are you kidding? That's all?*" Release swells in me like the flood of some hypnotic potion.

"Mr. Scribner, I've got to say," Dr. Frank replies, reeling back for emphasis while at the same time oddly amused, "I've never seen a patient quite so happy to hear he's got pneumonia."

"Think about it," I go on ecstatically. "It ain't the *bad* stuff! We all know pneumonia can be treated."

"See," Jane chimes in, beaming, tickled with herself, "told you so."

"Damn, damn, damn!" is all I can utter. In me, the news feels fiery, wonderful. "And to think, the only symptoms were the tightness in my lungs and those involuntary little breaths. Don't people usually have more symptoms with pneumonia—like fevers or something?"

"With the assortment of drugs you're taking, a lot can be masked."

"Okay," I say, feeling rejuvenated, "where to from here?"

"What I want to do—after going over your 'thousand questions' yesterday—is recommend a few drug changes, get you started on an antibiotic—for that pneumonia you're so proud of."

Dr. Frank goes on to explain how the oral adrenal steroid, Prednisone, more closely emulates the hormone the human body naturally produces, compared to the hydrocortisone I'm currently taking. "By switching to Prednisone," he explains, "we can not only reduce your daily intake of pills, but you should feel better too, more energetic."

Jane asks if he's including these recommendations in his report to Dr. Bristol, "Because," she notes, "local HMO doctors don't always listen to us patients." Smiling as if to say, 'I understand,' he assures us he will.

Now, all that's left is gathering up my films. No matter how conscientious M.D. Anderson and its people have been, I can't entrust anyone with returning something as crucial as the CT films to my local clinic by US mail or other means. In my hands is where I want those films before leaving Houston tomorrow morning.

Calling radiology and finding that the films are still listed as 'in use,' Dr. Frank suggests the best way to rescue them: go directly to fourth-floor radiology and personally pick them up.

Anderson's a monolith of meandering, look-alike hallways. Jane and I are on the fourth floor for but a few minutes before we're thoroughly confused. After we pass the same doctor twice, he smiles, asking if we need help. On hearing our predicament, he does an about-face, leading us to the door of radiology.

A young woman behind a glazed window invites us to come in and search for the films ourselves—she's by herself. There are only two doctors in at the moment, both busy.

We're led to an extended film viewing room where huge backlit walls revolve, with the push of a button by a radiologist, displaying prepositioned films. Two radiologists—one, a fleshy middle-aged man, the other, a tense-looking vernal woman—are each evaluating a series of films on their respective lighted walls and dictating quietly into hand-held microphones.

Both doctors nod a courteous greeting, then continue about their business. Finding my films seems impossible: the place looks like a teenager's bedroom—towering accumulations of film all over, some in envelopes, some profusely splayed on tables.

(Recommendation: Make an itemized list of all your effects—medical records, CT/x-ray films, pathology slides—that you transport to another clinic for a second opinion or other consultations. With some intuitive forethought, I'd made an inventory of my films [the quantity, their dates, numbers shown on the film, and so forth] before we left California in the event I'd have to later identify them.)

Despite trying to remain focused on my film hunt, I find myself occasionally glancing at the doctors' work: Illuminated images of anonymous lungs spotted with chillingly odd-shaped shadows . . . grotesquely twisted spinal columns . . . rib cages showing ominous perforations. The power of these images is profoundly disturbing: Real people—human beings—go with these heart-breaking films . . .

With films in hand—the search took almost an hour—Jane and I walk back to the hotel, taking a different route. Leaving the films in our room, we decide to hop in our rental car to go to Galveston for a bit of celebrating. In Galveston we stroll around in the humidity of old town, a nicely restored historical district.

Between Gaido's Seafood restaurant and the shoreline is a four-foot-high block rampart separating Texas and the Gulf of Mexico. Entering Gaido's by way of the gift shop, we wait to be seated. It's mid-afternoon, a balmy, sunny day. The nicely appointed restaurant is only about a quarter full. Each table is draped in white linen tablecloths and the flatware has a decorous, hefty look to it. By all appearances, we've picked a good place for a late lunch.

We're taken to a window table. The ocean remains visible over the seawall. This day the Gulf's at rest—only faint undulations. I recall seeing amazing TV accounts of violent hurricane winds and gargantuan waves exploding over this same seawall, flinging cars about and inundating this very roadway.

"What do we feel like eating?" Jane asks, picking up a menu.

"Whatever's good for a celebration. I may even bend the rules a bit and have some vino."

"Very good! Nice to see you loosen up, Mr. S!" she responds. Then, more pensively, "This . . . crab dish here (she's pointing to the item on her menu) looks interesting. Lump crab, they call it. What do you suppose that means? Ask our waiter."

In his sixties and very British, the waiter seems oddly displaced in a southern restaurant. With a shock of wiry gray hair, he's uniquely ceremonious. "It's a locally caught delicacy," he recites in a syrupy, but personable limey cadence, "in a rich garlic-butter sauce."

"That's it?" Jane asks abruptly.

"Oh, ma'am, it's quite decadent, I assure you," he replies with aplomb. "It does come with a fresh green salad—or jambalaya—and plenty of our robust bread."

"Why's it called lump?" I want to know, handing him our menus.

"Because," he goes on, "it is served out of its shell, ready to eat. The meat's been removed for you. No untidy fingers. Exceedingly fresh, I assure you. The chef does away with the shell just before the dish is prepared."

Savoring glasses of chilled white wine, snacking on bits of freshly buttered warm-crusted bread, we await the arrival of this uncommon meal.

After eyeing the near-calm Gulf for a period, Jane sighs, "So, you feeling better now? More relaxed?"

"Well, Dr. Frank didn't do like I'd secretly hoped and say everybody before him was wrong."

She nods, listening, sipping her wine.

"I'd be lying, though, if I said I wasn't relieved," I go on. "Having pneumonia's nothing to write home about, but it sure beats the other."

"Scared, were you?"

"Goes without saying."

"I am happy for you . . . for both of us."

"Bad thing is I've got to keep taking this damn Mitotane," I comment as the waiter appears carrying twin, copiously full sterling-silver bowls of crab meat submerged in a simmering, aromatic white sauce. With the first forkful, Jane and I gape at one another.

"Oh, my God," she breathes, "this could replace shopping as my first love!"

The symmetrical harmony of butter and garlic and whatever else is in the sauce releases a heretical flavor across the taste buds. There's perhaps a pound or better of this wildly delicious crabmeat in each of our dishes.

"This may be," Jane whispers, "the best meal I've ever eaten."

"Ditto," I reply, washing down a tasty piece of crab with cold wine. "This is good! The perfect celebration!"

Jane, glass offered in toast: "To cancer staying gone forever!"

"I think," I say, touching my glass to hers, beginning now to feel the warm radiance of the wine, "I'm going to start meditating."

"—Right here?"

"No. You know what I mean. But I have to do *something*—whatever I can. You heard those doctors . . . saying like everybody else, this cancer can come back."

"Um-hm. And I put it out of my mind . . . as you should. You talked before about diet—becoming a vegetarian. Still thinking of that, too?"

"Still a possibility."

We're truly enjoying this true bounty, this after-the-scare feast. But, I wonder as I sit eating, realizing the power of Mitotane will soon reverse these effusive feelings, is there truly a correlation between diet and the likelihood of cancer recurring? I have no real answers, save for the anecdotal tales I've read alluding to diet and cancer. But the question keeps popping up more and more now.

CHAPTER 22

MY TYPICAL DAY—
THIS IS ROCKET SCIENCE?

Back at home I return to working five days a week. Dr. Bristol gets a faxed report from Dr. Frank within days. She switches me from hydrocortisone to Prednisone as prescribed.

A couple of weeks later I undergo a follow-up CT.

The antibiotic Dr. Frank prescribed seems to have done the trick—no infiltrates noted! (Odd, how Dr. Bristol's able to get an HMO-authorized follow-up CT within weeks, while Dr. Drake couldn't get one—he said—within months after those mysterious shadows appeared in my left adrenal bed. Is Dr. Bristol that much more tenacious? Is she less intimidated by the HMO's bullying tactics?)

Dr. Bristol, following Dr. Frank's lead, sets up a thyroid blood test. My thyroid *is* found to be under-functioning—a hypothyroid condition. Daily synthroid is prescribed (yes, another drug I'll be taking the rest of my life) to bring the thyroid back on course. Dr. Bristol also starts me on daily Pepcid to relieve frequent bouts of painful Mitotane-induced indigestion.

Several weeks after getting home from Houston, I get in the mail an application to join M.D. Anderson's Patient Network. This, the literature says, is a free service that links like-diagnosed cancer patients via telephone, throughout the country, so they can talk, one on one, about issues important to them—cancer coping, success of treatments, test results, chemotherapy side effects, any other strange twists the disease presents. (See Appendix A for information on accessing this and other free telephone resources for cancer patients.)

Late 1991: I'm settling back into a pattern of working daily, taking Mitotane, trying to watch more closely the junk in my diet. Unconsciously, I'm moving closer to a major diet shift.

Going to and from work still requires that same nerve-jangling one-hour-plus freeway drive. Each way. At work, I'm a strategic figure in what's called Program Assessment, a function that entails my preparing an exceedingly thorough biannual report and slide presentation that executive management presents to NASA's executive management—a God-awful dance of overbearing peacocks.

This report and briefing on the status of the Space Shuttle Main Engines—a page-limited, program-wide summary covering everything from integral engineering changes to budget management and improved manufacturing techniques—is worth, to Rockwell, up to $20 million in pure profit, *twice* annually.

At any given moment, I'm under vice-like pressure from sundry high-level executives. It isn't unusual for me to find several ill-tempered vice presidents convening in my office, anxiously awaiting my return . . . from a restroom visit.

(My employer, Rockwell, has been given what the government terms an 'Award Fee Contract' to build the main engines for the Space Shuttle. Under this type of contract, every six months the company's given list of priority items NASA deems essential to the on-schedule delivery of these engines.

For each six-month period, NASA allocates a pool of money [award fee], often $10 to $20 million, which the company can 'win' all of or a percentage of. Usually, we achieve 85 to 95% of the pool. I detail for NASA how well we've done, or not done, against each criterion, via these all-important reports and briefings.)

This cash bonanza's said to go, in large part, for executive bonuses. So, to say my daily movements are under great scrutiny by executive management is putting it mildly. Me, the keeper of their purse strings.

(One time I was quite ill, at home, battling a 103-degree fever and God knows what else, when the president himself calls. "Eric, can you do it? We really need you here today." . . . Have you ever tried maintaining mental focus, concentrating, reading and writing coherently with a 103-degree fever? No easy task.)

For many months at a time I'm so sandwiched by schedule and deadline pressures that I am, admittedly, repellent to everyone, particularly Jane. She can sense from a distance when I'm in the jaws of a schedule crunch—with 'that damn report.'

Sleeping fitfully, if at all, I toss about, 'dreaming' of tomorrow's demands. (On more than one occasion, as implausible as it seems, I arose in the dead of night—having dreamed I heard the alarm—and proceeded to get ready for work, shaving, showering, and dressing, only to discover it was 2:00 a.m.!)

I'm ill-mannered. I eat a lot of the wrong foods. My stomach's often sour and cramped so tightly by the end of the day it seems an electrical current's shorting out across it—and, with the testosterone headaches hanging on, muscles at the base of my skull knot and throb to the point where I'm taking three Excedrin every couple of hours.

Much of this pressure is, admittedly, self-inflicted. Stress's frequently a curse we bestow upon ourselves. Too demanding of myself, I tend to be. The fact that my boss, this impulsive vice president of engineering, is grossly insecure and inefficient only compounds the issue. If he'd do things just once, maybe twice, *on time*, that'd been difficult enough. But this chameleonesque individual changes his mind, willy-nilly, from one minute to next like a wounded sparrow being stalked by a depraved alley cat.

And he expects me to respond to his unreasonable demands by providing extremely complex, updated material—we *are* talking rocket science here—in the blink of an eye. He believes I can create this out of thin air. We only stop making changes to a report or briefing when time runs out—the document has to be out the door.

Prior to this deadline, it isn't unusual for this paranoid VP to be at Cape Kennedy, awaiting a shuttle launch, and fax me some colossal mess at 2:00 p.m. outlining major revisions to every page of the project. This, just two days before the report's due in NASA's hands. No matter how extensive the changes, he wants the updated/revised material faxed back to him, pronto—usually by 10:00 a.m. the following morning.

These rapid-fire changes always involve me researching some nebulous rocket-engine manufacturing or test issue, at breakneck speed, and accurately rewriting that portion of the report while maintaining the proper slant. This involves my sitting down with extremely harried and often acrimonious engineering directors to reformulate information they'd input earlier. Often they'll argue that nothing needs to be revised—they provided their best originally. It's then my function to put on my PR hat and redirect this kind of thinking along the lines of the VP's desires.

Revisions, once I begrudgingly receive them from department heads, are usually crudely drafted; never in the proper context. This means I have to rewrite their text—eliminating the rocket-scientist jargon so non-technical NASA higher-ups can understand—before faxing the package back to the VP for his review . . . and, yes, further changes.

Many a morning I arrive at my office, expecting to deal only with yesterday's massive changes, but learn there's been a whole new, overlapping batch of changes faxed in by this indecisive VP—changes to everything from already-revised material, to confusing revisions to older versions of the project. And he wants this newly revised material sorted, rewritten and faxed back to him not at 10:00 a.m.—like he'd decreed the day before—but by 9:00 a.m., an hour from now!

Again this means racing about, contacting overworked departments heads to get their cooperation, making another round of complex data or financial adjustments, rewriting this highly technical material, making it understandable, putting all the words in the proper style, coordinating the clean-up of the material (getting it retyped in final format *without* error because this is the only way the VP will deign to read it), then faxing it to the VP—on time.

Whether it was pride or innate efficiency, never once did I miss these absurd deadlines.

The unreasonable demands of this job and the relentless high-dollar pressure—nonstop stress to the nth degree—contributed heavily to both my original and recurrent cancer. Because of the millions of dollars involved, these projects were literally written and rewritten daily, *all year long*. And I was squarely on the hot seat, the focal point of all wrath—all that could go wrong.

This job, instead of consisting of peaks and valleys as most jobs do, is one of incessant, non-stop boiler-room pressure. Seems I'm forever attending some high-level meeting and updating or monitoring the progress of some insurgent department's under-achievements relative to NASA's six-month requirements.

Keep in mind the adrenal glands' hormonal output, cortisol, is the body's stress hormone. Being that I'm not producing any cortisol because of Mitotane suppression, this all-consuming stress is literally wearing me away—taking its evil toll.

CHAPTER 23

THAT FEELING OF HIGH ANXIETY—
HOW OUR FIGHT-OR-FLIGHT RESPONSE
EFFECTS OUR DAILY LIVES

One of the primary reasons mankind's fared so well in this hostile world is that we have a profound sense of survival—fight or flight. Simply put, we've learned to intelligently perceive danger and how to cope with it. A million years ago prevalent stress probably amounted to having some voracious beast lurking too closely to you or your clan.

Today, we seldom have to fight or flee from physical danger. Most commonly our stresses are attitudinal or psychological—a threat we only perceive.

Whether a stressor impacts us physically or cognitively—we only *think* we're being threatened—the body's survival responses are identical. Explosive release of the hormones adrenaline and cortisol causes major shifts in gastrointestinal, endocrine, nervous, cardiovascular, immune, and respiratory functions. Though we may only think we're being threatened, these systems gear up for fight or flight as though a salivating saber-tooth were physically at our doorstep. (Further verification of that elusive mind-body connection.) The body then shifts from its usual anabolic mode (cell regeneration) to a catabolic mode where cells are broken down for utilization as quick energy.

A properly functioning immune system, something of great concern to cancer patients, can be broadly defined as an extremely complex process involving various organs and an army of white blood cells—T-cells (from the thymus gland) and B-cells (from bone marrow)—which gives the body its ability to decipher what is you and what is not you, and the ability to do something about it.

One of the immune system's principal functions is recognizing and destroying aberrant cells—cancer cells—that commonly arise in everyone's body. This amazing silent cellular security system is operating within us 24 hours a day. Without it we couldn't survive the unceasing onslaught of microscopic threats.

When the body's on fight-or-flight alert, an under-functioning immune system is oftentimes impaired to the point where this precise surveillance process is disrupted. A weakened immune system, though, does not necessarily cause cancer, but does create an assailable environment where cancer cells can flourish.

In long-term stress, where there is no release from the fight-or-flight mode, the body sort of seethes internally, while the endocrine and nervous systems remain fully armed, suppressing the immune system. Researchers in the field of breast cancer have established that women under heavy, long-term stress have lower levels of natural killer blood cells (T-cells), those that watch for and destroy cancer cells.

There have been a number of scientific investigations showing that the hormone cortisol, while serving many vital and positive functions in the body, acts also as a potent immune suppressant. It's reasonable, then, to suggest that infirmity in general—whether it's a common cold or cancer—can most easily attack the body in times of sustained stress, when the immune system is down. This may be an overly simplified interpretation of a little-understood medical phenomenon—the causative stages of disease—but with data gathered thus far by researchers in Psychoneuroimmunology (PNI), the picture's becoming ever clearer....

With the removal of stress and the correct mental attitude, theoretically the body-mind can re-establish a state of balance, and the immune system can resume its methodical surveillance, helping the cancer-plagued patient to move toward recovery.

So... as I continue to labor away at the same cortisol-laden, stress-ridden work environment, my viscera feels forever tied in knots, and I know, intuitively, that something not-so-good is bearing down on me.

Dr. Bristol, in her intuitiveness, questions my energy level in general. I am feeling somewhat overtaxed, I admit, more fatigued than normal. I think it unmanly to discuss stress reduction remedies with her. Because I'd felt healthier months before, she suggests I go back on hydrocortisone (instead of Prednisone), and that we step up my thyroid medication.

June 1991: I telephone Dr. Frank in Houston to see what, if anything, he can propose to boost my energy. (These calls I make occasionally without my local doctors' consent. This isn't to say I'm playing one side against the other, but I feel and still do, redundancy's good medicine: you give yourself the greatest chance of survival by talking to as many knowledgeable doctors as possible, then picking and choosing your course.

(In today's let-the-patient-beware world of cost-effective HMOs and managed-care medicine, the phrase, 'The Lord looks out for those who look out for themselves,' has never been truer. We, the patients, sadly must act in our own behalf... tirelessly, over, and over, and over.)

Dr. Frank—chuckling as I remind him I'm 'The Man of a Thousand Questions'—offers a major turn-about: Stop taking Mitotane for a week or two to regain energy and 'that feeling of good health.' (Odd, isn't it, how we have to *stop* taking a restorative drug in order to feel better.... Something doesn't quite add up. What kind of 'cure' is this?) He says I should resume the chemo in a week or so, starting at one gram a day, increasing one gram per week till I again reach MTD.

Telling Dr. Malone, my new oncologist, what Dr. Frank's suggested, she comes back with a curious statement to the effect she doesn't want me going above 4.5 grams per day . . . "Till," as she put it, "there's an apparent need."

This is a good news/bad news situation. Good news, because now I have an oncologist telling me not to exceed a certain dose of chemotherapy. Bad news, because I know in my heart, with my prior reading, Dr. Malone has no scientific basis for making this judgment. What does she mean by 'an apparent need?' . . . 'When I have a recurrence?' It's my understanding that Mitotane's not an after-the-fact drug. It is, for me, an adjuvant chemotherapy—an insurance policy to, hopefully, keep cancer far, far away.

I am, however, so appreciative of being rid of the morose Dr. Drake and decreasing my intake of this tempestuous drug, that I don't want to tax my alliance with this new doctor by questioning her critical faculties, though as I say, I know I should. All literature and logic tell me I should resume taking the maximum tolerated dosage—the MTD. Anyway, call it a matter of convenience or a relapse of TDKB, but I let the issue slide.

(With all cancer treatment there's one issue we, the patients, should keep in mind against which to weigh all things: Does the approach being recommended make *sense* to me? I've talked with many a patient about their intuitive notions and one thing we agree upon: we all know when something's seriously wrong—our bodies have a way of telling us when there's a recurrence, for example. This same sense of intuitive logic applies to all medical care offered to you. Ask pointed questions! Do not be intimidated; do not stop until *you* are satisfied with the answers!)

So here I am, sitting in this scanty exam room facing this mild-mannered oncologist. I've been fortunate enough to be referred to an outside (out-of-network, in HMO jargon) oncologist. In the puzzling and often perilous world of HMO medicine, this is a real plus.

No one's really sure, from all I've learned, what the right dose of Mitotane is for each person. Maybe . . . this doctor does know better than me. When I ask, diplomatically—and reluctantly—if she's ever treated another ACC patient or prescribed Mitotane for anything, she reservedly says no, then proceeds to a new subject.

I should have called Dr. Frank again, seeking his opinion on this permanent Mitotane reduction, but, as I say, I don't want to rock the boat. Being your own advocate's a remarkably stressing, full-time undertaking. Dr. Frank's my ace in the hole. Don't want to wear out my welcome. I'll save him for a better time. Maybe I'll never again require a high dose of Mitotane. Who knows?

About this time, to curb some the anxieties brought on by the oral steroids and an on-going concern the cancer may recur, I begin taking the drug Buspar, recommended by my new psychologist, Dr. McElliot. This is the only anti-anxiety drug I've found to be compatible with Mitotane. All others—Xanax and Valium, for example—literally leave me out in left field, mentally stalled for a minimum of 24 hours.

Ingesting a sand-sized chip of Xanax, I became unhinged—like listening to an uninterrupted time-delayed recording of myself speaking—for a least a day. Very, very strange. So, when Buspar is offered, I'm thrilled. This drug doesn't have the mind-numbing effect of a Xanax. It does, however, provide a subtle anti-anxiety effect once it kicks in, after a week or so.

My new shrink, is, well, a caricature of sorts—a stunted, thick-waisted guy in his fifties, balding, with feeble striations of demonic hair lashed across his glinting summit. He invariably offers a satiny, semi-wet handshake, and he possesses off-beat, almost Hitler-like facial hair. (Are these guys all spooky?)

For several months he and I trade beliefs every other Friday evening. We have our polite differences. He, for example, habitually wants to go rearward, to explore the litter of my adolescence. I make it clear I'm here as a medical patient with a physical ailment, who's been guaranteed by physicians he is going to have a recurrence and is being treated with a DDT-like oral chemotherapy for an uncommon cancer.

As we chat, I have to remind this Hitleresque fellow of my physical-only approach to psychology many times. He then becomes sulky and takes to contemplating the creases in his hands or the tiles on the floor . . . sort of pouting, if you will. He does this so often, I begin to feel guilt-ridden about making him feel . . . well, disappointed.

There is indeed something eccentric about this patient/doctor association: Aren't I the one in need? (Many folks in mental health occupations, it seems, tip-toed into the field originally to unravel uncertainties within themselves.)

In due time I inform Dr. McElliot, after maybe six months, that I don't feel it urgent to see him any longer on a fixed basis. Odd as it seems, I feel penitent, like we're some impetuous teenage couple breaking up, because he's *really* pouting now. For the rest of that session he barely mumbles a word.

He says he feels it necessary—for my well-being—that we continue meeting at least once a month. Standing firm, I tell him I'll return only if I require his professional guidance in dealing with tactile, real-life medical issues.

Over the course of our meetings, he did offer several effective ways to meditate. And, I have to admit, he didn't inflict the emotional harm Dr. Holt had.

CHAPTER 24

UNEXPECTED TWISTS—
TWO NEW DOCTORS ENTER THE SCENE

So we move into 1992. Not the best of years. It's been over two years since my original surgery. Things seem to be rolling ahead at an orderly pace, without significant warning signs. But anticipated Mitotane side effects are mounting: Often I find myself mysteriously losing my train of thought—in mid-sentence. My skin's becoming thinner, turning purplish in places and bleeding more easily. At 4.5 grams of Mitotane per day—as Dr. Malone's dictated—I'm experiencing prolonged bouts of diarrhea.

A chilly Friday evening, late April: Because I'm experiencing deep, stabbing pains that course across my upper abdomen—site of the original surgery—Jane and I drive once again to Urgent Care. For the better part of the evening, this painful sensation's been with me. After palpating the area in question and skimming my medical history, the duty doctor, a smooth-faced man, says he doesn't feel anything, but, with my history, he's going to try to arrange a chest and abdominal CT in the ensuing days.

(By now, I'd started compiling my own portable medical record—an abbreviated chronology beginning with the 1989 surgery [see Appendix B]. Over time, this condensed, simply worded record has proven invaluable. With it, an unversed MD can be brought up to speed in minutes. I still today update this chronology on my PC. This brief history—because my case's so unusual—goes with me everywhere.)

A week later: Dr. Malone, standing uneasily before me, is scanning the two-page CT report with me sitting anxiously on the paper-covered exam table. "They didn't see anything," she notes, seemingly relieved at not being the bearer of bad news. But, I tell her, the discomfort is still there in the stomach area.

"Probably adhesions," is her catch-all decree, "—from your surgery."

A lot of doctors are especially fond of this catch-all escape clause—this glossing over of a patient's concerns. Any distress or discomfort in the area of a previous surgery is the result of adhesions-internal scarring. It's as simple as that. Doctors will often offer this adhesion catch-all without ever physically evaluating other, more dangerous causes—like the very real possibility of a cancer recurrence.

FINDING HOPE WHEN DOCTORS SAY THERE IS NONE

A sunny June Saturday afternoon: Jane and I are on our way to a seaside inn in San Diego for a well-deserved, weekend getaway. After maybe 20 minutes on the busy freeway, I'm feeling . . . strangely woozy. My head's swimming. There's a detached-from-the-body feeling about me—cars all about me going 70 miles an hour. They seem feathery, hallucinatory.

Fifty some miles from home, I tell Jane we have to turn back. Pulling off the freeway, she takes the wheel. Though it's Saturday, I'm able to get through to Dr. Malone—her weekend on call. When I spell out the odd—and frightening way—I'm feeling, she hesitates a moment, asks about my Mitotane dosage, then asks if I've had my ACTH level tested.

Adrenocorticotropic hormone (ACTH), she explains, is the hormone our pituitary gland—the master endocrine gland—releases into the blood stream, commanding the adrenal glands to secrete their stress hormone, cortisol. My remaining adrenal gland, I remind her, is being suppressed by Mitotane.

Do nothing but rest for the remainder of the weekend, she advises. On Monday she'll try to arrange an ACTH test. I say *try* because this is a doctor who's made it obvious she doesn't in any way contest the HMO way of doing business—if the HMO says it'll eventually review the idea and decide in a month, she'll most likely not object.

This is a battle that she, a highly trained specialist, should fight more vigorously. But in the one-way world of HMO leverage, they, the HMOs, can fire a doctor without cause and that doctor will no longer be authorized to treat that HMO's patients. The doctor can find herself without patients—or earnings.

A week later the blood test comes back showing my ACTH level soaring—well over 1200 pg/ml (normal's 9-52 pg/ml).

"These results, Mr. Scribner," Dr. Malone concludes blatantly, glancing at the numbers, "are obviously a lab error."

Remarkably, having decided that, she's now going to drop the issue!

"Why have the test done in the first place, doctor," I persist, astounded, "if we're just going to set aside the findings as an error?"

Looking annoyed, she very hesitantly agrees to a retest, continuing to insist the numbers represent a lab error. She is, I perceive at this moment as we sit looking at each other, at least as intimidated by the opposite sex as by the no-frills HMO.

The next ACTH results come back the same. "So . . . what do we do now?" I ask a bit peeved, wondering: What would've happened if I'd gone along with your initial decision and *not* sought validation of the original results?

"Probably," the doctor replies ingenuously, never acknowledging she might've erred, "we should have you see an endocrinologist. I'll submit the paperwork."

Seeing a local endocrinologist was something I'd been wanting to do. A National Cancer Institute fact sheet on ACC stated that an endocrine specialist should be part an ACC patient's medical team. I'd intimated this to Dr. Bristol but, for some reason, she became surprisingly put out—one of the few times I'd seen her this way—saying in no uncertain terms she was in control of my medical care and she'd decide who I saw and when. Almost going toe to toe with her, and pulling out the NCI report, I instead bit my tongue. Staying on her good side proved wiser.

A month and a half later, I'm at the endocrinologist's office. Dr. Crandle is an abrasive, mad-scientist-looking guy, on the lean side, in his mid-fifties. Thumbing through my records—including my own computer-generated chronology—he remarks offhandedly: "I've only seen one other case like you . . . a case of adrenocortical carcinoma."

"You've actually treated—" I ask, suddenly infused with hope, "—another ACC patient?"

"Not exactly. I read about it. In a medical school textbook. People don't live long with this diagnosis, you realize. Your days are numbered." He's still thumbing through, reviewing my records.

"So I've heard. But it has been almost two years since the diagnosis."

A minute or two of quietude goes by. Startling me suddenly, he's now waving separate sheets of paper about: "What in the holy hell did he order these tests for?"

"First," I respond loudly, trying to sound as equally fanatical as he, "Dr. Bristol's a she not a he . . . and I have no idea why she ordered any of those tests. Pick up the phone and call her."

"This . . . is just ludicrous," he goes on, looking at me now with renewed respect, as if accepting me as one who'll shout back. Cracks in my TDKB orientation are starting to appear. "Look here. She's tested you for cortisol. Anybody knows you're not going to get an accurate reading when a patient's on cortisone." He shudders for effect. Despite this guy's audacity, the message that's coming through is 'It's you and me, kid—against all these non-endocrine know-nothings.' Take this guy with a grain of salt, I decide . . . humor him. He is all the HMO has to offer.

"Holy—" he remarks, looking over my latest blood work, "your ACTH is like rocket fuel!"

"Could that be what's making my head feel like it's swimming sometimes?"

"A slim possibility." His oddly matted hair—close-cropped, reddish-brown—looks like he scrubbed in the shower last night, then slept on it. His wide-set, fast-moving topaz-brown eyes stay on me.

"What now?" I ask faintheartedly, not knowing what to expect.

"Assuming you don't have a pituitary tumor—which, I see they've tested you for—a medication change might be all that's called for."

"You can adjust ACTH with drugs?"

"That's what I said. What we'll do," he's now riffling through pages of my record, "is take you off hydrocortisone and start you on Prednisone."

"I was on that a while back. I felt drained all the time. Like a cement truck was parked on my chest."

"Ah, but we have to use Prednisone," he persists, spiritedly. "It comes closest to mimicking your adrenals' own secretion—cortisol. What we have going on here, I think, is your pituitary's not recognizing the hydrocortisone your taking. And, by not recognizing it, the pituitary's pumping out an overkill of ACTH—no humor intended."

He's got my attention. I am fascinated learning more about this extraordinary endocrine system that influences so many of life's everyday conditions in elusive ways—and not so elusive ways.

"While I'm thinking of it, I want to ask . . ." I begin. "I'm getting testosterone shots every two weeks—"

"—What the hell for?" he interrupts abruptly, looking at me with a thin smile.

"Because the drug I'm taking," I reply, smiling in return, "Mitotane, interferes with testosterone production. But my question is . . . why, after each shot, do I get killer, three-day headaches?"

"Allergic reaction," he replies derisively. "What's the dosage? Frequency?"

"One-hundred milligrams every two weeks."

"That's not going to do it. How's your libido?" he asks, nodding with a mild sense of disgust—as if to say: 'Those other doctors, what nitwits.' "A man your size needs at least two-hundred milligrams every two weeks."

"Libido isn't the primary issue. The shots are to counter breast tenderness—and enlargement. Caused by the Mitotane."

"Whatever. Two-hundred milligrams—every two weeks—that's what I'm recommending. I'll stick that in my notes to Dr. What's-Her-Name."

"And what can I do about the headaches?"

"That, my good man," he says, smiling as though elbowing one of the boys after exchanging a bit off-color humor, "is the price one pays."

Another dead-end.

"I'm writing you a prescription," Dr. Crandle continues, "for Prednisone. Start taking it right away. We'll retest your ACTH again in about three months. Takes that long to see any real shift. If my hunch's correct, your ACTH level should drop as the pituitary recognizes the Prednisone."

Again, I remind him of my earlier negative experience with Prednisone.

"We'll play with it, okay?" he declares, pointing to the 7.5 mg written on the prescription tablet. "I want you taking at least two milligrams before bed. Your pituitary wakes up early, around 5:00 a.m., and it wants to see that cortisol."

So self-assured and brusque is this fellow that one might be inclined to lump him in a category with those bad-boy genius-types who're invariably on the money about their areas of expertise. Not knowing whether to be upset or amused, I decide to accept the guy with a grain of salt. Am I becoming hardened?

There was another endocrinologist in town—a professor of medicine from USC who'd actually worked with ACC patients. But she wasn't on the HMO's provider list. The HMO would not approve my seeing her. If I had seen her on my own and paid for the visit myself, any further visits, prescriptions, or testing she prescribed would've been denied by the HMO as well. Simply put: She was not on their list of approved doctors.

More good news/bad news materializes: Dr. Bristol's being promoted to director of the whole medical clinic. Good news: she'll oversee everything—a unmistakable plus for me. Bad news: I'm losing a concerned primary-care physician.

Time to search out yet another new doctor.

This is always a sticky predicament because, while HMOs tell you can choose your doctor and that's true, you can't actually interview them as you'd like, then pick one. No, in order to speak with a specific doctor you have sign on as a patient, then schedule an introductory appointment. You cannot schedule introductory appointments with more than one doctor at a time. The HMO system won't allow it. This doctor-choosing procedure—if you 'interview' more than one doctor before making your decision—can eat up months of your precious time.

Around the clinic I ask whoever—Dr. Bristol, her nurse, girls who draw blood, counter people, anyone who'll give an ear—who they favor as primary-care physicians. No consensus emerges. There are, however, some emphatic washouts: positively do not get doctor so-and-so, people insist in hushed tones.

Dr. Bristol's cherub-like nurse, Paula, informs me of a new doctor who's recently joined the staff. From all she's heard, he's pretty capable. The only obstacle, as Paula tactfully puts it: this new doctor's a newcomer to America. . . there might be initial communication difficulties.

Prior to my introductory appointment, I jot out a short list of essential qualities I want in a doctor. Inspiration for this came from a number of books I'd read on weeding out the right doctor.

This new guy, Dr.Tzu, bristles noticeably, taking great issue with my questioning, indicating his indignation by firing back mock inquiries of his own . . . in very flawed English: "Why you ask so many questions?" . . . "Where *you* go to college?" And so forth.

This, to him, has become not an introductory meeting but a showdown.

Two years earlier, he graduated from a distinguished New York medical school. That's in his favor. A bantam fellow with frowning eyes, English obviously is Dr. Tzu's second tongue. While awkward to understand, he seems capable. Dr. Bristol will stay on as my primary doctor until she takes over the administrative reins entirely.

Call it laziness or a growing belief I wouldn't need him in the near future, but I decide to give this doctor a try—become his patient; at least for a while. A real letting down of the guard, if you will. Bad, bad decision.

CHAPTER 25

STRANGE TWISTS OF HUMAN NATURE—
A RACING HEART LANDS ME
BACK IN THE HOSPITAL

Despite my previous experience with Prednisone, a negative experience, I feel oddly enthused about this Dr. Crandle's guidance—the endocrine system *is* his specialty. That night I start on the drug. Two days later . . . I'm getting up in the morning, or attempting to, when I discover my body strength's vanished, as if all vitality's been sucked away by some nocturnal vacuum. I'm wilted. All over. Each muscle's lost its reserve. Scarcely am I able to crawl from the bed to the bathroom.

"Sure hope . . . " Jane observes, sitting up in bed, "you're not planning to go work today, Eric."

The sun is just now illuminating the east window.

I couldn't get ready and go to work even if I wanted to—though I most likely would've tried had she not intervened.

"What you better do," she asserts, throwing off the covers, "is call the doctor, the one who put you back on this Prednisone. Let him know what it's done to you. I told you it was silly to try this drug again. Call him, please, as soon as you can."

I'm in no condition to argue. She's being rational. Often it takes the critical eye of a spouse or other family member to redirect logical action. Fortunately, I'm not in the midst of a nail-biter at work, so missing a day won't mean a lot.

A little after nine, I telephone Dr. Crandle's office. Even over the phone this guy's outrageous. I'm wholly thrown off when he retorts, quite cockily, "Stay on the Prednisone . . . double the dosage. Go to 15 milligrams a day. Five 5 milligrams after each meal. In the morning after breakfast, after lunch and so forth."

"But . . . " I ask, startled, calling to mind my prior adventures with this medicine, "shouldn't I stop taking it and go back on the hydrocortisone . . . if this is making me feel this way?"

"Hell no," he fires back. "You're not taking enough! That's the problem. Start more today. Take 10 milligrams after lunch, then another five at dinner. If you don't feel 100 percent better by this time tomorrow, call me."

The phone is back in its cradle. I'm lying in bed, staring out at the soothing Pacific, the peaceful turquoise horizon, attempting to fathom the logic of this approach. I'm thinking, in my layman's view, the prescription itself is to blame for my past troubles, not the dosage. In parallel, I'm also thinking, how lordly it is for physicians to presuppose their lowly patients have all the time in the world—like none of us work, have lives, or places to be—when they specify stay-at-home regimens.

Shortly after lunch: I'm feeling slightly livelier, even before the extra Prednisone kicks in. After putting away a peanut butter and jelly sandwich, I gulp the prescribed measure of Prednisone. In a den recliner, I start reading my newest acquisition on cancer survival: *From Victim to Victor*, by Harold H. Benjamin.

We cancer patients, Benjamin astutely emphasizes, should never view or speak of ourselves in the negative: As victims who're powerless to escape the tentacles of this disease. We should, instead, see ourselves as victors battling a war of survival. Intriguing, this is.

The following sunup: The moment the god-awful alarm starts its chafing resonance, I know the increased Prednisone has done its job. Without shifting a muscle, I can feel the power to move is there. Wow, that arrogant bastard Crandle was right! Thus, the new dose of Prednisone becomes 15 milligrams a day: five mg after each meal, with Mitotane.

For the next couple of months I feel tolerably good, almost healthy in my daily activities—if one can say that of a cancer patient on oral chemotherapy. The stabbing pains that had appeared in my side remained at bay. (Actually, I'm beginning to lose sight of what 'feeling normal' really means.)

Then something unforeseen materializes—something that causes a major shift in course direction.

Saturday night, around 11:00, a simple act: Dropping my comb on the bathroom floor, I bend to retrieve it. During the process of bending over, my heart, without warning, starts pounding wildly. Periodic palpitations are something I've grappled with since childhood. What causes this intermittent condition has never been determined. These palpitation episodes occurred fairly regularly, maybe once every six months or so.

So I know what this is, what to do. Or did I?

Because of the excitable feeling that accompanies it, this episode does concern me, but I'm not going nuts with worry. Yet. All this will cease on its own in a few minutes. On the floor, I push my head downward, toward my knees. Usually this brings quick relief.

But my heart refuses to cooperate. It's flailing so unpredictably that I'm feeling oddly nauseated, short of breath. Panic's now coursing through me.

"Oh, God, Eric... not your heart again," Jane says, almost blandly, walking into the bedroom, seeing me on the floor.

"Mm . . ." I strain to mutter, trying not to sound unduly pained, hoping the heart will suddenly slow to normal as it always has. (Why do people try to camouflage moments of suffering as though these were somehow an embarrassment?) "Been acting up now . . . about five minutes. Won't seem to . . . back off."

Standing near me, she's looking down, hairbrush in hand. Her recall is weighing things, I can sense that. "Head for Emergency, you think?"

"I hate that place. It's like retreating. Sign of . . . defeat."

"How long has it been this way?" she asks, looking at her watch. From her inflection it's obvious she's not eager about getting dressed, driving to ER. "Maybe . . . if you lie flat. On the bed. Someplace where you're comfortable," she offers, helping me up. "I'll get the water."

Hobbling to the bed, hunched over like some ancient creature, I know this time's different: the heart's become a rabid beast. I'm trying to sip water. Jane's got the phone to her ear watching me—she's following orders given us a while back by Dr. Zindler—and calling ahead to see if the HMO on-duty doctor agrees we should go to the hospital ER. (What if he says No—do I stay home and die?) As fluke would have it my new primary doctor—Dr. Tzu—is on duty. He'll meet us at the ER in 30 minutes.

At the car, down three flights of stairs, I'm totally breathless, near panting . . . and quite terrified. The heart's positively racing now, feeling like it has swollen to twice its normal size and repositioned itself at the base of my neck. A feeling of faintness zooms through me. I'm already in the car; Jane's leisurely pulling on a sweater.

"Can you . . . please hurry, dear?" I breathe emphatically. "This could be . . . a friggin' heart attack, I don't know."

"You don't have the right symptoms," she replies disdainfully, climbing in behind the wheel. "Being a little theatrical, Eric, aren't we?" she goes on, turning the ignition key.

"This time's different . . . " I groan, not understanding why she's adopted this blasé attitude. "People do have heart attacks at my age."

It's between midnight and one o'clock, a moonlit, wind-swept night. All streets are eerily uninhabited. The hospital is eight miles away.

CHAPTER 26

LITTLE DID WE KNOW—
AN INEPT DOCTOR REVEALS HIMSELF

Within minutes of describing my symptoms to a nurse through a round hole in a glass window, I'm in a gown, on an icy exam table. The room air's quite cool, smelling heavily of chemicals. Two youthful, crisp-looking doctors are floating above me, faces very near, seeking rapid-fire answers, barking directions to the nurse. Before leaving home I'd grabbed my two-page medical history. I shove it toward the nearest doctor—a well-tanned, dark-haired guy with a Clark Gable mustache. Also listed are drugs I'm taking.

Talking hastily, but not in a ruffled manner, the second doctor, a thin-faced man with coarse, straw-colored hair, suggests they have several options. After hearing the name of my HMO doctor, these two doctors glance at one another suspiciously, stepping away. Now deliberating, they're whispering, pointing to sections of my medical history. Nurse Wiggins, her eyes as earnest as a hawk's, is expertly hooking me up to several monitoring devices, including an EKG machine. In seconds, some sort of IV's spilling into my forearm.

From out of the blue, my undersized, brooding primary-care physician, Dr Tzu, looking altogether baffled, appears as noiselessly as a cat. This is only the second or third time I've seen him. The ER doctors, immediately recognizing this fellow, begin firing pointed questions at him about what he wants to do—since I'm his patient.

Noting Dr. Tzu's ever-so-slight hesitancy, the ER doctors, like neighborhood bullies, step up their pursuit. "What do *you* want to do?" they're demanding. Inordinately querulous, they seem, like maybe they'd observed—and not appreciated—Dr. Tzu's exploits on some prior occasion.

Dr. Tzu, reacting excitably to the ER doctors' feeding frenzy, gestures for them to step away, with him, out of hearing range. Sensing my doctor's irresolution does not give me a warm feeling.

Five minutes zoom by. A sense of composure, of restfulness, suddenly washes over me as the drug dripping into my veins begins taking effect. Whatever the drug is, it's slowing my heart rate dramatically. Relaxation suffuses me, slowly, like a warm Hawaiian wave. That earlier feeling of panic's disappearing.

Jane's light brown eyes calmly take in the chaos of apparatus plugged into me. "What are they doing?" she asks.

"Apparently, there are several approaches they can use. That's what they're talking about now—with that little guy, Dr. Tzu. He's my new HMO doctor. From God knows where. He barely speaks English. The ER doctors are pushing him to the wall for some reason. Maybe they know something I should."

Couple of minutes later: All three doctors are hovering over me. One of the ER guys, the one with the Gable mustache, is explaining to Dr. Tzu how they'd taken a gamble—based on my medical history—and started the drug verapamil. Seems to have done the trick, he notes. Dr. Tzu looks down upon me with the detached concern of one gazing at a moon rock. He nods a belated approval.

"Your patient, doctor, brought his own medical history," the second ER doctor offers. "Quite helpful and to the point, actually."

"What we'd like to do, is keep him here for the time being. So we can monitor him," the mustachioed doctor volunteers. "Beyond that, *Dr.* Tzu, it's your call."

Looking at the lighter-haired ER doctor, I ask what we're dealing with.

"Sure," he begins, folding his arms crisply. "Not only did you exhibit an extremely rapid heartbeat, like one-eighty, but a very erratic one as well. Chancy combination. What we did's not always the way to go, but based on your history, it seems to be working."

"This whole episode," I explain, hoping to elicit some answers, "started with me bending over. Like that simple process compressed something inside. Make sense?"

The doctor, shaking his head: "Couldn't really say at this point. Till we get more tests on you. But considering all the drugs you're taking, it could be anything." He's looking expectantly to Dr. Tzu for further elaboration.

"We get tests done next week!" Dr. Tzu intones briskly, throatily, as if he isn't quite sure what's cooking. Straightening himself a bit, he seems a shade taller.

"It's our recommendation," the straw-haired ER doctor goes on, "that we keep Mr. Scribner overnight. For observation."

"Yes, yes," Dr. Tzu effuses in a sort of growl, as if he'd already resolved this himself.

By now I'm feeling near normal—breathing and heart rate have relaxed notably. There is, however, a mysterious jumpiness, an anxiety haunting me. "Do I have a choice?" I protest. "I spend too much time in this place," I add, seeing my staying overnight as a major subconscious trouncing in this war to survive cancer.

"Be best," the straw-haired ER doctor submits sympathetically, putting a strong grasp on my exposed shoulder. "We can certainly understand your feelings. It is, of course, ultimately your call. We can keep an eye on you."

With that said, and after reassessing the dancing electronic monitors on all sides, the ER duo walks away in conversation. Jane and I: Alone with Dr. Tzu.

"You know about my husband, doctor, right?" Jane asks, she, too, recognizing this man appears to be out of his element. To give him the benefit of the doubt, though, maybe his apparent floundering is a cultural difference, or a language-barrier thing. But, one wonders, how did he get through medical school?

Furrowing his brow, Dr. Tzu gives Jane one of those vacant What-Did-You-Say looks.

"I asked," Jane repeats, "if you know about Eric's history—his rare cancer, the weird chemotherapy he's taking?" She's talking slowly now, like he's hard of hearing.

Dr. Tzu smirks, nodding sharply as if he's in control of the situation. For the next few minutes Jane and the doctor discuss my condition. Lying there, I'm listening to the internal feedback from various body parts. Jane's doing most of the talking, bringing Dr. Tzu up to speed. He's now glancing over my written medical history.

"If I remember correctly," Jane's saying, "last time Eric went through an episode like this, he had the cancer surgery shortly thereafter."

Looking up, Dr. Tzu has that deer-in-the-headlights look.

With that, Jane jams her arm through his, leading the little doctor out of my hearing range—at least she thinks it's out of range—and discusses the possibility of having a CT scan in the near future, maybe tomorrow, to see if something new has developed. Dr. Tzu's eyes are saying, 'Yes, this is a good idea. . . .This is my idea.'

Returning to my bedside, Jane explains that Dr. Tzu will try to get a follow-up CT scan in the morning, here at the hospital, just for good measure . . . since it's been about five months since my last.

Caving in to popular opinion, I agree to spend the night. Actually I can see the logic in this, in that no one can say what caused this arrhythmia—that's what they labeled this episode—and no one can tell when it'll strike again. What the heck, I decide, it's only one night and, by staying, I'm sure to have someone nearby who knows how to respond to heart problems.

FINDING HOPE WHEN DOCTORS SAY THERE IS NONE

CHAPTER 27

UNDONE BY SURPRISE—
A CT REVEALS *MORE* BAD NEWS

By the time I'm situated in a private room on the fourth floor, it's 2:30 a.m. With all that's taken place I'm pretty well beat, but don't realize it till I lie on the soft bed. Jane and I and the floor nurse are the only ones in the room. Dr. Tzu's long gone. The ER guys removed the IV, suggesting—after Dr. Tzu didn't contribute anything—I begin oral verapamil once I get settled in a room.

Actually, I don't so much mind being here, inasmuch as no one knows what sparked this prolonged bout of arrhythmia. Never had an episode lasted beyond 10 minutes, give or take.

The nurse is now gone. Jane says wearily, with some disappointment in her voice, "If you give me your billfold and your rings and stuff, I'll take them home with me."

I fall into an easy, deep sleep for the balance of the night. This night's stay is, overall, a piece of cake. In the morning a volunteer brings a lukewarm, but good-smelling breakfast. Just as I'm bringing a piece of bacon to my mouth, a perfume-smelling nurse blasts through the door, bellowing: "Don't take a bite of that! They've got your CT scheduled (she pauses, puffing, catching her breath) . . . soon as they can work you in."

Stealing away my fragrant breakfast tray, in its place she plunks down a pint of Readi-Cat, a barium-sulfate suspension all patients have to drink prior to an abdominal scan. Sipping the thick, orange-flavored liquid, I flip through the morning paper. Undergoing this CT doesn't trouble me enormously. In fact, it seems sort of standard procedure by now and, notwithstanding last night's heart thing, I've been feeling fairly decent.

Jane telephones close to nine, asking what they've decided to do, CT-wise. I tell her they've set it up for later that morning. "Your little discussion with the good Dr. Tzu evidently worked," I say, watching a pair of animated morning doves doing some sort of ritualized dance on my window ledge.

"Thought as much," she answers, yawning. "When push comes to shove, I think he got scared when I explained your situation. Like a little mole, isn't he? You feel safe with him?"

"A little late now to be thinking of that."

Chatting for a moment, we both agree there's nothing to be gained by her spending the morning sitting here while I'm off at the CT station.

Two CT technicians inform me that they're going to inject barium into my rectum, via enema, for the sake of further diagnostic clarity. Objecting, I tell them I've had numerous CTs and never had this procedure before. They maintain it's the way this facility executes all abdominal CTs. No alternative—my doctor ordered the exam.

Aside from the embarrassment of the female-administered barium enema, the CT goes smoothly as I lie there, for 45 minutes or so, breathing and not breathing. Once completed, a candy-striper wheels me back to the fourth floor: I'm supposed wait there for a doctor to discharge me. Word on the CT report will come days later, I reason, as they invariably do.

Close to 1:00: A very dour-looking Dr. Tzu struts into the room. Wearing a black leather sport jacket, a madras, open-neck shirt, he is. Evidently he's on duty all weekend, this being Sunday.

"Meesta Scrimna," he starts without fanfare, fumbling with my name. Jane glances up from her crossword puzzle. "Meesta Scrimna," Dr. Tzu blunders on without pretense, "we find new tumor." He thrusts his forefinger into the flesh on his left side to demonstrate. "Here. Adrenal."

"No. How can this be?" I respond disbelievingly, but all the same swallowing hard, sure this is some kind of new-doctor faux pas. "I feel great. No symptoms whatsoever."

"Yes," Dr. Tzu persists almost dementedly, nodding in haste. "New tumor. Here." Now he's pitched forward, aiming his thin finger at the corresponding spot on me.

"Have you . . ." Jane interjects wisely, "compared these films to the last?" A good deal of color's drained from her face.

"Yes, yes, yes. We check," Dr. Tzu goes on assertively, as if his professionalism is being challenged. "Small lesion there before."

"But . . ." I persist cautiously, "the last radiologist's report, back whenever . . . said everything was okay. Nothing to worry about."

"That doctor make error! Tumor there now," Dr. Tzu says, the squeaking noise of his leather jacket sounding like thunder, "—and tumor there then."

Two minutes ago I was sitting here, altogether content, chatting with Jane . . . now my entire world's imploding. I feel as if someone's thrown gasoline on me and ignited it. My sense of panic is in high gear. My surroundings surge forward in a swirl of madness, like swarming summertime gnats.

"What . . . do I do now, doctor?" I ask, reasoning grimly: Why was I so lazy as to allow myself to get stuck with this compassionless foreigner?"

"Surgery to remove," Dr. Tzu declares throaty, abruptly, in flawed English. "Surgeon down hall right now. He see you soon."

"Wait a second, Dr. Tzu," Jane says, "this is too sudden. We need time to catch our breath."

Taking several rearward steps, Dr. Tzu moves out into the hallway, anxiously looking for someone to turn this ordeal over to. "He still with other patient," Dr. Tzu observes haltingly. With a slight nod of his head, as if to say good-bye, he's gone.

The fatalism that seizes you—a cancer patient—once you're set upon like this, is unexplainable.

Jane, wondering after a moment: "Is there any way he could be . . . right?"

"Not in my book," I reply, feeling now a glimmer of confidence as I mouth these words. "I feel too damn good, aside from last night. With that first tumor—remember—I felt really bad all the time. This Tzu character's got to be all wet. He's new. That's it! They must've got my films mixed up with somebody else's."

"Why, why, why did Dr. Bristol have to move on?" Jane laments, nibbling her lip. "She was on our side. So good."

"God, this could open up so many creepy things," I mutter, my sanity racing. "Like, if the doctor's right, where do I have the surgery? Do I try for Houston, where they know what they're doing? Will the HMO buy it?"

We both fall silent. Minutes go by. Hearing voices outside in the hallway we look up. A pair of unfamiliar doctors strides in—a middle-aged man, a woman in her early forties. "I'm Dr. Kirk," the woman states, extending her hand sympathetically, "filling in for Dr. Malone this weekend. This is Dr. Hubbard, a general surgeon. We're sorry, both of us, for meeting you this way. We both happened to be on the floor seeing other patients when Dr. Tzu flagged us down."

Sitting there, I feel as if my will to go on has been severely damaged. Jane clears her throat. Things are becoming undeniable.

Dr. Hubbard shakes my hand. He's wearing faded Levi's, a western snap-button shirt. His hand, on the hefty side, doesn't have the silky texture of a doctor, a surgeon. "We've been reviewing your film . . . and those from last April. Dr. Tzu—who had to go home—has already discussed surgery with us."

"Hold on a minute," I respond. "This is all coming too fast. *Surgery?*"

"We can appreciate your shock, Mr. Scribner. But I'm afraid it's a necessity we have to discuss. We'll need to conduct a number of tests—bone scan, MRIs of both your head and abdomen—before we schedule anything. To make sure the cancer's not spread to either your brain or bones," Dr. Hubbard says matter-of-factly, looking me dead in the eye. "If either's the case, I won't do the surgery."

More good news topples on me with the weight of so many bags of cement: In a few words, this man's just walked into my life, advising me that my condition—a condition, I might add, that didn't even exist in my mind 10 minutes ago—might be inoperable. I feel myself losing control—my breathing, my vision, and my judgment. Can this be happening, or is it something from a repulsive dream from which I'll soon awaken?

The cancer's come back . . . It's growing again! The words dripping slowly . . . like an acid in me.

"You're sure . . ." Jane puts in weakly, "it was there in April?"

"We were with him—the radiologist—when he compared films. It was there."

My head's teeming with unruly, nonsensical thoughts, most of them rather hideous, morbid. I can't even bring myself to think about the reasons for the bone scan, the MRIs. Insanity reigns for the moment, saying there should be a consolation . . . some powerful neutralizing force should come down from above and enact something to the effect: Since the earlier radiologist missed this new growth, then, *he, not you* will undergo this troubling operation. Crazy thinking.

"What . . ." I ask quietly, "do I do next?"

"I'll let Dr. Malone know as soon as we're finished here," says Dr. Kirk, a slender-faced woman with haggard blue eyes. "Dr. Tzu, I believe, will be in touch with her regarding other issues."

"Other issues?"

"Surgery. Tests. So forth."

"My most immediate question is *when*?" I ask, resigning myself to their dire message. "I'm determined to be aggressive. Let's do it quick. Get in, get it done before this stuff grows anymore."

"We can't talk about *when*, Mr. Scribner, till we see *if*," Dr. Hubbard interjects. "A lot of tests and paperwork have to be completed. But I wouldn't rule out some time next week."

In the span of 15 minutes, my life's been indelibly changed . . . and I've come to abhor the brutal give-and-take of surgeons.

CHAPTER 28

UPON US LIKE THUNDER—
ANOTHER NEW HMO DOCTOR AND
FURTHER DELAYS

The two doctors are now gone. Jane and I are alone. An indescribable sense of emptiness permeates the room, each of us staring at different inanimate objects. Me, visualizing again that barefoot, worry-free boy roaming the warm summer shores of the Chesapeake . . .

"You think . . ." Jane offers softly after a few minutes, "there could be a mistake?"

"These guys seem pretty much on the money," I respond sluggishly, as if returning from a drug-induced stupor. "Not like What's-His-Face."

"You . . . able to think yet?" Sitting on the edge of the bed, Jane lays a feather-soft hand on mine. "I know how it must be for you."

"Numbness, yeah. Doesn't seem . . . a human being should have to go through this a second time. But maybe we're not talking about me here. We're looking at a black comedy . . . about somebody else's life.

"But you know what's truly weird," I go on, feeling an unexpected burst of mental energy, "you expect a major disease like this to be painful—to let you know it's there, killing you. Remember Drake? How he hit us with the news about me being dead in a little over a year?"

After a long, impenetrable silence, Jane, exhaling: "I really hate this."

Words that hang in midair—Is she referring to her involvement . . . or the sea of uncertainty I'm—we're—facing?

"Let's just get you the hell out of this place," she says abruptly, standing, as if having resolved something within herself. "They said you could go—that I could take you."

"This is the floor," I say just trying to be casual, to fill a void, getting dressed, "where they give IV chemo. You notice the special signs in hallway?"

"It's the only place this shitty hospital had a private room."

At home, feeling utterly depleted, I go upstairs and lie down. This new heart medication they've got me on adds greatly to my bone-weariness. Watching the unfeeling waves of the Pacific roll in and pound the shore, I wonder bleakly, simply: Is this cancer. . . strong enough to win?

Trying desperately to recall any of the uplifting things I'd read about overcoming cancer's dark side, my mind's rebelling as I try to focus it away from all the negativity. This simple truth I can feel with a shuddering reality: Hearing you have cancer a second time—knowing this wrathful disease has mounted another assault—is even more devastating than hearing it the first time. A colossal sense of vulnerability—of alone-ness—consorts with the simple words: "We found a new tumor."

All you thought you'd accomplished, all you thought you'd done to move beyond the ruthless grasp of this ruthless disease means . . . nothing; so much hot air, good intentions.

Jane is down in the kitchen. Hours have slipped by. I hear her preparing dinner. A great deal more clamor emanating from below than usual—a metal pan falls hard, rolling round and round and round on the cold tile floor. A cabinet door bangs shut, then another.

"I . . . " I begin inanely, standing in the kitchen doorway, "heard you. Down here."

"It's me. I'm . . . here," Jane breathes solemnly, not looking my way. "Decided I'm going to fix your favorite: meatloaf and mashed potatoes."

At the sink, Jane is languidly peeling potatoes. Late afternoon sunlight spilling in the window plays on the listless way her slender hands are moving. Watching a moment, I maintain my distance, sensing her thoughts. "Anything you need from me? A hand?"

She stops peeling, her mind sorting thoughts. She nods slowly, not turning toward me. She hasn't looked this way since I walked in.

"Really gets to you, doesn't it?" I offer.

In the solemn quiet of the lifeless kitchen, her nearly silent reply: "Mmmm."

"We're a team, though, babe. We can pull it off," I say, trying to sound confident, but not really sure of pulling off anything. Moving closer, I slide my arms around her. She turns.

"You *are* the one I love," she whispers. Her eyes are puffy, red. With half-peeled potato in one hand, the paring knife in the other, she dabs away tears with the back of her wrist.

Then, as she slides her arms tightly around me, we both, as if on cue, begin weeping aloud, profoundly . . . like terrified children. The tears—fiery, overflowing—feel almost immediately cleansing. But they're also accompanied by a loathsome sense of abandonment, of defeat.

My sister, Jennifer, three years younger than me, lives full time in Mammoth Lakes. She and my brother-in-law recently purchased a 48-foot sailboat they moored at the harbor, a couple of miles away. Jenny and Lloyd drive five and half hours each way, down from Mammoth, every other weekend to spend time relaxing in the sun, tinkering with the boat. Being an unfailing sister, she frequently checks on me to see how things are progressing. Whenever I have a CT or some other test, she's on the phone soon afterward seeing how things went.

So it made sense to go to the harbor the next day, Sunday, to give them the news about this latest turn of events. Seemed the brotherly thing to do. Not fair to them, really, in terms of inflicting emotional pain, but they should know. Don't want them hearing this news later, from some second-hand source.

After the initial hellos and hugs on the boat deck, I accept a canned soft drink. Sitting in a canvas-and-wood deck chair in the warm afternoon sun, I begin my latest story. Both Jenny and Lloyd look on apprehensively, listening. We humans, it seems, know instinctively when another of our kind's caught in an emotional undercurrent.

We reveal all Jane and I know up to this point. Mainly, that some form of surgery will be required. The damn cancer's back, I hear myself saying.

In Jenny's eyes, I can see her watching me, recalling our father's tortured death. She is, at that point, significantly paler then when we arrived. She offers to take a week's vacation to help. Since Jane would most likely be unable to be with me as much as she'd like (she's lately accepted a new job), this sounds like a wonderful and comforting idea. Jane and I head home feeling better, knowing at least someone who cares is going to be looking after my simple needs: I won't have to rely on the assistance of unpredictable nurses.

Calling the medical clinic the next day, Monday, to make an appointment with Dr. Tzu to get the necessary procedures rolling, I'm told he's 'out for a few days, maybe a week or more.' Another doctor is filling in for him, a very disturbing turn of events. Bad enough having to deal with the bumbling Dr. Tzu, but now, having to deal with an entirely new doctor . . . Square one.

Resigning myself, I ask for—and surprisingly get—an appointment that day with this other doctor.

Far exceeding my expectations, this new doctor's a vibrant, can-do, nattily dressed woman in her thirties who's just joined the HMO. Buoyant in spirit, she instantly grasps the magnitude of all Jane and I are telling her about my recurrence. Scanning my version of my medical history, the dark-haired Dr. Paravano says confidently: "Okay. We'll set up all your tests on a stat basis. We want you in surgery as soon as possible, right? That is your wish, isn't it, Mr. Scribner?"

Flashing back to the good old days when doctors took charge, I swallow and reply astoundedly, "If that's possible."

What this new doctor accomplishes in the next eight days is truly amazing, considering normal HMO procedures: I have a blood test (including ACTH), an MRI of my head and abdomen, a full-body bone scan, a CT of the chest. These tests are done at three different facilities by three different sets of technicians. Lots of paperwork. In the annals of HMO medicine this kind of rapid-fire testing is all but unheard of.

(Months later, once this doctor becomes my new, new primary-care internist, she reveals she'd gotten 'raked over the coals' for the stat handling of these tests. Seems she didn't 'understand HMO procedures.' The administrative powers at the clinic felt she'd gone overboard in my case. *Nothing, it seems, is really an immediate concern in the world of profit-driven HMO medicine.* The one element consistently absent from HMO reasoning is the emotional or physical well-being of the patient—everything is determined by dollars and cents.)

During this eight-day battery of tests, I find myself growing increasingly apprehensive: The law of averages, as I see it, has to be closing in on me. At least one of these tests will uncover something hideous.

For some reason, the test results are delivered via Dr. Malone, my oncologist. To say I'm rather fidgety waiting in her small seventh-floor exam room for her arrival is putting it mildly. (Seems all oncologists, at least those I've been exposed to, postpone till last the vital life-and-death information you're there to hear. They discuss myriad other non-essentials *before* getting to your true interest—the crucial test results.)

The docile Dr. Malone enters, proceeding immediately to look me over physically. After prodding the lymph nodes in my neck, she palpates the stomach. Her touch, as indicated earlier, is too delicate to really accomplish anything meaningful. It's as though she's gently applying a cooling salve to a sleeping infant's sunburned skin rather than probing for deep tumors. She's that delicate.

Little is said as she goes about this ritual. She does, however, congratulate me on the rapid-fire way which I, 'or someone,' had achieved the necessary pre-surgery tests.

Yes, yes, yes . . . I'm thinking. But get to the test results! (I don't come right out and ask for them because . . . well, you want them . . . but don't want them: negative results can change your world in an instant.)

Now, thumbing through the pile of paper that her nurse's paper-clipped to my file jacket, Dr. Malone's poker face shows nothing.

"Your ACTH . . . is way down, Mr. Scribner," she begins. "—420 as opposed to over 1000. And—" she continues, reading silently to herself. (Guess I can't blame doctors who don't read test results before they enter the exam room—they are busy people. But it'd be a nice, faith-building courtesy. Patients like to think their doctor has enough interest in them to have at least read these pivotal test results *before* he or she enters the exam room.) "Looks like everything else . . . is normal."

Instantaneously relieved, feeling as if I've miraculously survived a murderous, days-long gauntlet, I ask: "The MRIs . . . the CT . . . the bone scan . . . all are good?"

"Nothing out of the ordinary noted. The MRI of the abdomen does, of course, show the new lesion."

"So—" Jane puts in anxiously, "we can go ahead? Schedule the surgery?"

"After a fashion." Dr. Malone has her pen going, noting something in my file. Without looking up, she continues: "We should be able to set something up in . . . approximately six to eight weeks."

"You're not serious," I put in, now feeling crestfallen. "That's way too far off. I want to get this over quickly—like yesterday. Aggressiveness is my policy, and I thought it was the general policy in all cancer treatment. Doctors are always preaching about early detection, early eradication—if there's any hope of beating this disease."

"Mr. Scribner," Dr. Malone begins, exhaling audibly, "there are a lot of approvals, a lot of people involved."

"But six to eight weeks," Jane mutters. "That's an eternity. So many things can happen."

Dr. Malone grins wryly, as if to say: Now you'll feel the cruel jaws of the snail-paced HMO. One of the few times I recall seeing her smile at all. "Your husband did so well maneuvering these tests, Mrs. Scribner, maybe he can work that same magic again. I couldn't have arranged all the tests Dr. Hubbard insisted on any quicker, I assure you."

"Doctor," I say, "since you mentioned him—Dr. Hubbard—I noticed he's listed as a general surgeon. Do you think he is the best doctor for the job? Not that I doubt his talents," I add submissively.

"He's as good as I've seen locally, Mr. Scribner," she replies, seeming ever so miffed I questioned a colleague.

"Well, doctor, could we please do this?" I continue undaunted, figuring it's my life we're talking about here. "Could you call Dr. Saltz at M.D. Anderson and get her thoughts? I mean, would she recommend me going back there for surgery? This is an unusual cancer."

Looking not terribly thrilled with this request, Dr. Malone mutters unconvincingly, "Yes, I'll call, Mr. Scribner," as she leads us to the door.

FINDING HOPE WHEN DOCTORS SAY THERE IS NONE

CHAPTER 29

AN UNFORTUNATE CONCERN— A QUESTIONABLE SURGERY

Over the next few days I talk at length with Dr. Paravano *and* Dr. Bristol, now medical director of the clinic. Both feel as I do: surgery should commence as quickly as possible. They'll do all they can to ensure paperwork and approvals are in place. Truly, I'm grateful that Dr. Tzu, in his magnificent ineptitude, is out of the picture. At least for now.

Three days later: Dr. Bristol, though technically no longer my doctor, calls to say surgery's been sanctioned via the clinic's (or HMO's) Utilization Review process. She says little to indicate how instrumental she'd been in orchestrating this. Not revealing that I'd asked Dr. Malone to check with Houston regarding surgery there, I thank Dr. Bristol lavishly, telling her I'll telephone the surgeon's office and make the arrangements. Emotionally, I feel supercharged—everything's falling into place so well, so swiftly.

Before I call Dr. Hubbard's office, I put in a call to Dr. Malone to see what she's learned from M.D. Anderson. "Dr. Saltz," according to the unelaborative Dr. Malone, "feels that any good general surgeon should be able to handle this surgery. And since we don't foresee anything unusual," Dr. Malone closes with, *"Dr. Hubbard's more than qualified."*

Her firmer-than-normal attitude resonates her none-too-pleased reaction to my questioning, ever so slightly, a member of the brotherhood's medical (surgical) abilities. Never mind that it's *my* life. Again, the second-opinion mirage rears its head and takes a bullet. At any rate, I feel self-satisfied having at least *explored* other surgical alternatives.

With that off my mind, I arrange with Dr. Hubbard's office the pre-surgery consult in two days, and surgery six days after that, at 7:00 a.m. In all, setting up the surgical agenda takes five days—a far cry from the six to eight weeks Dr. Malone offered via the typical HMO paper mill process. A process, by the way, that I believe the HMO *intentionally* mans with young, under-trained employees, who, when they're unsure of your questions, will always answer with a No. By design, a large number of HMO callers will then fall by the wayside, because most patients aren't persistent enough to follow through, to demand to speak with a supervisor. When I call the HMO, I make it a practice to *never* speak with the first-line HMO defense: These I-Could-Care-Less, under-trained telephone employees.

Calling Dr. Bristol, I give her an itemized account of the surgery schedule. Very pleased, she says she'll take care of the remaining paper shuffling. We're now calling one another by our first names—hers being Sandra (pronounced Sondra).

Before surgery, I have one last rendezvous to keep—with Dr. Crandle, the endocrinologist—for an ACTH follow-up. While I can put off this outwardly superfluous appointment, I don't want to set anything aside in the normal flow of events, as if to say this surgery's an end in itself.

The free-wheeling Dr. Crandle's perched in a chair on one side of the exam table, me in a chair on the other. He likes using this table as a impromptu desk. Running his finger down the newest ACTH figures, he seems elated with them—*and* himself for drafting this strategy.

"But," I object to deflate him a bit, "things're still on the high side."

"Hey, bud, I could've told you that," he retorts, burping quietly into the back of his hand. "It takes a while to get ACTH to react. Stay with the Prednisone, like you're doing. Things are . . . on course. Maybe two months more, we should see some *real* change."

It does me a world of good, perceptually, just hearing a doctor of medicine —*any doctor*—proclaim things're going well . . . even if it's something as seemingly unimportant as my ACTH level. As we talk, I mention the looming surgery.

A contorted expression twists Dr. Crandle's face. He pulls back for emphasis. "You're actually serious?. . . *Surgery?"* he asks as if I'm pulling his leg. "You look so damn *good.*"

"Yeah, well, that's the insidiousness of this disease," I say, feeling silly explaining this to a physician. "Outside you look good . . . inside, another story. And to further complicate things—I *feel* great."

"What's the calendar date on this thing?"

I pass along the time, date, hospital, surgeon's name. "You know this guy?" I inquire, trusting he does and will say Dr. Hubbard's a genius.

"Chatted with him a time or two. What I'll do," Dr. Crandle goes on, scratching pensively the crown of his close-cropped mane with his thumb, "is write out for you—*him actually*—the steroid dosages you'll need." With great flourish, he scribbles several sparse observations on his pad, tears them free. "Here. Be sure our man knows you're on Prednisone and sees this."

Slowly, Dr. Crandle restates the date and time, pinching the bridge of his nose. "I think," he begins abruptly, in an *Ah-Ha!* fashion, "I'll make it a point to be there."

Glancing at his scribbled note, I'm suddenly taken by this case-hardened man's apparent concern. *"You're going to be there?"* I ask, amazed that a doctor not immediately involved wants to follow my surgery without being obligated to—and without remuneration. I'm thinking: Maybe I sold this character short. He talks a tough game, sure, but he's a caring individual.

"Normally, I make my rounds a little after that time. So what I'll do," he says, seemingly pleased with this game plan, patting my hand, winking at me, "is show up a little early."

Days later: At the pre-surgery consult, after a very thorough strong-handed physical, Dr. Hubbard spells out, step by step, what he expects to accomplish in surgery. He's a broad, easy-talking, red-cheeked, ranch-foreman type guy . . . as the Levi's and western shirt alluded to at our original encounter.

Slipping an expensive-looking ball-point from his shirt pocket, he draws a torso on the brittle exam table paper. Here's where and how he's going to cut—through the original scar. He talks about convalescence and the benefits of self-administered Demerol as pain relief. He's entirely unhurried, very personable.

He feels I'll be hospitalized four, possibly five days. Do not take any aspirin or aspirin-like products, he admonishes, such as Advil, prior to surgery. The diet he prescribes is vastly easier to live with than the clear-liquid regimen Dr. Lutes, the original surgeon, had required. When I hand Dr. Hubbard the notes Dr. Crandle scribbled, he politely accepts them. I gather from his face, however, that he's well aware of the needed steroid dosages.

With all pre-surgery transactions out of the way, I can breathe easier, hunker down to some serious old-fashioned, all-night, stomach-churning pre-surgery worrying. In an effort to refocus my mind, I drive over to the hospital, spend part of an afternoon with the woman in charge of patient self-help literature and audio tapes. Rummaging through the selection, she recommends a set of Dr. Bernie Siegel tapes, a surgeon who's created a number of superb books and tapes to aid cancer patients in getting through the unfamiliar territory of various cancer treatments, including surgery. These tapes, for me, prove to be a windfall.

Becoming my devoted companions during the 45-mile freeway commute to and from work for the next few days, I pop a tape into the car's cassette player and Dr. Siegel begins discussing the mind/body relationship in healing, in beating cancer. With the innumerable topics covered on the tapes—and he covers a lot: everything from chemo to dying with dignity—it's as though I have my own personal therapist, one who knows, who truly understands my plight. I cannot applaud Bernie's tapes and books highly enough. After listening to him and digesting all he has to say, I'm more able to focus my fight for survival, much like a boxer going through training camp.

The nerve-jarring alarm rattles me from a light sleep. It's 4:00 a.m., the morning of the surgery. The motionless ocean beyond the bedroom window's black as ink. It's one of those almost-mornings where the full moon's squatting like a ball of blue cheese on the horizon, refusing to disappear. Though the surgery isn't till 7:00, I have to check in at 5:00.

In the glum morning light, driving to the hospital Jane and I say almost nothing. This is by no means getting to be 'old hat.' In me are gnawing and very animated fears: Will they go in and find the situation inoperable? A point over which I've had innumerable nightmares. Will they find something unexpected? Will I be in excruciating pain again? Will they *this* . . . will they *that*? Worry on top of worry, on top of worry.

. . . . In the operating room a dominant white light, much like you'd imagine an alien spacecraft to emit, glows above as wakefulness slithers quietly away. That glare's the last image I have prior to waking. This post-surgery wake-up call's immensely different from the one I experienced in 1989 with Dr. Lutes.

Regaining a foggy degree of wakefulness, my partially open eyes deliver this message to my brain: You're in a nearly unlit, almost cave-like area, intensely quite, without windows. For some reason, I imagine I'm in the bowels of this facility, the basement. Glowing monitors abound—orange, blue, flashing red, dancing.

Realizing I'm back, a nurse leans near, asking quietly if I'm okay. Her voice balmy, unobtrusive.

Tubes going in, going out of almost every bodily orifice. Only minor pain at the surgical site. Nothing like the chain-sawed-open abdomen Dr. Lutes left me with. Maybe it's a delayed pain, I'm thinking, like when your toe snags the coffee table leg in the dark.

"Where . . . is this place?" I mumble.

"You're in ICU, Mr. Scribner," the nurse, a short-haired woman of thirty-five or so, whispers leaning nearer. "Dr. Hubbard wants to be sure you're stable. Before putting you on a floor."

I can see little lying there, not raising up for fear of awakening the pain. The ward's dim, but presents a soothing ambiance. Two other nurses are talking quietly among themselves maybe 15 feet away, near a central monitoring station: one male, one female. No doctors in sight.

"Time is it?" I want to know, having no idea how long I'd been under.

"Coming up on two," the nurse says. "Your surgery went well, I understand. Did all they expected to." She looks over her shoulder. "Dr. Hubbard's here abouts, somewhere."

"Why am I not feeling . . . more pain?"

The nurse smiles, patting fondly a blinking box-like device next to the bed. "He has you on a Demerol drip. *Wonderful* stuff. I'll show you later how to use it. Once the doctor's finished with you."

"When can I see people—my wife, my son?"

"Visitation in here, Mr. Scribner, is strictly controlled," she explains. "We only have a total of 10 patients—two for each nurse. Only close family members get in. And then only for short periods. We'll get your family in probably in about an hour." Touching my hand, she squeezes reassuringly. This simple touching feels wonderfully restorative.

My sense of awareness is, at best, extremely hazy. I'm drifting in, drifting out of wakefulness. Minutes later, a familiar male voice reaches out, grabs me.

Feeling the grasp of a powerful hand on my calf, I catch a glimpse of Dr. Hubbard's face. A welcomed face. It just *feels* comforting to see him standing there.

"Your surgery, Mr. Scribner, proved a little more involved than we anticipated," he explains softly. "Things went well, though. We did have to take the spleen, part of the left kidney, a portion of your diaphragm."

Instantly my mind jumps to those areas of my body, sensing for the loss. "But you got *it* . . . the *thing*?"

"And then some."

"So," I quip groggily, feeling a rush of relief, "then I can look forward to joining in at The Running of the Bulls this year?"

FINDING HOPE WHEN DOCTORS SAY THERE IS NONE

CHAPTER 30

WINNING THE BATTLE, LOSING THE WAR—
THE SURGERY'S A SUCCESS, BUT
THE NEWS IS NOT GOOD

"Mr. Scribner, I'm recommending follow-up radiation," Dr. Hubbard continues, not at all playing off my attempt at humor, his words rolling through me like a low thunder. "As soon as you're well enough."

This, I rationalize in my hazy state of uncertainty, is standard fare for him: All his cancer patients get radiation follow-up. Viewing everything at the moment through a sort of soft-focus haze, I'm not in the best physical shape to debate the idea's pros or cons. (Radiation, from what M.D. Anderson doctors said, is unproductive—even an accelerator—in treating ACC.) Nodding affirmatively, I smile weakly—just content to be back among the living.

A nurse—Kelly, her name tag says—is standing to one side. The doctor asks if she's had a chance to demonstrate use of the pain medication. Kelly says she's just about to.

"I'll return this evening, Mr. Scribner," Dr. Hubbard assures me, moving away. "It's my wish that we keep you here at least 24 hours till you're fully stabilized." Winking at the nurse, he adds: "These folks will treat you like royalty."

With near-transparent, well-veined hands, Kelly demonstrates the use of the self-administered pain-relief system. "This medication," she underscores, "is the crème de la crème. Better than morphine, in my book." She's gripping a plastic, syringe-type plunger I'm supposed to activate when I feel the slightest discomfort.

"You literally can't over-dose yourself," Kelly goes on. "This gadget's designed to discharge only a precise amount of drug, at programmed intervals. In other words, you can't keep working the button and get more. You have to wait. You're set for—let's see—10-minute intervals. What I tell my patients is this: press once for pain, once more for pleasure, then again if you want to drift off to la-la land. What I'm saying is . . . if things get too crazy in here and you want to doze off, use the three-hit method. Don't worry, none of this'll harm you . . . be addictive or anything. Did you catch all that, Mr. Scribner? I know you're pretty much out-of-it right now."

Squeezing the plunger, within seconds a euphoric flow of pleasure's speeding through every capillary of my being. The perception of pain dissolves and an incredible sense of bliss fills me. Though almost incoherent, I'm lying there, calculating how crudely I'd been treated following the initial surgery—given only periodic pain injections, made to lie in semi-agony in a sweaty, conventional room. Dr. Lutes' approach had been, at best, inhumane.

"Good thing about Dr. Hubbard," Kelly resumes some time later, "is he doesn't like seeing his patients in pain. Of any sort." Casting a quick glance over her shoulder, she goes on under her breath: "Used to be . . . he was a real prick."

Kelly's odd sense of candor catches me off guard, like a stream of ice water in the face.

She continues: "Then it was his turn to have surgery. Last year. I was assigned to him. Talk about a big wuss! Whoa! But the good thing is—now, he understands. But don't get me wrong: He's good at what he does. We encounter very little difficulty with his post-op patients. Probably. . . he's the best in this county. But before his surgery . . . a cat of another color."

Later—maybe hours, maybe minutes—having just floated off to some joyous, pain-free latitude after hitting the Demerol button twice, I'm vaguely mindful of an undersized human figure floating about the foot of my bed, flipping nosily through sheets of paper. Forcing my foggy thought processes to focus, I make out the silhouette of my bumbling primary-care physician: Dr. Tzu.

Oh, God no—he's back!

I hadn't counted on him or his alternate, Dr. Paravano, being here because he was away, and she said she's too new to have hospital visitation rights. She was going to have a third doctor visit me, and keep her posted. Unless, she said, Dr. Tzu returned. Then, of course, he'd take over.

So here he is in all his amateurish splendor.

"Meesta Scrimna," Dr. Tzu begins in his irritatingly distorted English, his facial expression utterly unexpressive, "surgery go good." He offers this observation self-importantly, as though he'd performed a hands-on role. "But you," he carries on throatily as a mildly irritated karate instructor might, "—not going to make it."

What? My mind, grapples clumsily with these annulling, these lethal words.

One minute my head's levitating in ebullience—and the next, unexpectedly, I'm being yanked back to the ugliest of realities. Is this doctor, with a single callous remark, intentionally trying to sabotage my convalescence? My life?

Maybe this is a drug-induced vision . . . Why would anyone awaken an ICU cancer patient and offer such a fatalistic observation? It's this Demerol! That's it—I'm hallucinating!

"Doc-ta. Hubb-ud," the voice at the end of the bed stumbles onward in ungrammatical syllables, the words still devoid of emotion, "cut tumor, make spill."

What has been up to this point an uneventful, remarkably pain-free recovery, now takes an abrupt decent into blackness. Still heavily befogged, not really totally conscious, I succeed in asking Dr. Tzu what in God's name he's talking about. Forcing my eyes open wider, I'm trying to see whether this is a dream, a hallucination.

He echoes his earlier words: about the cancer being cut into, its spilling. Despite the pain-killing fog of Demerol, a heavy wave of panic hits me. I'm almost totally sedated, but this man's managed to awaken in me an electric sense of fright—along with an intense desire to break free of these tubes and drugs and inflict upon him the same pain he's inflicting on me.

How dare he appear like some perverted god, announcing I'm not going to make it!

"Get away from me, you asshole!" I shout as forcefully as I can, feeling as I rise up an intense pain explode across my midsection.

Like an innocent child offended, Dr. Tzu retreats cautiously.

With him gone, I shut my eyes, attempting to push his grim prognostication out of my thoughts for the moment, at least. But doubt—and now understanding (I realize now why radiation is being considered)—burn in my gut.

"Mr. Scribner," a male nurse's voice murmurs quietly some time later, inches from to my ear, "your wife's here."

I've no idea how long I've been in ICU, how long I've been dozing when Jane appears. With her is my son Marc. (My other son, the 26-year-old, still hasn't spoken to me for whatever excuse. I'd hoped when he heard I was going to have another cancer surgery, he'd break his silence. That didn't happen.)

"Handling the cobwebs okay, hon?" Jane whispers, stroking my forehead, kissing me. "You really look spaced." Her fearful eyes surveying the flickering monitors above my head, at the foot of the bed. Marc pinches my big toe beneath the sheet. "Hey, dude," he says, forcing a smile.

"You guys run into that . . . idiot Tzu?" I ask.

"He . . . materialized toward the end of surgery," Jane answers, embellishing no more, her voice cautious.

"So . . . you caught his line of bull?"

"He was in here?"

"Long enough . . . . I threw his ass out."

"Damn, damn, damn!" Jane breathes sympathetically. "Wish we could've known and cut him off—him and that other worthless being, that Crandle jerk. What a heartless pair of jackasses!"

"No, no, Crandle's my buddy. That's him—that's how he is."

"No, honey, take my word for it, this person is not your buddy."

"He only seems obnoxious. Really he's not."

"Let's let this go for now, okay," Jane says, squeezing my cold hand once more. "We know what an ignoramus that Dr. Tzu is. Consider the source. So . . . did Dr. Hubbard see you?"

"He's talking about me having radiation. Just something, I figure—" I reply, seizing upon Tzu's ominous remarks, "—he recommends for all cancer patients."

"What's all this stuff, pop?" Marc asks as an obvious diversion, pointing to the Demerol drip.

I explain the device's function. Both Marc and Jane seem greatly relieved as they banter playfully about me—husband and father—becoming a junkie. I understand now, I tell them, how people get enslaved to this stuff—if the street version's this euphoric.

ICU, Day Two: Being in ICU, if one must be in such a compromising position, is much like flying first-class versus coach—coach being a typical private room. ICU nurses are assigned just two patients. They're watchful, compassionate, and very close by. They're the hospital's cream of the crop, the astute, proficient, thoughtful. A far cry from some of the gritty, regular nurses I'd been exposed to.

Kelly and a male nurse whisper that Dr. Hubbard wants me up, walking about as much as possible. Kelly's advises that I hit the Demerol a few minutes before this attempted walk. They hoist me gently, cautiously to a standing position.

With the two nurses' help, I move along with astonishing ease, actually propelling my own IV pole. Doddering, I cover maybe 20 yards, total. I trek around the small ICU area twice, amazing the nurses—and myself.

Again I realize how brutal my care had been following the first surgery when, upon trying to walk the day after surgery, I nearly collapsed due to profound pain. Remarkable how much contrast—humanity—there can be in a surgeon's follow-up care.

Approaching the close of day two, an orderly rolls me out of ICU—to a life with commoners, a private room. Reality: a vulgar comparison.

Chapter 31

Getting All Too Familiar With Disappointment— The Difficulty of Disposing of an HMO Doctor

Going from ICU to an everyday room is like, well, going from a suite at the Ritz-Carlton to a cheesy room next to the ice machine at the Big 6. Floor nurses seem, by contrast, somehow inattentive, aloof.

Dr. Hubbard's left orders to wean me quickly off Demerol. He wants me on an oral pain medicine called Vicodin. I don't comprehend just how effective Demerol is—till they slide the needle from my arm. A dull sense of pain, almost without delay, begins seeping in, converging in my upper belly, producing a stinging sensation. Not as hurtful as after the first surgery, mind you.

An especially gloomy disposition overtakes me as I withdraw from the Demerol.

Dr. Tzu's visits I come to dread. My guts actually start to twist agonizingly the minute this simpleton appears in the doorway. Never, in all his inane blathering, does he offer words that are heartening, positive. Always it's some aberrant paraphrasing of: 'You aren't long for this world, Mr. Scrimna.'

On one of his rounds Tzu casually mentions that, since I've had a splenectomy, Dr. Hubbard's ordered a Pnuemovax injection to boost my immune system.

"Will this be a permanent boost, or something that lasts only so long?" I ask, turning my gaze from the window, from my new friends—the two isolated oak trees standing atop a distant hill.

"Literature say five year," Dr. Tzu acknowledges, looking at me with cheerless black eyes that might've been in a snake's body in another life. "But, Mr. Scrimna, you not have worry about that."

So shaken do I become at Tzu's fatalism, I demand to see the hospital's resident patient advocate/social worker—the only recourse I can think of. Several hours later, I'm out of bed, resting very uncomfortably on a cushioned bench, when David Lopez, the social worker shows up. Reasoning that mine's an unusual case, one that'll enrage even a seasoned social worker, I detail Tzu's most cutting remarks.

Lopez, maybe 35, gaunt-faced, wearing a pale blue button-down shirt, yellow knit tie, turquoise-inlaid wedding band, comes off as more a PR type than an ally of the hospital-bound.

"Well, Mr. Scribner," he offers abstrusely, sounding like a taped message, casually turning a chair and sitting with his elbows propped on its back rest, "sometimes we've got to adjust. Take these little eccentricities with a grain of salt."

"Little eccentricities?" I respond, now feeling provoked. "This guy's telling me I'm not going to make it. And you see this as little eccentricities? This clown's a damn doctor, for God's sake!"

"Some of our newer physicians, Mr. Scribner—especially those from other cultures (he's whispering this)—bring with them views we haven't yet adjusted to."

"Oh, I see—it's us, not them?"

Lopez cringes markedly as if to indicate I'm edging into a sensitive area.

"I know this may be politically incorrect," I go on. "But I was brought up believing in doctors. Only recently did I realize they're humans—like you and me. The point is: I find myself dwelling on what he says. And I can't sleep because of it. If I felt better, I'd get up and loosen the son-of-a-bitch's teeth."

"There is a simple solution, Mr. Scribner," Lopez offers patronizingly, as though dealing with a rookie patient who's overreacting. "Just close your ears."

"David, we're talking my life here. I'd kind of like to look forward to getting well, getting back to a run-of-the-mill existence . . . maybe holding a grandchild in my lap someday. But this jerk, he's doing all he can to undermine that."

"Okay. Okay," Lopez continues, condescendingly. "I sense where you're coming from, Mr. Scribner. Let me suggest a couple of names. Different doctors you can look into." With a look of frustration, he volunteers his white business card. "Call me . . . once you're discharged."

"This is how you're going to fix things?"

"For the present, Mr. Scribner, I'm afraid you're pretty much in the thick of it. Dr. Tzu's in the driver's seat. We, unfortunately, have to work around that."

"That's a solution?"

"Such as it is, hospital politics being what they are. Among these doctors," he adjusts his yellow tie, looks about furtively, "things can get pret-ty sticky. Sorry."

"What about *us*, Mr. Lopez—the patients. We don't matter?"

He vacillates as if perceiving this reality for the first time. "Okay," he says under his breath. "Tell you what. When you can, shift to Dr. Yarrow at your same clinic. I've known him a good number of years—he's one of the actual physicians over there. This won't remedy things today . . . I don't know if anything can. With

HMOs now calling all the shots, Mr. Scribner, it's the way we're forced to do business."

As long as various on-going details relating to my in-hospital stay have to be approved by Dr. Tzu (my first-line HMO physician), and secondarily by Dr. Hubbard (a non-HMO physician), I can't fire Dr. Tzu—though I should do something drastic. But, if I fire Tzu, I'll be left alone in the testy world of HMO regulations, without the obligatory gatekeeper doctor to span the gap between the dictatorial HMO and my non-HMO surgeon and hospital.

Thus I'm coerced into enduring Tzu's savage prophecies, his innuendoes. But I vow to dump the bastard the second I can.

Because I don't feel at this juncture I can face the explicitness of Dr. Hubbard's likely response, I haven't yet revealed to him Dr. Tzu's prognostications. When I finally get up the nerve, Dr. Hubbard is stooped at my bedside doing a dressing check-over, listening to my stomach via stethoscope. When I explain Dr. Tzu's revelations, Dr. Hubbard at once seems wholly and rightfully disturbed—not at me, but at Dr. Tzu.

"He let you in on all that?" Dr. Hubbard replies, unmistakable displeasure twisting his face.

"Nothing he says sounds like I'm going to make it," I add.

Dr. Hubbard, nibbling quickly at his lower lip. "I was holding off," he explains genuinely. "There *is* a right time."

"As I'm coming back from the anesthetic, that's the first thing Dr. Tzu hits me with—this tumor spillage thing. For a minute, I'm thinking this is some kind of nightmare. Then he repeats the whole business. Since then I've gone from being reasonably hopeful . . . to seeing things as pretty bleak."

"Please understand, Mr. Scribner, it wasn't my intention to keep you in the dark," Dr. Hubbard explains. "In the margin where the mass and the diaphragm were attached . . . we did encounter some drainage. Clearly, we'll all have to wait and see—the consequence."

"It's my understanding, doctor, from reading and what have you," I say, dispiritedly, feeling his words slicing away all hope, "that radiation's basically of little benefit (I almost say useless) with this kind of cancer."

"I can't address that issue, Mr. Scribner. But I can say there aren't a whole assortment of options out there," he says, laying the bed sheet back in place. "Radiation happens to be one of the few tools we do have."

"Doctor, I'm kind of begging here . . . but is there something you can do to call off Dr. Tzu? He's just tearing me up. All this negative talk."

Dr. Hubbard deliberates, exhaling empathetically, patting my bare arm. "I'll see if I can work something out."

Seeing in his eyes that his hands too are tied (because of the medical brotherhood . . . HMO entanglements?), I can only nod hopefully.

Jennifer, my sister, remains with me during the daylight hours, helping me out of bed, and walking, washing my hair, occupying time with dialogue about arcane family matters—like the passing of our father, the severe pain, the misery he endured. (She was there.) One of my foremost fears, I disclose—certainly one of the foremost fears for many cancer patients—is the long, drawn out torture that will most likely fill our final days.

Repeatedly Jenny's confounded by Dr. Tzu's lack of polish. She thinks this dolt's way off center, I can read that much in her eyes—but, being that he's my doctor, she says nothing.

Among my occasional visitors is the ever-reserved Dr. Malone. Her style is entirely unlike the other doctors: She never advances more than a foot or two into the room. She, instead, prefers to stand just inside the door, discussing what she's come to say.

She is—I have to give her credit for this—more upbeat than either Drs. Tzu or Hubbard. We discuss my staying on Mitotane, the feasibility of radiation treatments (I hope she's already up to speed on this). Finding out she isn't, I ask that she again call Dr. Saltz at M.D. Anderson to get her take on my continuing Mitotane and the proposed radiation treatments.

"So you're taking how much Mitotane right now?" Dr. Malone wants to know.

Four grams per day, I tell her.

"I'd like you to stop all together. Till you've recovered, and your convalescence's more final. In the interim, I'll check with Dr. Saltz."

That she's agreed to check with Anderson's comforting. I nearly ask her feelings about the tumor spillage issue and her prognosis, but don't: I don't feel up to watching those dark walls closing in any further on me.

Advice: To further impersonalize the in-hospital doctor-patient relationship, HMOs have of late come up a new medical specialty—called the 'hospitalist.' This is a physician whose job it is to *remain at the hospital full time,* only seeing patients there. He knows *nothing* of your medical history other than what he reads in your chart or what you or your primary-care doctor tells him.

This 'cost-effective' measure is supposed to further reduce the expense of hospitalization *and* free your primary-care doctor of the laborious job of seeing patients in the hospital. With this approach the primary-care doctor can stay in his or her office all day, seeing an HMO-dictated number of patients, and not be 'bothered' with visiting his patients who're hospital-bound. HMOs want to eliminate those time- and cost-wasting trips your doctor *used* to make to the hospital.

Who cares you'll be seen by a physician you've never met before, who doesn't know your medical history, who has no personal interest in you, who has never treated you, and whose primary function it is to get you out of the hospital as quickly as possible so the HMO can save money. This may be the epitome of impersonal medical care.

FINDING HOPE WHEN DOCTORS SAY THERE IS NONE

Chapter 32

The Tangled Web We Weave— Telling the Most Negative Doctor Where to Get Off

With a doomsday picture of my future overriding my thoughts, everyday things during the ride home assume an extraordinary air of concreteness: The lush green of the fields seems wonderfully vibrant, alive. Something I can actually feel. The light of day, detonating through the windshield, feels delightful on the skin.

Keeping an eye on the familiar panorama of gray-green trees, the broccoli fields, the reedy beach dunes that sweep by, mother earth seems startlingly new—fragile at this moment and very much mine to soak up. Four days after the surgery. I'm going to my sanctuary . . . (this thought reverberating in my head) not as an ebullient cured cancer patient by any means. After going up against the realities of cancer therapy, I at no time anticipated a cure—but I had hoped for a more heartening prognosis.

Settled warily in the front seat of the car, I'm finally on the way home. Jane's at the wheel. Once in the upper floor bedroom—where I feel immediately more unassailed and sheltered than I have in days—I ease down onto the king-size bed, my nest, and sit, braced by one arm, watching the simple-hearted Pacific beckon.

In the discordant light of day, away from the mental sterility of the hospital, I realize I have to face specific disturbing treatment decisions. Welling in me right now is a newborn recognition of despair. Will I give way and let the doctors decide for me, or will I decide the course of events for myself? These questions, falsely distant at the moment, gnaw at me.

"Anybody talk about what's next?" Jane asks, tossing back the bed covering, reading my thoughts.

"I'm supposed to . . . check in with Dr. Hubbard in a couple of days. The stitches. But, as soon as I can," I respond, watching a black-and-yellow wet-suited body-boarder grab a curling wave, recalling for a split second the days when I was out there, worry-free, "I'm heading for the clinic, and telling Tzu where he can shove it."

"Don't you think that sort of thing can wait?" Jane is now raising the blinds on other windows, allowing afternoon sunlight to fill the room with an soothing, care-free radiance. "There's got to be more important things to occupy your thoughts."

"First things first," I say, gingerly lying back on the bed, now smelling the comforting aromas of home—coffee from the kitchen, freshly laundered sheets. "It's a man-thing, maybe. But this SOB is going to get his."

"In that case," Jane begins emphatically, placing hands on hips, "you might as well include that other SOB. What's-his-name—your favorite endocrinologist—on your hit list."

"How's he figure in this?" I ask, Jane's emotion-filled observation catching me unawares.

"Oh, never mind, " she sighs compassionately, as if letting the cat out of the bag. "It's just . . . something. Probably shouldn't even mention it. Not right now, anyway. But let me say this: Your favorite endocrinologist—if that's what that quack is—might be more unfeeling than Dr. Tzu. In my book."

Watching Jane flow about the room—a human without visible pain—fitting various articles of laundered underwear in dresser drawers and sorting and stacking the over-sized bandages I'd been sent home with, I can, with a stretch of the imagination, see this is one of those times it's best not ask what she's talking about.

The rest of the afternoon's spent with Marc, my son, stretched out on the bed, the conversation focused on me—getting well, further treatment, going back to work. This unaffected talk feels particularly satisfactory: Your kids most often dwell on their lives, their problems, themselves. Marc too, I later learned, was privy to what Dr. Crandle had donated to further blight the hope accompanying my surgery, my recovery. But at this point, he too, says nothing.

With the stitch-removal appointment out of the way, it's time to zero in on Dr. Tzu. By now a week and a half has passed. I'm feeling fairly good, strength-wise, but not sure how to plunge into this encounter, emotionally. From my point of view I feel justified in taking any action—a swing at him or bluntly expressing my dislike for the guy.

Waiting in the small exam room, I flip tensely through a timeworn, pleated journal, biding my time. What little adrenaline I can generate has me edgy. This encounter could escalate into a no-holds-barred street fight, so angered am I. I don't feel I owe this demoralizing little bastard anything—not reverence, not the time of day. . . not even civility. Nada.

"Mr. Scrimna," Tzu mutters impassively as he enters, a new air of self-possession about him. He even seems taller for some reason. My now half-inch-thick file's tucked beneath his arm. "Make announcement, Mr. Scrimna," he continues throatily in his chopped-sentence, karate-instructor manner.

His odd demeanor is holding me at bay for the moment. 'Oh God, no,' I'm thinking, 'he's cutting me off at the pass—with more negative news.'

"I leave . . . quit. . . . go away," Tzu resumes brusquely, with a strange sort of proud finality, dropping my file on the counter with a loud thud as if it were some sort of statement. "Leave clinic, one week. Go, yes—San Francisco."

He's . . . leaving? My battle plan's suddenly lost some steam. I'm wondering: 'Does he expect me to feel bad or say I'm sorry to see him leaving?'

"You're actually quitting," I ask redundantly, reformulating my approach, still seated awkwardly on the exam table, "leaving this clinic?"

"—Take assignment with prominent research biotech firm," he goes on exaltedly, throwing up his impatient little arms.

"That, my good man (I'm not about to call him 'doctor'), is the best news I've heard in years!" I interject, offering a cruel smile. "Better than anything I could've ever dreamed!"

"I . . . " Tzu pauses at length, looking at me strangely. This spineless little man has yet to open my file—and apparently he's not going to. "No want be doctor. Do very well in college—in biology, mathematics," he offers, as if he knows he owes me an explanation for his aberrant behavior. "Professor say he no allow me go into anything but medicine. He say I too smart. . . . But I no like this," he says, flourishing one arm in a circular motion, looking about the modest room with clear loathing. "No like all this . . . politic (he spits the word). Everyone tell me what do—like baby."

Notwithstanding the repulsiveness, the negativity he's brought to bear, a fraction of me, maybe one tenth of one ounce, feels a pang of remorse for this wretched, unknowing little man. But this isn't about to prevent me from having my say.

"Friday, my last day," he continues, nodding his head, lapsing again into his earlier self-possession. "No practice here anymore."

"Okay, you little bastard, like I said . . . this is the best news I've heard in ages. I am de-lighted, as I'm sure are many of your other patients," I begin, sensing the stage's mine. "You know. . . I can only agree with your assessment of yourself as a physician: You don't belong; you stink. You've got no sense of what bed-side manner is, no business walking around, telling sick people they're going to die . . . . You don't know the first thing about the psychology of people. You're not even close to being a real doctor. You're one shallow, insensitive little prick. You know what prick means, doctor?"

A strange sense of fear dominates his black eyes.

With these purging words spewing forth, feeling good, I sense an unhindered hostility developing within me, which I know I must curb before I hurt him. At the same time I realize I'm endorsing the reasoning he's using to move on. Through my head zips the thought that maybe Dr. Bristol, now medical director and his boss, has somehow recognized this fellow's serious flaws and pressured him to leave.

With a sort of righteous anger, as though my convictions have added to the crush of his suffering, Tzu inflates himself like a courting bullfrog, stating loudly, indignantly: "I required to recommend new doctor, Mr. Scrimna."

"Don't waste your breath, you jerk," I respond, trying to sound cynical, but probably failing. This pitiful out-of-place man's taken much of the wind out of my sails. (Actually, I knew I wouldn't really be *that* offensive—he has the title doctor, after all, and I'd been brought up to venerate them. TDKB, remember?) "I've already decided on a new doctor," I tell him. "That's one of the reasons I'm here. To tell you: I don't ever need to see you again. For any reason—thank God."

One strange turn of events—here's a man who didn't want to be a physician at all, but had it forced upon him, and it was my misfortune to link up with him. Now I'm stuck with the flawed hope he dumped upon me.

Prior to this appointment with Dr. Tzu, I'd tried to set up a visit with the real doctor the social worker at the hospital had recommended, but found that doctor's practice full. No waiting list. So I make another introductory appointment—as the HMO mandates—with the same doctor who'd substituted for Dr. Tzu while he was out of town, Dr. Paravano. She becomes an important component of my long-term survival team.

During the ensuing weeks I try to extract myself from the gloom and doom of Dr. Tzu by continuing my studies into conventional and alternative cancer treatments. Seems everything I'm reading homes in on lifestyle (principally stress or lack of it) and diet as major elements affecting the course of cancer. While admittedly anecdotal, writer after writer keeps driving home the point: How we live, what we eat does absolutely affect cancer's outcome. Many people, it seems, have been cured of this disease—in combination with conventional medicine—by these simple, yet not-so-simple lifestyle changes.

Also about this time, I begin a more passionate program of meditation and visualization in an attempt to rid my body of cancer cells by perceiving them as helpless and deformed little blobs being vaporized by a powerful beam of light.

CHAPTER 33

AS ALIENS AND SOJOURNERS— LEARNING THAT RADIATION WILL DESTROY A WORKING KIDNEY

Physically, my healing seems to be coming along well. I can actually now trudge a quarter mile or so along the shoreline without faintness, without plopping down breathless on a rusty-legged beach bench. Being near the Pacific and its mesmerizing sands proves uniquely rehabilitative.

Insignificant, commonplace stuff I chance upon during these rehab hikes, everyday things I'd once taken for granted—fine-spun orange and violet native flowers waving in the breeze, gray-toned lizards poised with aplomb on the walkway like sunbathing vacationers, platinum sunlight rippling on the ocean's ever-changing surface (one of my most-loved mental pictures), the merriment of bottle-nose porpoises carrying out aerial feats above the turquoise waves—stir deep and unfamiliar primitive awakenings in me. Like I can *see*—and comprehend— now that I'm an essential member of . . . everything.

With my mind often drawn to morbid thoughts of the tumor spill, and the melancholy that engenders, I begin acknowledging, feeling, living, truly treasuring the moment—the here, the now. There is in me now an unseasoned insight, an explicable converging of ordinary things, a growing consciousness for the way things are . . . . An unmistakable admiration for life, the planet at large . . . .

October 1992: My medical team embodies Drs. Malone, the oncologist, Paravano, the internist, and at a distance, Dr. Crandle, the endocrinologist. Tzu, the doctor from hell, has been forgotten—almost. Because of the surgery, I've been off the job now for a few weeks.

To focus solely on getting well, on getting in touch with my innate curative powers, I'm going to remain at home—in a stress-free environment—till the radiation treatments are finished, maybe another five or six weeks. Rockwell, my employer, has been more than generous.

My boss tells me to take all the time I need. A poster-size art-department-created card comes from the gang at the office. Lots of friends have scrawled poignant messages—including a revitalizing note from the big guy, the president—all of them wishing me well, God's speed.

Though I spend many hours hibernating—reading, listening to cancer self-help tapes (Drs. Carl Simonton and Siegel)—there dwells in me a disturbing sense that radiation isn't the way to go. At my next visit with Dr. Malone I ask if she's checked with M.D. Anderson about the success rate of these treatments. (Maybe, I project naively, something's been discovered of late and radiation's now a potential treatment. Me, ever the dreamer.)

Dr. Malone's evasive, won't say whether she's called. She suggests I talk with Dr. David Goetz, the radiation oncologist who'll begin treating me in a few days. "When you talk with him," Dr. Malone says, "get his feelings. He's a straightforward guy. He'll tell you."

She's passing the buck, I know. Again, because of TDKB and not wanting to rock the boat, I don't press her about calling M.D. Anderson . . . though I know I should.

Also, at Dr. Malone's suggestion, since the surgery, I haven't resumed taking Mitotane. She wants me to reacquire as much strength and weight as possible before continuing the chemo—in that it tends to subvert energy. She's even gone so far as to recommend staying off Mitotane the whole time I'm undergoing radiation. These treatments, she feels, will hit pretty hard. Mitotane will only worsen an already bad situation.

Intuitively, I know I should ask her—challenge her—about the advisability of this approach (not taking any chemotherapy), knowing there's often only a small window of opportunity during which to attack cancer. But again TDKB rears its head. I don't confront her. Hindsight's always 20/20.

It's an unusually humid weekday morning. Eleven o'clock. Jane and I traverse the near-vacant parking lot of the treatment center. The morning sun is stinging my forehead.

Coast Radiation Treatment Center, while possessing an impressive title, is quite the antithesis.

It seems disappointingly—well, rundown. This doesn't augment my wavering confidence or endear the whole idea in general. Sitting in a disorderly 12x8 waiting area, adjacent to the appointment counter, in back of which three young girls are typing, answering phones, and discussing future appointments with patients, I look for anything that'll make me like this place.

The office staff seems quite ingenious, appearing to know what they're doing. The slow trickle of other patients, ones who've clearly just returned from treatment, doesn't communicate much. Most look unruffled—some brooding, some not, some bandaged, some with heads shaved in odd patterns.

A white-coated doctor, youngish, with ill-mannered red hair and flowing Bolshevik mustache, holding a clipboard, looms in the doorway, announcing my name. We file into a cramped office that's plainly being remodeled. Immediately the reason for the chaos, the rubble, strikes me—the whole place is being restored, modernized. A positive sign—in a place where there haven't been many positive signs.

First thing you notice about Dr. Goetz is his effortless smile (a cancer doctor who smiles?), the conscious way he makes eye contact. He opens by saying he's examined in detail my most recent CT scans (pre-surgery scans) and has put together a regimen calling for six weeks of radiation—five days a week, with weekends off to recover. My God, a doctor who's prepared—done his groundwork *before* the patient arrives! How novel!

Treatments, he explains, speaking, it seems, mostly to Jane, are to be aimed in a highly focused manner at an isolated site about the size of a cantaloupe, just beneath the left ribs. By using lead shielding, the technicians will minimize radiation damage to the rest of the torso. Opening an anatomy manual, Dr. Goetz indicates with his finger the margins to be irradiated, positioning a pencil to show the intended angles of treatment. Throughout, he remains strikingly cocksure and, at times, even entertaining. A very personable man, he is. Salesman-doctor, if you will.

"I need to know something, doctor," I say, interrupting his delivery. "I've been led to believe that this type of treatment's essentially, well . . . ineffective. In treating adrenocortical carcinoma. Doctors at the Anderson Cancer Center in Houston say that, anyway. But you see it otherwise?"

"Mr. Scribner, nothing's absolute," he replies, with a sort of crisp candor. Handing me a brochure illustrating what a patient can anticipate during therapy, he's come prepared. "Admittedly, adrenal cancer isn't something we see everyday. So, having questions of my own, I called several colleagues at Sloan. In New York."

"Sloan-Kettering?" I ask, having read ample cancer literature now to be acquainted well with some of the principal cancer centers in the U.S.

"Um-hm. Spoke with a few of the guys I went to med school with . . . at Yale. Other radiation oncologists who've favorably treated this cancer."

"Using radiation?"

"So they say."

"But the doctors with a fair amount of experience in treating this cancer," I persevere, "at Anderson, say—"

"—These doctors, Mr. Scribner," Dr. Goetz proceeds with a hint of exasperation, "I'd venture to say . . . are not radiation oncologists, true?"

Coerced, I compromise. Jane, watching this interchange like a ping-pong match, offers little, choosing a watch-and-see approach.

"Everything, Mr. Scribner," Dr. Goetz continues, "is radio-sensitive. Permit me the use of indefinite radiation and I'll terminate any cancer in its tracks. Any cancer. So the real issue becomes: How much radiation can we safely use and not otherwise cripple the patient? Our staff radiation physicist and myself have worked the numbers and propose, for your treatment, we go the limit for that region of the body—in the neighborhood of 6000 rads."

Having spent several years as an industrial x-ray technician (x-raying metals on aircraft, not flesh and bones), I have a feel for what rads are, or the amount of radiation he's proposing to 'shoot' me with. "What kind of side effects does that mean?" I ask.

"Reasonable question," Dr. Goetz concedes, as if this has become a polite debate. "There'll be some days of nausea. But we have drugs for that. And, there'll be an appreciable decline in stamina. Also," he says, hesitating noticeably, looking for a instant at Jane, then me, "there's good chance—you'll lose permanent use of that left kidney."

"Wait a minute, doctor—you're saying *I'm going to lose a kidney?*" I ask, amplifying the words. The upper portion of my left kidney had been sliced away during the recent surgery, so I'm already running on impaired renal function.

Radiation's supposed to be a relatively non-toxic, somewhat benign treatment. I thought there would be some vomiting, maybe some minor scarring down the road in years to come, but nothing as foreboding as destruction of an essential organ.

"With the dosage we're proposing," the doctor replies, chewing unconsciously at his mustache, "your left kidney will almost certainly be destroyed."

This bombshell dazes me into near speechlessness. "So, in addition to all the other BS this disease has laid on me," I assert slowly, dejectedly, the office around me suddenly seeming much colder, "now I have to consider losing an *organ*?"

"Comes with the territory, I'm afraid, Mr. Scribner," Dr. Goetz replies a little too cold-bloodedly for my liking, as if this were supposed to have been explained to me beforehand.

There is a soft tap on the doctor's door. Grasping a dripping sheet of film, a slight, dark-haired technician asks the doctor to step into the hallway. With Dr. Goetz out of sight, Jane and I gape at one another close-mouthed, pitifully. She shakes her head. "Like . . . can things get any worse?"

"You freezing, like me?"

"We need a champagne night—real bad."

"Am I hearing things right—" I mumble, gazing up, ruminating on the millions of petty perforations in the sound-deadening ceiling, "they want me to scrap a perfectly good kidney?"

"Not like what you're led to believe on Marcus Welby, is it?" Jane comments.

"Too many . . . ugly as hell choices."

"It's your *kidney* we're talking about, for God's sake! Part of you that you were born with!"

"I should just leave. Say to hell with this. But I can't . . . I've got to stand and fight."

"Too, too scary." Jane's grimacing ungratefully, pressing her foot against mine.

Exhaling, I go on: "I've got to run this by Dr. Bristol. Kidneys are her thing. Maybe she'll have some ideas."

Jane's just said, "Good thing we've got her in reserve," when Dr. Goetz re-enters.

"Sorry," he says with a earnest exasperation. "Techs—they can't be held up."

"Did you expect us . . ." Jane pipes in with, "to commit to something today?"

"We've created a slot for your husband next week," Dr. Goetz resumes. "The sooner we start treatment, Mrs. Scribner, the better."

"I'm going to need a day or two. To think this over," I say, reasoning aloud. "If I'm going to be voluntarily donating a perfectly good kidney . . ."

"Doctor," Jane interjects, expectantly, "can you be more specific—about Eric losing that kidney."

"I've put all my cards on the table, Mrs. Scribner," he says, folding his ghostly hands passively on the desk. "What normally happens, when we irradiate that area, four months or so later the kidney will start to waste away . . . shrivel up. After about a year, it will have withered to the point where it's not functioning at all."

"—Why didn't I just have the damn thing removed during surgery?" I interrupt dispiritedly.

Smirking curiously, Dr. Goetz shrugs. "Had you only known."

"What I'm bothered with, is . . ." I go on, now that I have his attention, "what if I'm unlucky enough to have another recurrence? And it pops up in the other kidney. Leaves me pretty well up the creek."

"Does the shriveled-up kidney . . . have to be taken out?" Jane wants to know.

"It'll only atrophy to a point," Dr. Goetz explains, shaking his head. "Then cease to function. Basically, it'll end up (he grins as if relishing this) looking like an apple core left out in the sun. It'll still be there, in the body, but it won't be functioning."

"Man, we're talking a major decision here," I volunteer, visualizing my kidney as a shriveled apple core. "Once you get caught up in this cancer avalanche, it's one depressing decision after another."

"Life, Mr. Scribner, is never easy," Dr. Goetz replies philosophically.

Thinking rather bitterly to myself: 'This guy's too damn youthful to really know what it's like dealing personally with cancer,' I begin again: "So . . . you want to start when?"

He says he wants me to return in a couple days so the technicians can take a sequence of alignment x-rays. Then minute marks will be permanently tattooed on my torso at which they can direct the daily beams.

"There'll be a baseline CT?" I inquire. "Before we start?"

"Not likely your insurance will okay that," Dr. Goetz remarks peculiarly, as if using this as justification for not doing a CT. "Besides (he grins again), I don't recommend scans so soon after surgery. The images would scare the hell out of you."

Chapter 34

Abandoning The Straight Road— Saying Goodbye to a Kidney

"What do you mean—the images would scare the hell out me?"

"The anatomy, Mr. Scribner, requires time to stabilize," Dr. Goetz goes on, aligning various sales tools—thick manuals, color brochures, a waiver form of some sort—by tapping them repeatedly on the desk top. "Invariably, after a major surgery, we see a lot of internal scarring. The area would not appear unblemished, I guarantee you. There'd be many more questions than answers."

Failing to see how not having baseline CT is logical—but then again, I am just a layman—I question how we'll oversee the efficacy, the progress of treatments unless we compare before-and-after scans.

"Mr. Scribner, you have to keep in mind," he says, "this is adjuvant therapy. We aren't treating anything specific—yet. Let's keep it that way." He grins as though complimenting himself at having arrived at this altruistic explanation.

Again, by virtue of being raised in the TDKB culture, I feel myself caving in to this doctor's learned assumptions. Still, I'm extremely wary of this whole, outwardly inconsistent, no-measurement approach.

"Never seem to give you any slack, do they?" Jane comments pensively as we wait at a red light, each of us mired in our own thoughts.

Radio's playing softly—a harmless old rock and roll tune from years back when cancer, even death, seemed indefinable. "You're beginning to see now," I ask, "how this is something that you've got to stay ahead of?"

"Meaning?"

"All the reading I've been doing."

"It seems to have helped you, yes," Jane responds vaguely, as she might in a debate with her sister.

"Not ready to concede that I'm on the right track?"

"One can overdo anything."

"How could reading about other patients and their plight not prepare me for the unknown—psychologically, if nothing else? Without this vicarious experience, I probably would've been a basket case by now. 'Course, one never expects to be negotiating away an internal organ, either . . . 'Patient, heal thyself!'"

"It all gets to be . . ." Jane says dismally, after a pause, "too much to think about. I don't know how you do it."

Though not an inflexible deadline, I have roughly two days to choose—whether to undertake the treatments or refuse. The only feasible other option, should I refuse, would be to press Dr. Malone to resume Mitotane, or to initiate some other chemo. But there are no other chemos I'm aware of through my reading.

At any rate, the ball's in my court.

Late that evening, lying in bed, feeling profoundly alone, musing on the Milky Way splashing its way across the blackened sky, I sort, agonizingly, through the pros, the cons, of sacrificing yet another vital body part to treatment of this disease. Feeling light-years from any intimacy with anything, I find myself yearning again for the bliss of childhood . . . that little boy on the beach, for whom a higher authority—adults—always made decisions. With the Pacific droning peacefully, rhythmically, in the night, a mysterious sense of detachedness grips me.

For the first time since grade school, I find myself attempting a short, unsuccessful dialogue with . . . God.

Why, I go on, hadn't Dr. Goetz or Dr. Malone been charitable enough to walk me through the pros and cons of this barbarous treatment, giving me *their* thoughts? Wasn't that within their professional responsibility?

When I appeal to Jane the following morning, she won't—can't—render an opinion. "The decision's too . . . hideous," she declares, a disturbed, faraway look in her brown eyes. "How can anyone be expected to make such a choice?"

"We're in this together, I thought," I persist. "You're supposed to be my helpmate."

"I am," she insists almost listlessly. "And you I love more than anything, but—it really hurts thinking about this. Like giving someone permission to . . . cut off part of your kids. Last night I had this dream . . . about those coyotes you see on TV chewing off their legs to get free of those steel traps. We're human, we shouldn't have to make these terrible decisions. This disease is making us . . . despicable."

"But I'm really in need here. Where the hell am I supposed to go for answers?"

Recoiling, she wrings her hands as if shaking foul dirt from them. I'd trusted that she'd offer at least something. The crush of all this—this agonizing stalemate—remains squarely, heavily on my shoulders . . . pounding downward like some gloomy, endless waterfall.

One thing for certain: Cancer brings a sense of wasteful isolation—even with good-meaning people nearby.

The next day, on the phone with Dr. Bristol, I characterize my deep anxiety, while trying not to sound too wimpy. Pressed for time, she volunteers fleetingly: "All sorts of people, Eric, are living quite normally with one kidney."

"That I realize, Sandra—but that's not my concern. I'm asking . . . what do *you* think about a treatment that's going to kill off my left kidney, leaving me with only one to fall back on in the event of another cancer recurrence?"

Murmuring voices in the background, I've interrupted some office event on her end. "Eric," she says hurriedly, "this, I'm afraid, has to be your decision. It's your body."

Square one again: Isolation. Is there no one I can turn to? For an instant I consider sitting down with a priest. But I don't even know how to arrange this anymore. I'm no longer a member of any particular parish. It's been ages since I've been to Mass.

Next minute I'm contemplating a call to Dr. McElliot, that tedious shrink. But, calling to mind his habit of burrowing in the past, I decide to abstain.

Two days later: I'm again sitting again with Dr. Goetz in his small glassed-in office. He's pulling idly at his red mustache, appearing unsurprised by my go-ahead decision. To arrive at this conclusion, I'd weighed every what-if proposition I could dig up. And, ultimately, I'd fallen back on the cornerstone of my basic approach to attacking this disease: Act promptly *and* aggressively—*always*. Cancer's never as treatable as it is this minute.

Over the next hour or so, a pair of radiation technologists twist my torso in a variety of awkward positions on a flat table, taking a succession of alignment x-rays. With purple felt-tipped pens they sketch an array of cris-cross lines on my bare chest, indicating already exposed areas. These films, I'm told, are to authenticate the angles specified by Dr. Goetz and will allow unerringly the fine-tuning of the radiation angle each day.

At the completion of this session, Dr. Goetz breezes in, an armful of 14x17 films. Jamming several up on the lighted wall, he indicates the beam angles they've been trying to achieve. With his index finger, he traces where the left adrenal would be—if there were one. This is the sector they'll be concentrating on.

"This has to be a repeatable process," he emphasizes, snatching the films from the light board. "We've got to be sure we hit the same mark day after day, after day."

"What would you do, doctor," I ask, still unable to get out of my mind the idea that I'm donating a kidney to this process, "—if this were you . . . sitting here?"

"I'm afraid that's irrelevant," he says, grinning oddly. "Because it's not me."

"Still, you know, I'd feel better if we had a baseline CT . . . " I persist, restating my earlier position, "to see how things are looking right now. Before we start."

Dr. Goetz once more declines—with a trivial grin, a parental, We've-Already-Gone-Over-This look.

Two days later, a Wednesday, in the cool of October 1992: With various pin-head-sized specks tattooed on my left chest, I commence treatment. This is a procedure that does not cause your hair to fall out, unless your head's being irradiated. In my case, the radiation's confined to a modest segment of the chest, encompassing the lower three ribs on the left side—and the stomach. I'm admonished: Expect nausea after each session.

To make these daily sessions more palatable and, hopefully, more effective, I glean a helpful hint from Bernie Siegel's books and try my best to envision the buzzing radiation beam as a golden stream of healing sunlight. Since I've bought into the treatment plan, I also force myself to look forward to the daily sessions—they are, I reason, designed to make me well.

Each day, Monday through Friday, I have treatments at 3:30 p.m. I arrive, sign in, and sit for several minutes in the waiting room, skimming magazines or talking with other patients—those who will talk.

At each treatment, the techs position me—always awkwardly—on the cold table using laser alignment beam to hit the tattoos, slip special lead blocks (focusing devices made especially for me from earlier x-rays) into the radiation machine's aperture, scoot from the room, then zap me.

Ordinarily, I'm only at the radiation center for a half-hour or so. The first few days I experience some rather potent stomach cramping. The predicated nausea, however, hasn't arrived . . . yet.

CHAPTER 35

THE FIRST PROPHETIC SIGN— A MYSTIFYING FALCON APPEARS

At the first follow-up exam, one week later, Dr. Goetz's delighted with the way I'm responding. No gut-wrenching nausea, no rampant side effects.

I find myself getting more comfortable with this doctor, won over by his I'm-Your-Pal manner. He's phoned Dr. Crandle, the endocrinologist, and gotten an adjusted Prednisone dosage since I'm no longer taking Mitotane. (Why hadn't Dr. Malone instigated this?) Dr. Crandle's advised reducing Prednisone from 15 mg per day to 10 mg per day, till I see him again, sometime in December.

The principal radiation nurse, also a doctor (Ph.D.)—who advises patients on everything from emotional concerns to nutrition—suggests that I maintain at least 2000 to 3000 calories per day. This is a cinch, I'm thinking, having always been a generous eater. When I try consuming that amount of food, however, I find that (1) I'm spending too much time at the table, and (2) that volume of food now really fills me up. The nurse-doctor suggests one of the nutritional-supplement beverages, like Ensure, to conveniently add calories, to cut down on my at-the-table periods.

The biweekly testosterone sticks continue. These, I trust, remain the chief cause of my benumbing headaches. Now, though, the headaches seem ongoing, crowding together. Almost every day they're there. I'm popping two to three Excedrin every four hours or so, almost around the clock. While frowning on this practice, none of the doctors—Paravano, Malone, or Goetz—come up with a practical headache reliever.

Second week of treatment: Standing in for the vacationing Dr. Goetz, a woman radiation oncologist, in reading my file, notices I've in fact gained weight. Almost three pounds! Theoretically, I'm supposed to be dropping pounds. This doctor suggests cutting caloric intake. She also gives me a skin cream that'll alleviate radiation 'sunburn' (8x8-inch cube of crimson flesh) that's now become visible on my back.

Side effects to this point include exhaustion (a bone-deep sensation of being tired—to the point where I don't care if I move), tenacious headaches (no doubt the testosterone injections again), and stomach spasms and swelling. Queasiness, popping up now and then right after therapy, is controlled reasonably well with Compazine. Part of the cause of the bone weariness, I suspect, is the effect of decreased Prednisone intake.

In another closed-door session with the Creator, I'd ask Him, if He isn't too occupied elsewhere, to dispatch an omen—a sign—to indicate I'm heading in the right direction here. I'd likewise appealed for some sort of sign while trying to determine whether or not to yield to this whole kidney-killing procedure in the first place. No sign appeared.

In any event, this entire send-me-a-sign notion had subsided to the recesses of my mind. Then one day, in the middle of the third week, I'm casually driving to an afternoon treatment, when, at the outer edges of my attention, I become aware of a large bird perched on a power pole beside the road. The image amounts to no more than a dark shape against the sun.

But next day, the bird's there again.

Third day: The mystifying bird appears once more, poised sublimely in the precisely same spot, on precisely the same pole. A random event? And strangely—is this my imagination—the bird appears to be regarding me with great interest as I drive by. One of the things that makes this creature so eye-catching, so unusual, is it's a peregrine falcon; not your everyday variety—but a silver-white one.

Long about the fourth afternoon, I pull off the road and get out of the car. The falcon and I are making eye contact. Staring down, he exudes an unnatural sort of boldness, curiosity. That evening, on a whim, I call a friend of a friend, an esoteric fellow, one Polo Marquez, who lives alone in a trailer in the foothills—keeper, trainer various birds of prey.

I start by asking if he's ever seen, even heard of a white peregrine. This strange bird, I explain, seems to be watching only me for some reason. "He's just sitting there, Polo, day after day, in exactly the same spot . . . looking at me."

"Falcons can be really weird, man—" Polo begins obscurely, as though he'd had a beer or two or might actually be caught up in a sense of the unreal, "doing things that don't make no sense to you and me. But I never seen no . . . white one. 'Less maybe he's come down from the snow country. But you're living out there by the ocean."

"Polo," I go on, knowing this man has a passion for raptors, "this bird's never there at other times—only when I'm driving to and from my cancer treatments. Other times—weekends, for example—the pole is bare. No falcon is anywhere in sight."

"Got no explanations, man," Polo replies regrettably. Then, after some thought: "Reminds me, kind of, of them stories the old guys used to crank out at our bird meets . . . about the Chumash—Indians that used to live in the area—how they used to talk to falcons."

FINDING HOPE WHEN DOCTORS SAY THERE IS NONE

The bird's daily presence I now begin seeing as a sign—of something. But what? Perhaps I'm doing the right thing with these radiation treatments. Perhaps that God is listening? What could the bird's presence mean?

The very day the radiation treatments ended, the white peregrine disappeared, never to be there again.

Toward the end of week four, the radiation machine goes on the fritz (there's only one available due to renovation of the facility). This continues for three days. Calling Dr. Goetz, I express my concern. I'd been led to believe, that you aren't supposed to go more than a few days without treatment, once you've commenced. Dr. Goetz agrees, suggesting I drive to their sister clinic in a nearby community for continued therapy. He'll have their messenger take the essential films, paperwork ahead.

At the sister clinic, I link up with a radiation oncologist, who, like Dr. Goetz, is convivial, unrestrained. (Are these characteristics of radiation oncologists?) He goes over one more time, in labored detail, the films Dr. Goetz's sent, explaining the process, the purpose of radiation. (As mentioned previously, I always heed the words of new doctors. This, almost always, results in new information.)

Dr. Wellman is a more mature, more experienced radiation oncologist. When I ask about the likelihood of injury to the left kidney, he grins sheepishly. "Yes, yes," he says, poking one finger in the air. "Contemporary literature will lead you to believe such. But in all my years, I've never seen this actually happen."

Am I dreaming this? Did this guy say . . . what I think he said? You mean I put in all those sleepless hours for naught?

"But," I object, playing devil's advocate, "Dr. Goetz's assured me that kidney will die. May take a year, he said. But it'll look an apple core in the sun."

Dr. Wellman, a plump, red-cheeked fellow, wearing expensive buckskin suspenders and a large grin, not unlike an out-of-season Santa, chuckles . . . as if to say: 'Oh, that rascal Goetz!'

"I, personally, have never seen this," says Dr. Wellman. "And, over the years, Mr. Scribner, I've treated a lot of cases like yours."

"Wait . . . adrenocortical carcinoma cases?"

He nods yes.

Without weighing what I'm asking: "And . . . how'd they turn out?"

"Generally, quite well. Been a few years, however."

Good tidings, indeed! The jaunt here's been more than worthwhile. I don't want to push this Dr. Wellman too far, however, having him dump on me some gruesome itemized account of his ACC patients who're now pushing up daisies. Not really burying my head here, but I leave it at that.

Two morsels of unimaginable good news emerge: He doesn't expect the kidney to waste away, and perhaps most meaningful, he's successfully treated other ACC patients using radiation. (This sort of illuminating information's what I was referring to earlier when I said it's always good to rehash old notions with new doctors.)

Now I'm better than halfway through the course of treatment. Significant side effects persist: headaches, immense fatigue, and transient nausea. Radiation-induced weariness is vastly unlike what you ordinarily experience when tired. Entirely emptied of energy and wholly without vitality, is the feeling. The fatigue's such that I literally have to lie down—on the floor, even—to recover, whether I want to or not. This means I often find myself, at any given moment, lying on the floor in the living room, in the kitchen, elsewhere.

Much of the fatigue and loss in stamina is attributable to the reduction in white blood cell count that radiation provokes. Dr. Goetz has me taking weekly blood tests to monitor my white count, other markers for kidney function. Also, for my upcoming visit with Dr. Crandle, I have specific hormone tests run as well, including ACTH.

With two weeks to go in my radiation treatment, Dr. Goetz shrinks the exposure field to about fifty percent of what it's been. Now it's roughly 4x4 inches. This, he says, should result in fewer side effects, less fatigue.

When I tell Dr. Goetz about Dr. Wellman's assessment of kidney damage, he says almost playfully, "Old Wellman actually said that?"

"He's never seen a case go so far as to kill off the kidney, he said."

"That guy," Dr. Goetz says, nodding his head.

"Well, was he on target?"

"His experience is vastly different than mine. I doubt that he was being serious."

The appointment with Dr. Crandle ultimately arrives. I'm slightly suspicious, unnerved, in light of what Jane'd said about him being more inhumane than Dr. Tzu. With hair looking uncivilized, Dr. Crandle bursts into the scanty waiting room. He seems instantly taken aback, startled even, as if seeing a ghost.

"Whoa, you could've knocked me over . . ." he says, plunking down on a tiny stool. "You sure didn't look like this the last time I heard about you."

I ask about his impression of the surgery.

"No, no, no. I wasn't actually in OR," he replies, uncomfortably, as if cornered. "Dr. Hubbard and I conferred right after."

"And what did he say at that point—Dr. Hubbard?"

CHAPTER 36

CONDEMNED IN THE FLESH—
DR. CRANDLE SAYS MY DAYS ARE NUMBERED

Dr. Crandle, this squinty-eyed, wild-haired fellow, is now scanning my lab work—as though evading me.

"Hubbard was troubled . . ." he begins, running his uncalloused forefinger down a column of numbers. "Concerned since he'd lacerated your adrenal lesion . . . allowing a bit of leakage. That, as you can imagine, is not good news for you. Frankly, that's why I'm so amazed seeing you, looking so robust." Crandle, now having retrieved his doctorly composure, adds flippantly: "'Of course it's only been a matter of weeks. So what we're seeing here *won't* last."

So that's what you did, you egotistical bastard! I'm thinking, watching his serpentine eyes. You fed my wife, my son, my sister some hopeless scenario about how Eric wouldn't pull through, didn't you?

"We'll see about that," I challenge him, forcing a insolent grin. "I plan on sticking around for a long time—no matter what." This last comment is a mutinous statement of bravado. My allegiance for this guy's hastily dissolving.

"Your numbers," he says, returning to the lab work, "look good, though."

"You expected less?" I say, powerless to resist one more provocative remark.

"Thyroid and testosterone are on the money. Your ACTH's still running a tad high . . . about 550," he responds, eyeing me quizzically. "Maybe that's a number we'll have to live with. Your norm."

"That's higher than last time, right?"

He's leafing hastily through my file. "Correct. I see 420 in September. And this (he glances at a wall calendar displaying a grinning Tom-Sawyer-like kid and his puppy crossing a wobbly log bridge) is mid-December. Don't really see any real worries here, though. But let's do a recheck in . . . say, three months." Adding with a distorted smile, as though I'll find this amusing: "—If you're still among the upright."

Truly, it's unnerving to sit eyeball-to-eyeball with a doctor—or any other mortal, for that matter—and feel your faith in them seeping away, to the point where you don't care if you ever deal with that person again.

Here he is, though, simple-mindedly carrying on about me scratching at death's door—as if he were funny, or omniscient. Since I'd discovered eons ago that you can't *unsay* something—you can never really withdraw the spoken word—I bite my tongue, not burning any bridges.

With this being the sole endocrinologist in my HMO's referral catalogue, if I elect to toss him aside, go with another, I'll have to foot the bill—all of it. So I reason: What the heck, I'm a thick-skinned, innovative soul who can utilize this oddball for what he is—an endocrinologist—and not get pulled down by his gloomy forecasts.

The final days of radiation treatment tick by. Each day, in mid-afternoon, as I travel to the appointment, there's my comforting guardian, the peregrine. Eyeing this pale bird of prey, I laugh derisively, feeling a growing sense of determination. If only these merciless doctors knew!

Dr. Malone I've seen a time or two during these radiation treatments. Surprisingly, she wants me to start a new chemo. Once the radiation's complete. Hearing this, I volunteer to embark at once, in keeping with my 'most aggressive—action approach.' No, she decides, it'd be overly draining—going through radiation and chemo simultaneously.

When I ask about the type of chemo, she says it'll be intravenous. No more Mitotane—ever. This startles me, that I'm totally off Mitotane . . . that there *is* another chemo. Has she discussed this proposed IV chemo with the doctors at Anderson?

She has, she says.

". . . And they're going for it?"

"Dr. Saltz says since you've broken through Mitotane, yes. Next-phase chemo should entail some sort of intravenous cisplatin."

I'd heard and read things about this scary cisplatin. This is the drug they make teary-eyed TV movies about—frail, toilet-hugging patients, saying they'd rather dead than carry through with more chemo.

"I haven't decided yet what to use," Dr. Malone continues. "Cisplatin might be too damaging for your kidneys—after radiation. You're going to need all the renal function you can summon. I need to do more digging . . . checking."

This amounts to good news/bad news. Bad news: I'm about to go it alone—without the one drug I'd been led to believe is the best for combating ACC. While not something I covet by any means, Mitotane has become something of a crutch. Good news: I won't be gulping down up to 12 bulky, stomach-upsetting pills every day. And all the side effects, I won't miss either.

"When do we start . . . this new chemo?"

"Week after radiation," she responds with an usual intensity in her voice. I'm impressed. For the time being at least, she's stepped out of her mousiness.

She explains I'll be coming to her office for IV treatments. And I can most likely go on working during these treatments. Each treatment cycle will be spread over five days: I'll start on Monday and continue getting the intravenous drugs, after work, every day for a week. The next month, if my white count's okay, I'll resume another cycle for five days. This pattern will repeat itself for six months.

"And my hair—it's going to fall out?"

"Good chance," she offers, modestly folding her lean arms. "Everybody's different, though. Hair, for you, is a big concern?"

"I suppose not," I respond, falling back again on the Be-Aggressive approach. "I'm just happy to hear there's another chemo out there."

Radiation treatments end a week later than planned. No ceremony, no celebration . . . just a couple of radiation technologists shaking my hand, hugging me, wishing me well. That last day I'm sitting with Dr. Goetz, thinking this is the final time I'll see him. He says he'll go on seeing me every three months for two years. (At least this doctor is talking in terms of *years* concerning my remaining time on earth.)

Post-radiation treatment follow-up, it seems, is standard practice: Sometimes, he says, patients come up with ambiguous indications that regular doctors often misinterpret and resolve improperly—with needless invasive procedures . . . like surgery.

When I ask what specifically he's referring to, he says: "After treatments like you've had—we hit you with roughly 5900 rads, by the way—patients can develop anything from painful adhesions, to stomach ulcers, to fused bowels. And, unless a doctor's aware of what you went through, there can be a misdiagnosis."

"Yet another cheery round of long-term side-effects," I say with a touch of sarcasm. "Don't seem to recall you talking about this."

"Oh, we covered it. You were probably too absorbed in something else. So—" he concludes, shaking my hand affably, "congratulations. You made it with flying colors. Took all this like a teenager, no less." (He never did side with Dr. Wellman about the kidney atrophy issue.)

I take this opportunity to lean on him for a little extracurricular guidance.

"This chemo business Dr. Malone's been talking about—" I begin, knowing he and she talked about this.

"She hadn't decided. Last time we spoke."

"She's pulled me off the Mitotane. Going with some intravenous drug, she says."

"Cisplatin, most probably."

"What do you think about this drug? You seem to stay on top of this stuff."

(Again, not to sound like a broken record—but it's my policy to ask questions or opinions of *other* doctors—even if this seems repetitive or nonsensical. *You never know what new doors they're going to open.*)

Dr. Goetz sort of smiles. His tongue emerges idly, touching the edges of his red mustache. "Always rocky decisions—for doctor and patient. But as I see it, you have three ways to go: One, be aggressive as hell and go with the unconventional—the cisplatin; two, try to talk her into letting you go back on Mitotane; or three, do nothing and let Nature take its course. One thing to keep in mind, though—and this'll probably only muddy the waters—chemotherapy's not a science. It's an art."

"I don't like the sound of that. Coming from a doctor."

"Especially in cases like yours. Ground rules are nonexistent. Your type of cancer, remember, only shows up once in every two million people. Not much to go on."

"Which is why statistics aren't particularly relevant," I insert.

He nods, choosing not to enter a statistics debate.

"You used one of my pet words a while ago," I go on, after a moment's thought.

"—How's that?"

"Aggressive. I find that apropos. It's helped me get here, to this point. A while back I decided to do all I could to remain healthy . . . to be as aggressive as possible."

"Yes, well," he says, smiling broadly, getting up, signaling an end to our meeting, "sounds like we've finalized your decision for you."

CHAPTER 37

MY FIRST IV CHEMO—
SHATTERING MYTHS

I've been off work now for over three months. Like many aerospace companies, Rockwell grants a two-week paid holiday at Christmas. Four days before this two-week furlough rolls around, I'm back on the job. Promptly I sift through what's transpired during my absence. When I return after the holidays, I want no surprises, no upset VPs camped in my office.

Christmas this year looks hopeful—but less hopeful than many others. As a cancer patient, everywhere you go, you take with you a troubling onus: The intensely real understanding that cancer can be spreading in you at this very moment. As you relax with well-wishers and family, talking, celebrating the Yuletide . . . when you're driving to the store . . . while you're making love in the quiet of night.

Some cancer patients never get to a point where the disease does not dominate their intimate thoughts, fears. Braving your own death, when death has been scheduled for you by some unthinking physician relying on statistics, is a personal agony not easily ignored. Those who live with and care for cancer patients must work at perceiving this reality.

Linda Ellerbee, TV news personality and breast cancer survivor, in *Coping* magazine (May/June 96), in expressing her appreciation for the advice of other cancer survivors: "It's very encouraging, and nobody can quite give you that support but those people. Nobody but us really knows what it's like."

A cancer survivor, according to the National Coalition of Cancer Survivors, is any person who's still alive after contracting the disease.

Christmas, 1992: I'm getting increasingly immersed in alternative cancer treatments, specifically meditation and visualization, spirituality, and trying—at last—to eat appropriately (vegetarianism). Many of the books I've been dabbling in (Deepak Chopra, Bernie Siegel, Carl Simonton—physicians all) argue that meditation's an extraordinary way for cancer patients—anyone, in fact—to open their minds, defuse stressful situations, permit the body mind's own healing mechanisms room to operate.

Practically all cultures have practiced meditation since time began. The experience can be either secular or nonsecular. You can appeal to God or an unspecified higher power, or simply ponder nothing, allowing your body-mind to seek its own level of contemplation. Meditation is shutting off all the mental chaos we customarily live with, and bringing the mind home.

We're continually besieged by noise, mental pictures, introspection, subconscious feelings, and thoughts of people around us, worries and what have you. The mind's invariably racing about, going over this or that. Understanding how to meditate, to be selfish enough to lay these nuisances aside, takes some doing. But the venture's worth it.

In the beginning I use breath-watching (you actually watch your breath going in, going out), then guided imagery (visualizing some suitable energy devouring your cancer cells, liberating you of the disease), and finally I attempt Zen meditation (you free the mind of all thinking, lingering in an infinite nothingness). The process, whichever you choose, is empowering, giving you the positive feeling that you, the patient, are participating in your own survival. Meditation is, however, only a tool—it is not a cancer remedy in itself. (See Appendix F for meditation methods.)

Making this a once-a-day practice, I come home from work, do a few stretching exercises, then lie on the bed, in a semi-darkened room, observing in my mind waves of white blood cells washing over the surgical area, purging all those foul, malformed malignant cells.

With Christmas two days behind me, I drive to Dr. Malone's office to embark on this new chemo, not knowing what to expect. It's 11:00 a.m. Panic on my part's fairly intense. Will I get violently ill? Will I be cognizant enough to drive myself home?

Once I check in, a lab technician beckons. She draws blood—an unassuming finger prick. A gregarious blond with distinct facial features, the technician, outfitted in a starched lab coat and two-tone cowboy boots, explains that blood counts are necessary before each chemo session so the doctor will know if my immune system will bear the onslaught.

(Never refer to chemo or radiation as poison. These treatments were created by medical scientists to make us well. Cancer treatments *must* be perceived positively—with hope, trust, and belief—in order to garner all the goodness they have to offer. . . even when these treatments are unpleasant or inconvenient.)

"What did we decide on?" I ask the quiet-spoken Dr. Malone, as I uneasily take a seat in one of the well-worn naugahyde recliners she utilizes for out-patient chemo. There are three of these hot seats, side by side, in a very small, pale green, chemical-smelling, windowless room just down the hall from her office.

In the recliner nearest the far wall's a wrinkled, gray-haired man. His heavily lidded eyes are shut as if he's—dead. Above him hovers a single bag, dripping a deep-purple liquid, reminding me of grade-school fountain pen ink.

"What we're going to go with," Dr. Malone begins, wrapping a blood pressure cuff about my upper arm, "is a drug called carboplatin. And another called fluorouracil (pronounced floor-oh-YOUR-a-sill), more commonly known as 5-FU."

"Any reason—for those two?"

"Your left kidney, Mr. Scribner, I'm afraid, couldn't withstand cisplatin. This is next best—carboplatin. The other—5-FU—comes from my reading and talking with other physicians."

"—Anderson doctors?" I ask, though hesitantly, because I'd noticed of late she's seeming a bit thin-skinned about my allusions to Anderson doctors.

"Among others," she replies tersely.

"Doctor, I've been considering a shift—in diet," I begin prudently, watching her rewind the blood-pressure cuff. "Cutting out meat all together. I wanted to get your thoughts." I don't use the word vegetarian—it daunts people, carries a mystical or kookish nuance.

"Well," she says crisply, apparently still bristling from my last Anderson-related question, "while you're on chemotherapy, I don't want you undertaking any silly fad diets. I want you eating only good, balanced meals—plenty of meat and protein—to maintain strength."

Having tested the waters, I let the topic drop. I secretly hoped she'd reply in this manner—allowing me to go on eating what I intuitively knew was an unhealthy diet. Pushing on, I ask what I can look for today—during, after this first IV session.

"We're starting you with Zofran, a relatively new anti-nausea drug. I don't envision much stomach distress. But that remains to be seen. We told you not to eat this morning, right?"

A young, thin-armed nurse makes an entrance, carrying several plastic bags of fluid. Suspending each on a chrome pole alongside my chair, she says, "'Morning. I'll get you set up in a moment. I'm Rosa."

Putting on half-frame glasses, Dr. Malone inspects the bags' labels. She tells Rosa she's going back to her office. I'm on my own—with the ancient guy, who's yet to stir a muscle, and Rosa.

"First," she explains, unwinding some transparent plastic tubing and readying a tiny, green-winged butterfly needle, "we'll run a little saline solution through . . . to be sure we have a good vein." Swabbing the back of my hand with alcohol, she spanks the flesh sharply to bring up a usable vein. "Ever had chemo?"

"Only oral," I say. "No IV stuff."

"Sometimes," she explains, "people who've had chemo get really bad veins. Ones that roll or collapse when you try to stick them." She inserts the tiny needle beneath the skin, an almost imperceptible sting. Once she's run some saline solution through, she connects the first bag of fluid.

"—And that'd be?" I ask restlessly, feeling a mild stab of panic.

"It's an antiemetic. Zofran. We give it first to block . . . sickness. Used to be patients got very, very, very ill, vomiting everyplace." Rosa gestures grandly, taking in the entire room. "Now, very few get sick."

"But some still do?"

"A few. Yes. . . .Try not to look so worried, Mr. Scribner."

"How long is this drama going to last?"

"Usually about an hour or two," she says, gently squeezing my fingers. "I'll get you a magazine, if you want. We have the new *People*." Rosa's about thirty with pitch-black hair, remarkably thick, drawn back in a concise ponytail. Her precisely manicured fingernails are half pale pink, half lipstick red. Her walnut-colored skin's taut, appearing to glow.

With me I brought a Walkman and several tapes, a cancer self-help book. Listening to a classical FM station, I find myself transported to a peaceful land—for a moment. But very quickly, I'm back in this cramped little room, concentrating on the beads of fluid writhing down the tubing.

Twenty minutes pass. Rosa starts the carboplatin. "Let me know," she cautions, "if you feel anything at all. Especially in your vein or around the needle."

To say I'm not anxious would be lying. As drop after drop wriggles down the clear tube, I wait. Scenes from movies zip in before my eyes . . . wasted-away people, miserable with chemo, vomiting uncontrollably.

A minute slips by . . . and nothing. Ten minutes . . . still nothing. Gradually, when there's no gut-deep cleaving, my anxious concern begins to fade. Warily, I breathe a sigh of relief. Rosa's still sitting nearby, poised like a watchful cat. Grinning, she says, "See? Like clockwork."

"This drug, does it make a person's hair fall out?"

"With carboplatin, sometimes. But usually not," she replies, inspecting closely the green butterfly needle in the back of my hand. "It's six years now, I've been doing this. Everyone is different."

As the minutes tick by, this chemo business is becoming less fearsome. I'm not queasy—and apparently, not going to be. Rosa, standing, goes over, disconnects the old guy, neatly sliding the needle from his heavily veined forearm. The old guy—like a robot—just sort of comes awake, not showing a trace of emotion. This is old-hat to him. Laboring to his feet, he shuffles out. Not uttering a sound.

Rosa and I: now alone in the confines of this cramped, chemical-smelling, windowless room.

"What dosages am I getting?" I want these facts to update my computer medical record. "Let's see," Rosa begins, reading the label on the plastic bags, "400 milligrams of carboplatin and—" she picks up the other bag, "500 milligrams of 5-FU."

With carboplatin bag drained, Rosa starts the 5-FU. This, she tells me, is less likely to cause nausea. This drug may cause, in weeks to come, uncomfortable mouth sores. But, she explains, gargling with water and baking soda a couple of times a day will minimize the sores.

The low point in my white blood cell count, Rosa goes on, should appear in about 14 to 21 days. Most likely I'll feel more fatigued than normal, be more susceptible to infection during that time. So, she advises, be prepared to (1) take time off work, (2) go to work later in the day, (3) take longer, more relaxing lunches, or (4) leave work early during those days.

Departing the doctor's office, after two hours of chemotherapy, I feel oddly ebullient.

There's no immediate indication the chemo's going to cause any nausea—or anything else. Feeling quite bold, I head for a fast food joint to get a cheeseburger with all the trimmings. The doctor—the supreme authority figure for those of us who live by TDKB—said this food was okay.

An hour later I'm standing in line for a matinee with Jane. During the movie, a string of recurring hot flashes wash over me, bringing on a thin, body-wide sweat, a deferred reaction to the chemo . . . or the stuffiness of the theater?

FINDING HOPE WHEN DOCTORS SAY THERE IS NONE

CHAPTER 38

WITH KNOWLEDGE... COMES DOUBT— LEARNING THE UNSETTLING RATIONALE FOR MY CHEMO

Day one of chemo seems to have gone reasonably well. Sweats at the theater never amounted to much more than that. Next day I'm again sitting in Dr. Malone's stuffy, little chemo cubicle. Rosa's doling out another 45-minute cycle of 5-FU. (Carboplatin's dispensed once a month, on day one. The 5-FU is given in divided dosages over four days—the first dose being given with the carboplatin, the remaining three doses on successive days.)

Day two winds up as day one had—without discernible symptoms. I'm pleased, to say the least. Day three's dose of the 5-FU goes well, too. "Looks like this IV chemo business is going to be a piece of cake," I comment to Jane, lunching on red snapper Vera Cruz, rice and chilled chardonnay at our favorite marina-view restaurant.

"Could prove easier—" Jane offers, pointing out the window at a young couple hoisting their mainsail as they motor out of the sunless marina, "—than taking that three-times-a-day Mitotane for the rest of your life. Don't you wish they had lump crab here?"

"God, that was a meal, wasn't it?" I respond, watching a brown pelican light on the dock.

Though it's only been a matter of weeks since my final radiation treatment, later today I have my first follow-up with Dr. Goetz. Palpating my midsection and various lymph nodes, the ever-chatty Dr. Goetz says the new medical director—Dr. Bristol—over at my clinic's informed him the HMO will no longer approve payment for post-radiation follow-ups. Not for me, not for anyone.

He argued long and hard, Dr. Goetz says. But the director reasoned that any HMO doctor's capable of doing these follow-ups. Dr. Goetz, however, says he feels so solidly about the proper doctor performing these exams that he and other radiation oncologists at the treatment center have decided to perform them free of charge.

"The director made it quite clear she thinks this is a smoke screen," Dr. Goetz says candidly. "That we're using these follow-ups to line our pockets."

"Not a shy woman."

"You know her—this Dr. Bristol?"

"She was my primary-care doctor. Till she got promoted."

"Tough cookie. Set in her ways."

"She's great if she's on your side," I observe, feeling cheated that my former physician had selected now to institute her disapproval of follow-up exams.

As we talk, by virtue of his being in tune with chemotherapy and its side effects, I ask in passing, while buttoning my shirt, if he knows why Dr. Malone's selected the particular chemotherapy she's using on me.

Dr. Goetz draws a long breath, smiling peculiarly. "You don't really want to hear."

This flagrant dodge catches me off guard. "Try me."

"Now remember," he emphasizes, "you brought this up . . . Okay?"

Apprehensive, I say, "Understood."

"Okay," he resumes almost cautiously, fingering his red mustache. "How do I put this? It's in vogue."

"It's," I say slowly, "—what?"

"Remember I told you chemo's not a science, but an art?"

Nodding yes, I feel a new sense of muddledness.

"This happens to be an example. Carboplatin's the hottest thing on the market. In everything you read."

You're kidding me! I'm thinking, my confidence in Dr. Malone waning. "You mean . . . she's giving me what other people're getting—just because it's popular? I thought you were going to say . . it's the latest drug for treating ACC."

"No such luck."

"You're serious—aren't you?"

Shrugging blamelessly: "No reason to make this stuff up."

"She told you this?"

"Indirectly."

In the silence of the newly remodeled, paint-smelling office, I let the issue die—wishing, like Dr. Goetz'd cautioned, I'd never asked. Exiting the radiation center, I feel emotionally estranged, and vow to telephone Houston to get their reaction to this craziness. (This a superb illustration of how the body-mind works: The mind in this case perceived troubling news—words only, mind you—and suddenly the body feels infected, unsound.)

The following day: I call Dr. Saltz at MD Anderson. Had she advised Dr. Malone with respect to a chemo regimen in my case? Yes, she says reassuringly, offering immediate relief. Had she advised that carboplatin *and* 5-FU are the drugs to use? An ominous quiet.

"We discussed the application of a cisplatin-like drug," she goes on. "Now —what she'll use in conjunction with that, we didn't cover."

"So then . . . 5-FU's not a drug you routinely use. For treating ACC?"

"We don't, no, but I suppose you could."

The 'medical brotherhood' won't allow Dr. Saltz to pass judgment on Dr. Malone. Standing there, with the phone in hand, looking out at the quiet Pacific, I realize this may've been a case of asking too many questions of too many doctors. But not really—I simply heard things I didn't expect to hear. Now the dilemma: What to do with these revelations?

More than anything, I want to maintain an abiding trust, a genuine confidence, in my oncologist's treatment plan. Again, it's been documented that true belief in the curative powers of a particular therapy contributes greatly to that therapy working. (An example of the placebo effect in action—when you believe something will make you well, chances of it doing just that are positively enhanced.)

But how can I put my full faith in this regimen—this carboplatin, this 5-FU? Is this the way medicine's inner circle decides critical treatments? Via popularity contests?

When I mention this disturbing finding to Jane, she sides with Dr. Malone, saying only that I'm again over-reacting. Finally, with nowhere to turn, I take the easy way out—the TDKB route—reasoning that since there are no other drugs to treat ACC, maybe Dr. Malone's taken the right road. An educated shot in the dark, if you will.

Within the boundaries of the HMO framework—a structure that offers few, if any, patient options, save for paying for a new oncologist yourself—what alternatives do I have? Time will answer these questions.

While watching late news one night, a week or so after my last chemo, I notice a distinct, burning sensation in my left heel. Seeing this as no big deal, not related to anything of any consequence, I decide to tell Dr. Paravano about it, if it's still there, when I see her for a routine visit in a few days. Also, of more concern—I'd discovered a small patch of fibrous tissue on one of my testicles.

Following a thorough physical exam of the foot, an impeccably attired Dr. Paravano dispatches me to the x-ray department. Relative to the more intimate issue, she's noncommittal. Subsequent to feeling the thickening herself, she decides that Dr. Sugarman, a urologist, should review things. She'll submit the necessary referral to the HMO Utilization Review Committee. (This process can take weeks. Then I'd still have to make an appointment with that doctor and wait further still.) The condition, she believes, isn't a real danger. But, considering my medical history, she wants a specialist's word.

Nothing in the heel x-ray appears irregular. But, dammit, it positively aches—like somebody's driven a nail up through the bottom of my foot. Dr. Paravano suggests we let it resolve itself, look at it again in a few days. Little do any of us realize this is a red flag, a true warning sign.

Next day, as I'm getting ready for work, the relentless throbbing in the heel all but prevents me from placing any weight on it. Also about this time—a couple of weeks after chemo—I'm growing remarkably overtaxed and winded doing even the simplest tasks—like walking up the stairs to the bedroom. Afterward, I have to lie down, recuperating on the bed. Suddenly I'm quite fragile. Maybe this chemo isn't a piece of cake . . . what with the onset of drowsiness, lack of verve, constipation—and, little did any of us know this heel business would soon surface as a major medical issue.

Advice: In the HMO 'modus operandi,' it seems, never do HMO doctors speak with one another regarding your case or treatment. *You* become the conduit, the courier between physicians. It's up to you to convey important medical concerns from one doctor to next. Maybe 'the good old days' aren't what I remember, but this seems the outright inverse of what patient-oriented physicians used to be. Do doctors see too many patients today?

The '90's HMO doctor is, for all intents and purposes, a salaried employee of that HMO. Little more. He or she is not unlike the It-Ain't-My-Job civil service worker. Not all HMO doctors adopt this uninvolved approach, but a good many of them seem to. The current state of medicine—HMO medicine—is especially unsettling because elderly patients, those who're steeped in TDKB, are the ones who're most frequently given inferior care. Why? Because HMOs know they won't challenge the system—or, what their HMO doctors have told them. Always challenge HMO irregularities.

CHAPTER 39

BAD MEDICINE—
THE DOCTOR ADMINISTERS CHEMOTHERAPY

For the next week or so I go to work, limping from meeting to meeting, praying this bothersome heel pain will go away. Wearing leather dress shoes seems only to aggravate the problem—after going a couple of months in slippers, tennis shoes. A pair of Dr. Shoal's soft rubber insoles provides some relief. In the evenings, adhering to Dr. Paravano's most recent instructions, I down a couple of Advil and elevate the foot, draping it in a heating pad. This seems to help.

Eight days later, as strangely as it first appeared, the pain's completely gone when I wake up. The heel, mysteriously, overnight, has healed itself—gone from being extremely painful, to now quite normal, painless.

A few days in advance of the second round of chemo, there's a routine visit with Dr. Malone. When she asks about post-chemo problems, I mention the constipation, the tiredness. Run-of-the-mill, she declares. The sore-heel issue, I don't go into. Doesn't seem applicable.

Again, being that I advocate the 'most aggressive approach' to treatment, I ask about increasing the chemo dosages—to heighten their cancer killing abilities. Since I hadn't endured any incapacitating side effects, I figure we should push the therapy to its limit. When I ask about this and a follow-up or baseline CT—to track my progress—Dr. Malone's guarded, saying she'll look into it. Checking me over, she once again pokes around with the delicacy of a child. How can she detect questionable lymph nods or anything else with that soft-touch approach?

Days later I'm back in her office for my second round of chemo at 3:00 in the afternoon. A cherub-faced receptionist slides her frosted window open, smiling, telling me to take a seat. Seconds later, the sunny lab technician appears in the door to the exam rooms, motioning for me. It's blood-letting time. Minutes after I've returned to the waiting room, she pokes her head out the door again. I get the thumbs-up sign: my blood's okay.

A short while later a silver-haired chemo nurse appears in that same door, apologizing profusely. She'll be with me in a few minutes. Things are crazy today, she says. No problem, I say, returning to last month's *Sports Illustrated*.

A lite-rock FM station's playing in the tiny ceiling speakers. The phone rings time and again. Other patients come and go. An hour trudges by. About 4:30, from behind the frosted glass, I hear the chemo nurse quietly telling the receptionist good night. Not a good sign. Alone in the waiting area am I. Getting up, I slide the frosted window aside, asking what's up.

"Oh, Mr. Scribner!" the surprised receptionist exclaims. "You must've heard Marilyn, your nurse. Something's come up. She has to leave. Dr. Malone will do you herself."

Returning to the hard-cushioned couch, I find myself growing more restless, more rankled.

The door to the exam rooms, which hasn't been closed tightly, now swings open—unexpectedly, silently, exposing a down-the-hallway view of Dr. Malone's office. Perched at a bulky mahogany desk, the doctor's leafing through a K-Mart mailer (the logo's obvious) . . . while talking, laughing on the phone.

I pretend not to notice. The wrath festers in me. I had, after all, left work several hours ago to complete this still-unpleasant event, my second round of chemo. Feeling my eyes on her, Dr. Malone glances up. Nonplused, she leans forward, nudging her office door shut.

My watch says 5:05. I've been sitting here now for over two hours.

Another ten minutes go by. The receptionist, after unsubtly banging closed her metal file drawers, and making other close-of-the-day noises, skims open her window, leaning out: "Mr. Scribner," she says in a near-whisper, "we need to have you come back tomorrow. Too late for chemo now."

I want to bellow: 'Well, if the damn doctor would get off her ass!' . . . But I hold my temper.

"I'd like to oblige, miss, but, " I reply instead, feeling a rage just beneath my skin, "I took off work early to get this done. I've been sitting here for hours. I'd really like to at least get some of my chemo today—understand?"

"Well, if you're going to insist," the fleshy receptionist replies in a huff. "Lemme check."

Again I resume waiting. Minutes pass. In the still-open door leading to the small exam rooms, the receptionist appears. Her scowling, hunch-shoulder manner says she's one pissed-off young lady. Motioning me to the tiny, windowless chemo area: "The doctor will be with you in a minute."

Twenty minutes later: Dr. Malone enters, not offering any manner of rationale or regret. Gripping my file beneath her slender arm, she embarks abruptly: "Mr. Scribner, I don't have time today for a lot of inquiries. (She's referring to the typed questions I regularly bring.) What's today's visit for?"

"Dr. Malone," I reply, trying to remain calm, "I'm supposed to be getting my second round of chemo."

Glancing quickly at her black digital wristwatch: "It's after five."

"I'm well aware of that, doctor. I've been sitting out there for almost three hours."

"We're in transition, Mr. Scribner. There's not much I can do," she remarks brazenly, dropping my file on the counter with an emphatic thud. "I will give you your 5-FU. For the rest, the carboplatin, you'll have to return tomorrow."

Rather than argue, I agree—thinking something's better than nothing.

Rummaging through numerous disorderly drawers and cabinet shelves, the doctor pulls together the necessary items: a packaged butterfly needle, transparent bags of fluid, a length of sterile clear tubing. She has not bothered to don latex gloves. She swabs the back of my right hand with alcohol.

Her initial jab fails. This doesn't produce a lot of pain. But all the same it smarts—and produces a fair amount of blood. Without saying anything, she jabs again. Same outcome. Still no apology, she wipes away the blood, saying, "Give me your other hand."

After two more bungled stabs, and rivers of blood, in the back of that hand—is she retaliating?—she finds a vein on her third attempt. Keep in mind, this is a total of five times she's jabbed me! As my eyes follow the chemo drops spilling down the clear plastic tubing, I have a hard time seeing this as a healing potion.

I want desperately to yell at her—for her ineptitude, for the pain she's so callously inflicted, for all the time I've wasted here. But again I keep my trap shut. I've got too much time invested at this point to create a scene, to lose out entirely on today's treatment. Maybe she's just rusty, I tell myself, struggling to redirect my hostility, my doubt in her abilities.

"Shouldn't we," I suggest after a moment, with due precautions, "be running some saline solution through first—to see if it's a good vein?"

"That's not necessary," she says curtly, sticking a piece of tape on the back of my hand to hold the needle in place.

Again, I don't disagree. But I can feel turmoil growing inside. "When I was here the other day, doctor . . . I asked about boosting the drug dosages—can we do that?"

"I'm upping the strength on both," she replies, coarsely blotting blood from the oozing holes in my right hand.

I hope she'll sit with me, like Rosa, then, at least, I can run some cancer concerns by her at a leisurely pace. Maybe even experience this person as a human being. But once she gets the 5-FU started, the flow regulated, she stands, scurrying back to her nest—back to that ever-important K-Mart flyer? Her absence at least gives me the opportunity to read the dosage label on the 5-FU bag. She had upped the dosage. Thank God for small favors.

Thirty minutes later: Pulling the needle from my hand, sticking a cotton ball and some tape over the oozing blood, she asks, "Has anyone told you about our new chemo center?" There's an element of civility in her voice.

"Not a word."

"In that case, I want you going there tomorrow. Downstairs. First floor. We think you patients will like it. We've brought everyone together in one state-of-the-art center—pharmacist, chemo nurses, patients."

"Downstairs, you say?" I ask, watching her unfeminine little hands wrap the tubing and stuff it in a near-full bio-hazard bin.

"Yes. It's easy to find. Come in at your regular time. They'll take care of you."

Rolling down my sleeve, I ask: "Any news on my CT scan—when it might be allowed?"

"After this chemo cycle, looks like."

That night, roughly four hours later, while watching TV, something strangely familiar happens: my right heel (not the left as before) starts tingling. Pulsing blood I can actually feel—or a pulsing-like sensation—going through it. The same sensation is there at daybreak. There's no pain associated with it—yet.

At the new ground-floor Infusion Center the following afternoon, I ask my new chemo nurse, Abbie, if other patients experience tingling in their feet after getting 5-FU. She says some do, indeed. Some patients, she says, notice it to a greater extent—and longer—than others.

A sharp-featured woman in her fifties, Abbie seems to take pleasure in her work. Comforting it is to hear she has, over her career, administered chemo to thousands of patients. After last night's debacle, I hail someone with experience. Once I sink into one of the new black naugahyde recliners, Abbie—sporting sterile gloves—slips a needle into a good vein the first time, almost without pain.

When I describe last night's three-and-a-half-hour disaster, Abbie chuckles oddly. "You poor thing. That lady hasn't administered chemo in years. Surprised she even volunteered."

"'Volunteered' isn't exactly the word I'd use. Maybe that's why she had to stab me five times."

"Only five?" Abbie repeats, still seeing this as mildly humorous. "She is improving."

With my Walkman plugged into my ears, playing a soothing piano tape, my eyes begin meandering. As impersonal as a small gymnasium, this Infusion Center has a pharmacist's window, nurses' counter on the far wall, and a row of ten recliners facing *away* from a windowed wall. Suspended overhead are five remote-controlled TVs. The bank of ceiling-to-floor windows behind the recliners reveals a treeless parking lot—so much for Bernie Siegel's ideas about a pleasing window view assisting a patient's recovery.

All and all, the new center seems patient-unfriendly, barren of spirit; a rather uncivilized, impersonal, assembly line-mode of administering chemotherapy. A shame something so incredibly important to the patients' well-being—chemotherapy—is so lifelessly doled out.

Advice: Drive-Thru Chemo—Not bad in and of themselves, these highly impersonal, HMO-spawned Infusion Centers are becoming all too common in the world of cost-effective, out-patient oncology. Operated much like barber shops, these centers do provide an efficient means of dispensing *some* kinds of chemo, for *some* patients. But there are other types of chemo—e.g., those that require the patient get hours of IV hydration *before* chemo starts—that should only be administered in a strict hospital setting.

A person who's been told he or she has a life-threatening disease should not be required to sit in a recliner for up to eight hours at a stretch, with the distraction of strangers milling about, coming and going, while chemo's being dripped into them.

Prior to the birth of HMOs and cost-effective medicine, these out-patient assembly-line chemo centers were virtually unheard of. (Cost-effective and out-patient: two terms HMOs dearly love—because, translated, they mean *more* money in the pockets of already over-paid, limo-chauffeured HMO executives.)

At least one patient I'm acquainted with received very high-dose cisplatin (250 mg) at an Infusion Center. For five months her HMO resisted putting her in the hospital overnight for proper hydration and nursing care—it wasn't necessary, or *cost effective*.

This patient, because she'd been given the cisplatin at an Infusion Center *without* adequate hydration, had to be hospitalized for several days after each out-patient session: Predictably her kidneys began malfunctioning. Finally, for her sixth and final chemo cycle, her HMO conceded, allowing her an over-night stay in the hospital. Result: No post-chemo kidney complications and the HMO actually *saved* money. So how do we define cost-effective medicine?

FINDING HOPE WHEN DOCTORS SAY THERE IS NONE

CHAPTER 40

DEPTHS OF THE ABYSS—
TWO MONTHS INTO CHEMO AND
A CT SHOWS A NEW MASS

Over the next few days, assorted minor side-effects pop up: a tenacious headache (these still appear after each testosterone injection), seriously loose bowels, then constipation, then nausea, then the sensation of being bloated after each meal. My chemo nurse, Abbie, says all of this is pretty much expected. She forewarns, however, that I should not be taking aspirin for headaches or other aches, pains. Aspirin, she says, tends to induce a decreased platelet count.

Middle of the second week: I awaken, feeling both heels throbbing. By now I'm putting two and two together, suspecting that 5-FU's the culprit. Seems a strange coincidence that whenever I have this drug, my heel—or in this case, heels—throb painfully. This heel issue, though, doesn't seem worthy of a great deal of concern—a minor price to pay for the long-term benefits of chemotherapy, if it is the chemotherapy.

Feeling pretty washed out, overall, I get out of bed each morning, eat, shower and trudge off to work—vaulting headfirst into a raging river of paper shuffling and fragile personalities. Generally, that's how I see my day: A whitewater river into which I leap, swim as hard as I can, and, depleted of all stamina at the end of the day, crawl out and head home.

Long about this time, I discover three nickel-sized sores in my mouth. And my legs are feeling oddly heavy from the knees down. When Jane telephones that morning to check on me, I mention this. She'll call Dr. Malone, she insists, and run this by her. Arguing, I say I hate getting hysterical about every little sign.

Another doctor, filling in for Dr. Malone, suggests I leave work right away and come to his (and Dr. Malone's) office. A thick-necked, swarthy man with bejeweled gorilla-sized hands, Dr. Pateras, after looking me over, seems satisfied that we're seeing standard chemo side effects. He wants me to start dousing my mouth with baking soda and water on a fixed schedule.

What about this mysterious heaviness in my lower legs, this throbbing pain in my heels . . . does he think this is linked to the 5-FU? These issues are new to him. No one's ever reported heel pain or leg heaviness following 5-FU or carboplatin. He scrawls a prescription for Darvocet for headache, leg discomfort.

The irritation in the right heel again disappears one morning—again, for no apparent reason. Pain in the left heel, however, is furious, now generating a dull throbbing up the back of my calf and in the hind portion of the knee. Both areas, interestingly enough, seem to respond well to vigorous exercise—pedaling a stationary bike, for instance. I conclude it's feasible to work off some of this discomfort with physical activity.

Over the next couple of days, I'm taking more and more Darvocet, not so much as a headache remedy (which it isn't), but to kill the heel and leg pain. Since the heel's become such a prolonged problem, I arrange to see Dr. Paravano. It doesn't seem an oncologist's concern. Again she examines closely both feet, finding nothing unusual. Again, she has me get x-rays of both heels, which show nothing. Because the knee pain's new and seems independent of other aches and pains, I overlook mentioning it to Dr. Paravano.

While at her office, she provides a newly approved authorization for my CT scan. Now I must call the CT center, provide them with the authorization number, schedule an appointment, then go in and pick a CT prep kit.

What's the status of the referral to the urologist, Dr. Sugarman, I ask. She seems puzzled I haven't yet received the paperwork—it's been weeks. Must've fallen through the cracks, she says. She'll send through a new authorization request.

The CT's not for a week yet. In the meantime I find getting around at work on the very painful left leg to be more and more strenuous. In my office I sit with the leg propped up. That seems less hurtful. But here's a Catch-22: If I'm up and about, walking it off—exercising—so to speak, the pain's diminished. So I try not to sit for extended periods.

One of my colleagues—truly a conscientious lady friend—confesses she's concerned: "Maybe you've got a blood clot, Eric," she offers. "You actually should see a doctor with that in mind. You know, sometimes you have to point out the problem before they actually recognize it."

Giving this some consideration, I do feel a mild sense of alarm. But reject the idea—only old folks get blood clots . . . I'm only 50.

Lying in the CT scanner, I'm not overly concerned about the results. After all, I recently had surgery, radiation and chemo—cancer treatments' three big guns. What could go wrong this soon?

Days later: Jane and I are waiting for the CT results in one of Dr. Malone's exam rooms. Entering, Dr. Malone offers a careless little smile. Clipped on top of my file are recent blood counts. She looks them over.

This waiting is never effortless. As I've said before, it seems oncologists have an agenda—and furnishing you with the all-important information on your CT comes last. After she probes my stomach in a cursory fashion, Dr. Malone gets to the meat: the CT results. Her solemn eyes scan the printed pages. She's not studied them beforehand. That's nothing new.

"Well, everything looks . . . pretty much on-course," she says, not looking up as she reads. Then, vacillating, she squints, mutters: "Hmm . . . . They've indicated a new, 8-cm soft-tissue mass. In the stomach-spleen area."

Without warning, the exam table beneath me, like a trap door, falls away. My emotions nose-dive that suddenly. Hastily, I look to an equally stupefied Jane. "What're we hearing here, doctor? That there's already something growing in me?" I manage to say, feeling my throat constrict.

"After all my husband's been through—" Jane puts in incredulously, "—how can this be?"

In a flash, the doctor's become more circumspect, more attentive. "I have a hunch," she proposes with little persuasiveness, "that your film's been over-read."

"*Over-read?*" I repeat, at once unable to see how a eminently trained radiologist—an MD—could 'over-read' a set a films. Either the mass is there or it isn't.

"That'd be my judgment, Mr. Scribner," Dr. Malone goes on, still unconvincingly. "Whoever reviewed these films—let's see, Dr. Doyle—undoubtedly saw your previous scans and became, I think, a little overly cautious. I'll ask Dr. Goetz to go over them." She offers this as though I'm expected to breathe a sigh of relief.

"So . . . if there is something there . . . " I ask, disconsolate, wondering still how a expert film interpreter—a radiologist—can see something (a mass) that isn't there, "what're my options?"

"Not much at this point," Dr. Malone replies, exhibiting what seems a feigned smile. "Unless . . . you elect to undergo another major surgery. But I doubt you'll find a surgeon willing to do it. This soon after radiation."

"What could this represent—" I persist, feeling my up-to-now static world collapsing around me, "—in your opinion?"

"I believe," she states firmly, as if now defending her choice of therapies, "we're seeing a huge piece of scar tissue. Nothing more. A chunk of meat, if you will . . . . Considering the combined effect of surgery and radiation, I'd bet on it."

"How large are we talking about, doctor?"

"Roughly, Mr. Scribner, the size of your closed fist."

"How can we tell—for sure—what it is?" Jane interjects.

Dr. Malone, gazing out the 7th-story window at the swarming 101 freeway: "We could biopsy the area—which I don't recommend. Or we could go with something less invasive. An upper GI and small-bowel series, for example, might tell us." Paging through the rest of my CT report, she goes on, "Or, a third option, we could do nothing—simply watch it." She uses the term 'watch it' as if this were a time-honored oncological procedure. "They've also noted a slightly enlarged prostate—and," she turns a supplementary page, "the x-ray of your left foot—you had your foot x-rayed?—was normal."

"That reminds me, I've been having this throbbing pain . . . in my heels. Usually after chemo," I offer dully in response, recalling now the fear my at-work colleague had revealed. "Dr. Paravano's been looking for a cause."

Dr. Malone simply nods: All this is between your internist and you. "All else's normal," she goes on, folding, inserting the reports in my file. With some persuasion on my part, I convince her to give me a copy of the CT report. She agrees to submit paperwork to the HMO to see if they'll sanction an upper GI series to help resolve this mass question.

"Do you think, Dr. Malone," I ask reluctantly, not wanting to sound like I'm over-reacting, "this heel-pain business is being caused by a . . . blood clot?"

"The chemotherapy you're on, Mr. Scribner," she responds sternly, not offering to look at the foot or calf, "does not cause clots."

Leaving her office I feel almost nauseous—vulnerable again to everything. Why am I enduring this damn chemotherapy if it's not deterring the growth of new cancer? Seized again am I by chaos . . . . What is this new *thing* the CT showed? How'd it get there so quickly? If it is indeed there—and grew this fast—this presents a whole new concern: A very aggressive and perhaps deadly cancer.

"This is exactly the reason I wanted a baseline CT before starting radiation," I say angrily, as Jane and I drive home. "That damn Goetz. Then we'd know what was there—from day one. Now we've got nothing to fall back on. No post-surgery scans to compare anything with."

"Eric, you heard your doctor," Jane says protectively, apparently siding with Dr. Malone. "She's convinced it's just scar tissue."

"That's great—if it is. But how do I *know* that—unless it's proven? I'm the one, remember—who has to live with this shit inside him."

"She's an oncologist, Eric, for heaven's sake. You're over-reacting. She's probably seen a hundred cases like this. You said at one point that you liked her better than Dr. Drake, remember?"

"Sure, before going through this—and that chemo fiasco. I'm not sure she has any idea what the hell's going on. We are talking about a rare cancer here, Jane, one she's had little or no experience with."

"She's going to have Dr. Goetz review the film. Can we please relax till then?"

"Jane . . . " I say, looking up at the same high-power pole where the white peregrine had been as we drive by, "this crap's in me again."

"Dr. Geotz'll straighten this out, you wait."

"Sure," I remark sarcastically, visualizing again the well-schooled radiologist who read the film, "like some trained specialist is going to see something that isn't there. And Goetz is going to fix everything. Sure. Do we believe in the Easter Bunny, too?"

FINDING HOPE WHEN DOCTORS SAY THERE IS NONE

CHAPTER 41

THE SOLUTION'S THE PROBLEM?
SOURCE OF THE TESTOSTERONE HEADACHES IS FOUND

In the next few weeks I find my life being yanked in many directions. First, and perhaps most unexpected, the HMO approves the GI ultrasound test within two weeks. Unbelievable! Most likely Dr. Bristol had become involved, propelling the matter through Utilization Review. But maybe I'm giving her too much credit.

With half-glasses low on his nose, the gray-haired, gray-bearded radiologist languidly doing the GI procedure has a look of befuddlement—like he's seeing something, or not seeing something, he's never encountered before.

A rather unsociable soul, this distant radiologist volunteers little. Unable to see the TV screen he's contemplating, I ask if he'll swivel the monitor so I too can see. "Not possible," he replies tersely, "considering your position."

As he's approaching the end of the procedure, I ask what he's found.

"Small bowel loops high in the upper left quadrant—that's what my report will say," he offers vacantly. "No definite mass."

This, I cautiously construe as good news. My innards feel like cheering. "You didn't see any . . . big chunk of something?"

"Only what I said," the radiologist acknowledges coolly, passing the slickened probe to a reserved female technician who's stoically waiting nearby.

While I want his to be the final word—his *is* good news—logic, as if it'd left the room for the time being to answer the phone or something, charges back in, asking: How can one doctor—the radiologist who read the CT films—see a fist-sized growth, and another radiologist, doing a less precise procedure, see zilch?

For the time being, though, I'm exhilarated with gray-beard's conclusions. Now, for a third opinion, I have to await Dr. Goetz's re-review of the films. Next rendezvous with him isn't for a couple of weeks.

So, in today's soulless world of HMOs, uninvolved doctors, and patients who must fend for themselves, I take it upon myself to call Dr. Goetz. Has Dr. Malone approached him about reviewing my films? She has, but he hasn't received them yet. He'll be ready with a judgment, he pledges, by the time of my next appointment. "Sit tight till then," he advises casually.

Sure, I'm thinking, if we'd done a CT *before* the radiation treatments, then we might know what we're looking at today!

Several weeks after Dr. Paravano submitted a referral for me to see Dr. Sugarman, the urologist, it's finally approved. No mention made of what happened to the earlier-submitted paperwork. Sitting with Dr. Sugarman, a prematurely gray man of about 45, with inordinately green eyes, we chat briefly about my cancer diagnosis, the recent surgery, the eight-week radiation course, my past use of Mitotane (he seems surprisingly conversant in this drug), and my current IV chemo.

After examining me extensively, including a prostate exam (because I mentioned the CT'd revealed an enlarged prostate), he concludes the spot on the testicle's nothing more than a common condition, called epididymitis, a benign thickening of tissue. But, he admonishes, let's continue to keep an eye on it. If anything changes in any way—gets larger or firmer—return to see him. He also says, scratching a note in my file, that CT scans, in his judgment, are a poor diagnostic tool for defining the size and condition of the prostate.

If this is true, I'm saying to myself . . . then conceivably a CT's not as accurate a diagnostic tool as I'd thought. Maybe the radiologist who saw the 8-cm soft-tissue mass was in error.

Breezing through my file, Dr. Sugarman notes I'm getting bimonthly testosterone injections. I explain that Mitotane, to my understanding, knocked out my ability to manufacture that hormone—among other things. Reminded of the topic, I take this occasion to ask (remember: always ask 'dumb' questions of new doctors) if he has any idea why terrible headaches set in following every testosterone injection. Is this an allergic response to testosterone, as other doctors suggested?

Shaking his head: "What's more likely, is you're allergic to the fluid base in which the hormone's suspended."

Baffled, I ask him to elaborate.

"Okay," he says, hastily, "there are various oils—suspensions—used for injecting hormones. That's so these—the hormones—can be assimilated properly within the body. What I recommend is finding out what suspension they're using and have your doctor change it. You may have to experiment a bit, but that's your problem—the fluid. You're not allergic to testosterone."

I can't believe I'm hearing this. Was this mystery that easily unraveled? And if so, why hadn't other in-the-know doctors come up with a similar—and self-evident—conclusion?

That night at the local drugstore an amiable, very understanding pharmacist and I have a quiet discussion about injectable hormone suspensions. Leaning on her counter, she listens attentively to the urologist's reasoning. Leaving for a moment, she returns with an immense pharmaceutical guidebook. Flipping pages, this 30-ish druggist says, "This fellow knows what he's talking about. There are several different suspensions available." She very plainly writes out the various types, numbering each. Actually, there are four.

"So, you've done most of the homework," she says, folding the paper, handing it to me. "Now see which suspension your doctor's using—and ask him or her to experiment. Keep trying new suspensions till you find one that's compatible. One that doesn't give you those awful headaches."

This seems . . . too damn easy. After all I've been through . . . years of enduring killer headaches.

Now my chief concerns, things I can take to bed at night, become: The controversial lump in the left adrenal area (will this or won't this kill me?), the recurring hypersensitivity in my heel or heels—and, on the plus side, the good news that a change in testosterone suspension might well eliminate the headaches.

The following day, on the phone, Dr. Paravano and I discuss the various hormone suspensions. I didn't really anticipate much opposition on her part, because—unlike many other doctors—she's not afraid to admit that she doesn't know something. Once I outline what Dr. Sugarman had suggested, she says she'll investigate the idea. While I'm on the phone, she gets the vial of testosterone her nurse's been using, and reads the label.

"What we've been giving you," Dr. Paravano states, "is a cotton-seed-oil based solution. Do you sometimes have reactions to that?"

"Not that I'm aware of."

"We'll order that first suspension you mentioned," she goes on. "Which was, if I recall, sesame-seed oil. Correct?"

Feeling exalted by her cooperative manner, and not knowing what else to say, I offer facetiously: "Sounds like we're throwing together some sort of hormone salad, doctor."

Finding this mildly amusing, she says her nurse will have the new testosterone on hand for my next injection, the following week. Still, I can't believe the resolution's this easy—and, that the explanation came from an improbable source. Why hadn't someone like Dr. Crandle—a damn endocrinologist, for God's sake—known this?

Back at work: Always, like a rippling reflection on a watery surface, is the overriding mental doubt—What *is* this mass they're seeing? Is this frightening cancer growing again that rapidly? A constant sort of panic courses through my veins as I ponder these nonstop thoughts.

I'm still limping about the endless hallways on an increasingly sensitive left heel. Frequently it literally seems on fire. The woman colleague who works with me in shaping the company's ever-hectic biannual report card for NASA (actually, I credit her with much of the tangible drudgery—had it not been for her, I would've keeled over from shear mental depletion long before cancer laid me up), remains tenacious in her hypothesis: The heel pain originates from a blood clot.

"Is the leg red," she asks, "or swollen at all?"

"Swollen a little, maybe," I admit reluctantly.

"If it *is* a clot," she asserts discreetly, "and you don't get it looked after, you could just keel over dead. I know someone that happened to. After all you've been through, Eric, you owe it to yourself."

Male-driven skepticism forces me to gently dispute her inkling. Somewhere in my memory banks, though, I recall an adolescent friend's father who'd developed clots in his leg. It seemed so irrelevant to me then—something old folks got. My friend's father's leg, an angry scarlet hue and all swollen, had him laid up, immobile in bed. To my surprise, late one night, he simply quit breathing.

My leg *was* swollen. But not really that swollen . . . or was it?

I hadn't considered the swelling to be a warning sign, figuring the pain caused that, not the other way around. But then . . . surely all the doctors I'd talked to would've recognized that—a clot. (In actuality, doctors get caught up in a sort of diagnostic trap. If certain conditions are present or *not* present, and if the patient's blah-blah age, and looks a certain way, he or she probably does or does *not* have . . . . See Appendix C.)

In reality, I didn't have to wait long to ascertain whether this is or is not a clot.

That Friday night: After work, the heel's grown so sore I can't put any weight on it, period. I can't walk. The knee refuses to bend. The region behind the left knee's become extremely painful. At Jane's insistence, I grab my self-prepared medical history and head with her to the HMO's Urgent Care Center (you can't reach your primary-care doctor after hours in an HMO) to see a new doctor . . . . God willing, he can shed some light on this intolerable predicament.

CHAPTER 42

AS CHILDREN FEAR DARKNESS—
THE HEEL PAIN'S FOUND TO BE A BLOOD CLOT

After about 40 minutes of suspenseful waiting, I'm seen by a schoolboy-looking doctor with a glossy appearance. Briefly digesting my self-prepared medical history (doctors love this to-the-point chronology), Dr. Neilsen asks several questions about my current physical state, the heel and leg pain. Then has me remove my shoe, my sock, roll up the pant leg. I'm sitting on an exam table. His fingers are cool on my naked foot as he delicately pivots it this way, then that, asking about discomfort. Squeezing the calf lightly, he rotates the foot forward, then back. Much of this maneuvering does sting.

"Pain there?" Dr. Neilsen asks.

Indeed, I tell him, wincing.

He now has me stand, hiking the other pant leg for an eyeball comparison of the calves. With me still standing, he's checking the diameter of each calve using a fabric tape measure. Twice he does this before having me sit back down.

"I'm going to call over to the hospital, Mr. Scribner," he explains almost apologetically, pinching the bridge of his nose, "and have them prepare a room for you. You don't like hearing this, I can tell. My guess is that we are looking at a deep-vein thrombosis—a clot. And you should not be on that leg—at all. I'll have the duty doctor meet you."

No, no, this can't be! I'm thinking morbidly. Not again! I can't go back in the hospital!

"Can he at least walk over there, doctor—to the hospital?" Jane asks, already abdicating to yet another surge of gloomy news, the hospital being a block away.

"We should send him in a wheelchair," Dr. Neilsen replies soberly. "I guess, though, it'd be acceptable if you drove him."

"It's that bad?"

"Potentially."

Nearly 10:00 p.m., March 1992. Going back in the hospital's profoundly distressing . . . a hugely invalidating step in the *wrong* direction. Bad, bad recollections of the bleak Dr. Tzu in Intensive Care. Reeling, I implore the doctor—"Is it really necessary to be hospitalized?"

"In good conscience," he replies charitably, sensing my aversion, "I couldn't let you go home. It's not absolute, but I'd say you have something serious going on in that leg."

"But," I argue—thinking, My God, I've been walking around for weeks with a deadly clot—"it's been like this since I started chemotherapy, back in December. The heal pain started almost immediately. No other doctors have seemed concerned," I add, hoping it'll dissuade him.

"We may find you don't have a blockage, Mr. Scribner, but better safe than sorry."

After checking in at hospital admissions, I'm assigned a private room on the 5th floor. Within minutes a tall, smiling nurse shows up. The on-duty HMO doctor's in the hospital, she says. But he's tied up at the moment and has told her to start an IV. For maybe another half-hour or so Jane and I sit talking quietly. Will things ever improve, we both wonder gloomily.

Being hospitalized again makes me feel . . . contemptible—a spiritless medical bankrupt. I fear myself edging ever closer to the outer fringes of experimental cancer treatment . . . that scary zone, inhabited only by the emaciated, the terminally ill. . . . Oh, God, am I terminal?

The on-duty doctor, a grandfatherly man, leathery flesh, slow blue eyes, comes in, at once moving an armchair near my bed. Extraordinary, this is. Perchance he's a get-involved-with-the-patient, old-school breed of physician. Asking a few questions about the heel and leg pain, he looks over both, feeling the warm of the calf with his open hand, swiveling the foot.

Settling back, crossing his legs comfortably, this doctor seems not in the least bit rushed despite the late-evening hour.

Accepting my computer-generated medical history, he dons half-glasses, studying all three pages for a good 10 minutes. Occasionally he pauses to pose incisive questions about various therapies, my trip to Anderson.

At once, I'm wowed with this guy's thoroughness. Suddenly, seeing his name tag, it dawns on me: Dr. Yarrow. This is the doctor the hospital social worker recommended as 'being one of the good ones.' So here he is, in the flesh—the doctor I couldn't make an appointment with because his practice was full.

His first observation, an offhand remark after reading my history, strikes an icy chord. "Mr. Scribner," Dr. Yarrow comments, pocketing his plastic-framed glasses, "people with a history of malignancies are often prone to deep-vein thrombosis."

So now I'm lumped together with those who have a history of malignancies. The words land ominously in my mind like a flock of ugly vultures . . . a history of malignancies . . . again and again the words resound. Is that now me? Someone in that diffuse category: people with a history of malignancies? I, by this time, know I'm in an infamous pool of humanity, but hate accepting it.

"Why do you say that, doctor?" I ask skeptically, not sure I want to hear the answer.

"No one's precisely sure. It's just something we often see."

"Can you say (I hesitate again, not wanting to heed his response) that this is definitely a clot?"

"Certainly checks out that way," Dr. Yarrow responds, folding my medical history carefully, handing it to me. "I'm going to set you up for a venagram in the morning. Then we'll know for sure."

"—A what?"

"A test where they inject dye into your foot, then follow it through your leg veins. No one's available now, at this hour, to do it. Morning will have to do. In the meantime, I'm going to start you on Heparin, an IV blood thinner."

This whole mess's becoming more and more haunting. The reverberating fear fostered by the new CT findings—that new mass—has become a bacteria-ridden wound within, pulling in other contagions.

"Is this . . ." Jane asks, barely above a whisper, "the kind of blood clot that's . . . dangerous?"

"It's capable of serious consequences," Dr. Yarrow acknowledges benevolently, patting my arm reassuringly. This man truly has a likable style. "Mr. Scribner," he goes on, "from now on you've got to keep that leg elevated. And get some movement down there. Wiggle your toes for circulation, even."

"So this is something he'll have to contend with . . . for a while?"

"A precarious situation at best, Mrs. Scribner. In fact, tonight—and as long as your husband's here—I want him using a urinal. No getting out of bed for anything."

"*It's* that serious, doctor?" I ask, feeling a new stab of panic, thinking of all the times-days, weeks, months—I'd hobbled about, even forced myself to exercise, on this ominously painful leg. Had there been a clot there, or forming, after each chemo treatment? This is becoming increasingly disheartening: Till now, I'd assessed my physical well-being positively, as going well, improving . . . not going down hill.

Within minutes after Dr. Yarrow leaves, the nurse returns.

"I understand—" she remarks cordially, suspending a new bag of fluid on the now-familiar IV pole, "he thinks you have a clot."

Jane, taking my wallet and keys—this has sadly become a ritual—says she'll see me in the morning. With Jane kissing me good-bye, I say to the nurse, "So they tell me," trying to sound unalarmed about the entire affair, but all the same tormented.

"You can't do better than Dr. Yarrow, if that's any consolation."

"Heparin's a cure? I mean, it dissolves clots?"

"Heparin, you should know," she responds, "is a very dangerous drug. One that can induce internal hemorrhaging."

"You're saying—I could still die from this thing?"

"Heparin's very good at what it does," she replies, "thinning blood. But your coagulation has to be monitored regularly."

"This drug dissolves clots that are already there?"

"I apologize, Mr. Scribner, I shouldn't be saying this much. That's the doctor's territory. Better ask him," she says, begging the issue. "They get upset when we get too involved."

Out the window are the city lights, looking butterscotch yellow in the hazy night; beyond them a dense blackness that is the Pacific. That night I eventually fall asleep, with the aid of sleeping pills, hearing echoes of Dr. Yarrow's initial pronouncement: Mr. Scribner, people with a history of malignancies are often prone to deep-vein thrombosis. . . .The disturbing words 'history of malignancies' refuse to leave me.

This insidious disease . . . is attacking on a new plane. What else *don't* I know about this subversive illness? With a whole new vista of fear spreading before me, I fall into a light, uncomfortable sleep.

In the morning, after breakfast, a male technician takes me, via wheel chair, and my squeaking IV pole, down to Radiology. For some reason—perhaps the Heparin dripping into me all night—I'm feeling really nauseous as we enter and exit food-smelling elevators, roll along chilly hallways.

God, I'm wondering, refusing to make small talk with the technician, how much bad luck can one person have?

In Radiology, two technicians help me onto a table. The six-foot-plus, middle-aged doctor asks how I feel, while at the same time explaining he's going to inject a radioactive dye in my foot and follow it up the leg to determine if there's a clot. I'm feeling pretty woozy for some reason, I tell him.

"We're going to bring this table—with you on it—to a vertical position," he explains, not appearing to hear—or wanting to hear—what I'm saying about nausea. "So we'll have you in a standing position while we perform the test." With that, the motorized table begins whirring, rising my head, lowering my feet.

"Let us know how you feel," the doctor advises intolerantly, stooping to make his initial examination of my bare foot. Now in a near-vertical posture, I'm gaping down, feeling queasy, but confidently noting several veins bulging prominently across the top of my foot. He'll have an easy time finding a good vein. (Seems all of a cancer patient's life doctors and nurses are looking for a 'good vein' to jab.)

No sooner do I get to a vertical position when I feel powerfully ill, my stomach clenching violently. Usually not susceptible to nausea, this time I feel myself fading in and out . . . the likelihood of everything in my stomach coming up is very real.

"Wait! Wait! Hold everything!" I manage to bellow, grabbing the nearest tech. "I'm going to be sick!"

Standing at once, the doctor commands the table be returned to its horizontal position. Once lying flat again, the feeling of faintness, of nausea, passes fairly quickly.

"Ready again, to try?" the doctor asks brusquely, as though he has maybe a hundred patients waiting.

With me again in the upright position, the crouching doctor swabs the foot with alcohol and attempts to start the needle. The initial stick, an intensely painful failure. "Damn!" I grunt. Second stick, another blunder. Nausea, like a foggy blackness, surges around me with each incompetent jab. With these blunderous needle pricks—reminiscent of Dr. Malone's careless stabs—comes an exasperation.

"Doctor, damn it!" I snarl through clinched teeth, "Can't you do any better? I'm getting sicker by the minute and you aren't helping things with that needle!"

"This isn't as easy as it seems, Mr. Scribner!" he replies, his passion matching mine. "Your veins are not cooperating!"

My head back, my eyes trying to focus on the billions of black holes in the ceiling, I pray he'll quickly locate a good vein. After two more sharp jabs—the needle pain seems more acute in light of the nausea, the exceptional sensitivity on the upper foot—he finds a vein that suits him.

Stifling the powerful impulse to vomit numerous times as the radiologist is tracing the dye up the leg, I try centering my concentration on a dead fly inside the fluorescent ceiling light. Twenty minutes later I'm being wheeled back to the 5th floor. The radiologist says my doctor will have the venagram details in an hour.

As weird coincidences would have it, on the way back to my room, I chance upon Dr. Malone in one of the endless, frigid hallways, making her morning rounds. Seeming lost in amazement—she's invariably uneasy seeing me—she says she heard about my current crisis, asking what tests I've undergone. Venagram results, I tell her, should be available soon.

Again, I ask if she's ever seen a patient end up with a blood clot as a result of chemo, or more precisely, 5-FU. As if called on the carpet, she pulls back, maintaining if it is a clot, it's not chemo-related. Her It-Ain't-My-Fault temperament addles me. In parting, Dr. Malone remarks—obligingly—she's had my CT films sent to Dr. Goetz. I praise her, biting my tongue. God, how I'm getting to loathe the fragile politics of medicine.

Several hours later, in my room, Dr. Yarrow reappears—a kind face—telling me the venagram has disclosed a clot. Pulling back the sheet, he indicates a point about midway up the calf.

"This Heparin, doctor, that'll do the trick—dissolve it?"

"That's a frequent misconception," he confides. "It'll work on it, but it won't necessarily dissolve the clot. We're trying now to keep new clots from forming. I want to keep you here another day or two (Jane exhales disappointedly for both of us) till we're fairly certain you're out of the woods. On day three, we'll mostly start you on an oral medication to keep the blood thinned. And let you go home."

Sensational, I'm thinking sarcastically, just what I friggin' need—another worrisome issue to heap on the swelling pile, another drug to take on top of the Prednisone, the florinef, the arrhythmia pill, the thyroid medication, a handfuls of vitamin supplements. "How long will I be taking this drug?"

"Usually," he says, his eyes flaring, "we prescribe it for a couple of months. But in the case of cancer patients . . . well. . . ." I don't hear his words beyond that.

CHAPTER 43

OF DOUBT AND SORROW—
DR. GOETZ DECLARES THE MASS TO BE SCAR TISSUE

After three days in a hospital bed, Heparin dripping continuously into me, reading, and watching shadowy March clouds drift across the horizon, they let me go home . . . with yet another bizarre drug to take—Coumadin, an oral blood thinner.

Before being discharged, I'm presented with white knee-high stretch socks (stockings?), and told to wear them religiously to ensure proper circulation in the lower legs. Everyone—nurses and doctors—exhort me to take it easy on the leg, exercise lightly, do not to sit for long periods. (Sure, how am I supposed to get to work?)

Thus I'm off work for yet another week with cancer-related complications. This newest adversity has struck like one of many ground swells forcing me rearward. I've been working unbelievably hard, in my judgment, at overpowering and containing this dark disease. I even had myself believing I'd done it: Cancer was behind me, under control. But a very real sense of deterioration is now setting in . . . on all sides.

Later that week I again find myself sitting with Dr. Crandle, the happy-go-lucky endocrinologist, for an ACTH follow up. Once again, he's all hustle and bustle. My file is under his lean, hairless arm. His outmoded crew-cut needs pruning.

Looking at me—doing a cartoonish doubletake—he smirks wryly. "Still hanging on, I see."

"In the flesh," I respond sarcastically, pinching an inch of skin on my forearm as confirmation. "Going to be a while before they shovel dirt in on this boy."

Dr. Crandle's thin, whitish fingers dance around the ACTH figures. "Looks like," he remarks, eager as a seven-year-old with a new tooth, "we've done it. Your ACTH's cooperating. Now down to . . . well, actually below normal. Still taking Prednisone?"

Eight milligrams per day, I tell him.

"Why?" he fires back unexpectedly, as if having tricked me.

"Why the hell shouldn't I be?" I reply just as bluntly.

"Because, for God's sake, you're not on the Mitotane anymore! You don't need the steroids. And you're taking on . . ." he pats his cheeks, underscoring the fleshiness he sees in my cheeks, "a bit of a Cushionoid appearance. Your face's rounding out."

"I've always had a little chubbiness in my face. Even as a kid."

"You don't need steroids any longer, is my point."

"They make me feel good. Give me energy."

"That may be, but physiologically they're uncalled-for. I want you tapering off them."

"I can't just keep taking a little?"

"You don't need them," he repeats, shaking his head. "Your body will adjust in time."

"I've only got one adrenal gland left," I protest.

"One's plenty," he retorts snippishly. "It's just sleeping right now. It'll bounce back, given time."

(What I don't comprehend in my medical naiveté is that this doctor, this endocrinologist, is handling me as he would any patient with adrenal insufficiency—not as a patient with adrenal insufficiency compounded by adrenal cancer. Big difference. If he'd seen me first as an adrenal cancer patient, he would've most certainly tested the function of the remaining adrenal gland. Mitotane could've permanently shut it down, requiring that I continue taking at least a physiologic dose of Prednisone. This'll be clearer as I falter yet again.)

"But . . . I need the energy."

"That will return naturally," he insists. "Admittedly, it may take several months. I want you to begin tapering off—immediately. Cut down two milligrams every three weeks." He stops, thinking a moment. "Then, when you get to where you get down to three milligrams, slow it a bit and cut one milligram every two weeks." As he speaks, he's writing this out on a prescription pad. "You'll probably start noticing some muscle soreness and creaky joints. That's perfectly normal. You'll work through it."

"No other options?" I ask, tucking the paper in my shirt pocket.

Nodding, he eases back. "Damn," he remarks, chuckling to himself. "I'm still amazed at how good you look."

Knowing precisely what he's alluding to, I say nothing to spawn any further fatalism. Instead I take his wisecrack as a backhanded compliment. Somehow it's strangely reaffirming to lock horns with your own views on life, on death, though obliquely, through this sort of antagonistic human dialogue.

That day, I begin cutting down on Prednisone. My TDKB orientation tends to make me a dutiful patient. Within days, I'm noticeably more sluggish . . .

walking, getting out of a chair, moving about is much more laborious. At least the leg and heel pain are all but gone.

Days later: I have an appointment with Dr. Goetz. "See? I told you," he begins derisively, with respect to the 'over-read' CT scans, "you wouldn't like what you saw on your first CT—didn't I?"

Already, I want to believe him. I may be deriving some sort of twisted contentment from this apparent validation of his original prophecy. Sliding a weighty bundle of 14X17 film out of its protective envelope, he sticks several sheets on a light board. Putting on his glasses: "Dr. Malone tells me you're agitated . . . about this area." He's pointing to grayish oval on the film.

"Wouldn't you be?" I come back with.

He shakes his head, taking off his glasses, amused.

"And why's that?"

"Call it experience, but I don't think it's anything to worry about. It's almost impossible for cancer to have grown that fast."

Not true. In my reading—and experience with other cancer patients—I've encountered extremely aggressive cancers that almost propagate over night. "But," I offer placidly, "how do we know for sure?"

"You had an ultrasound, right? And it came back negative." Dr. Goetz is now looking over a copy of that report. "Bowel loops, they talk about as being the source of this image. (He again points to the gray oval.) With your spleen now out of there, your intestines—those rascals—saw that area as a low-rent district and moved in."

"But couldn't you, or the other radiologist, determine that—if that is the case? That these are only bowel loops and not new cancer—from these CT films?" I persist. "Wouldn't bowel loops appear on this film as just that—bowel loops? The other radiologist is saying it's a recurrence. That doesn't sit so well with me. Presumably, he's not some backwoods medicine man."

"Protecting his butt, is what he's doing," Dr. Goetz remarks haphazardly. "I can tell you, Eric, this is not a recurrence."

Desperately wanting to believe this, I force a thin smile: "Dr. Goetz . . . how do we know that?"

"A biopsy's an option," he suggests malevolently. "I wouldn't recommend it."

"The reason being?"

"Possible hemorrhaging. Then we'd have to open you up, on the spot. Take my word for it—it's nothing."

To say I'm annoyed with Dr. Goetz's hunch, his unscientific judgment, is putting it mildly. What am I to do? Should I, as a patient, place myself in Dr. Malone and Dr. Goetz's apathetic care and *not* worry, as they suggest . . . or should I become more persistent, demanding a more investigative approach to quantify this questionable mass? Remember: This is the unsympathetic world of HMO medicine where the patient's allowed little or no demanding power.

These thoughts gnaw deeply, further eating away at my trust in these doctors. It's probably here, at this point in my treatment, I begin cynically seeing medicine as a business—and doctors, no matter the physical or financial cost to patients, do stick together.

Dr. Goetz, noting I have another CT due in about six weeks: "We can use that to better define what we're seeing. Maybe, if we're lucky," he goes on with a forced optimism, "the mass will be gone. Or least be smaller. Then we'll know it was scar tissue."

At night, I can't go to sleep without rehashing this again and again. The perception something's physically wrong—really wrong—won't leave me. If there is something amiss—a recurrence—I know we should be countering it aggressively now with treatment of some sort. There's no more opportune time to begin treating your cancer than today.

By the time I go for my first sesame-seed-oil based testosterone shot, a week or so later, I'm feeling fatigued, worn out due to the steroid reduction. Dr. Paravano, being a pragmatic physician (two years later she was released by the HMO for just this reason: being too patient-oriented), notes that reducing my Prednisone by 2 milligrams per day amounts to a 25% reduction in this energy-giving steroid. A significant drop. She suggests while I'm on chemo, I continue 8 mg a day of Prednisone to bolster my energy. Concurring, I snicker at Dr. Crandle and his recommendation for the time being.

Analyzing Dr. Yarrow's file notes relative to my most recent hospital stay, Dr. Paravano says she's going to begin strictly overseeing my coagulation because of the new oral blood thinner, Coumadin. This has to be done to ensure the blood still clots sufficiently and yet remains thinned enough to hinder new clots from forming. This new blood test will be done every 10 days so adjustments can be made in my daily Coumadin intake.

If this drug is not adjusted appropriately and regularly, you can bleed to death internally, she admonishes. (Coumadin, she explains as an aside, began as a rat poison. It caused internal hemorrhaging, killing the rodents. It has since been modified as a blood thinner for humans.) I ask about taking something safer in its place, like aspirin. While aspirin does thin the blood, she says, it's a dissimilar class of drug and not sufficient for my needs. So we add yet another troublesome blood test to my already discouraging repertoire.

I don't ask myself 'Can things get any worse?' because I now know they can . . . and will.

The following day, after the testosterone shot, I awaken to the unnerving alarm clock, and glance out at the mauve-colored morning sky, realizing . . . my head's clear! No headache! At last, something's going my way! Over the next few days I await suspiciously the silent torture to arrive. But the headache never does materialize.

The antidote is that elementary—a shift in the injection's base solution. Again, I wonder why other doctors hadn't recognized this glaring variable. To repeat: This is an excellent reason to ask seemingly dumb or superfluous questions of new doctors.

Back on the job, I'm outfitted in new leotard-like, knee-high support socks. These, I have to admit, are comfortable and do feel as if they're improving circulation in the lower legs. While driving the nerve-jangling 101, I frequently reposition my legs, wiggling my toes.

In my office, I prop up the left leg whenever possible. Also I have the maintenance crew fashion an elevated wooden footrest under my desk. And lowering the level of my chair improves the incline of the leg.

There is, however, an unmistakable trepidation associated with the damn leg—is a new clot going to abruptly appear, causing more life-or-death problems? Dr. Paravano says a clot, once broken free from its primary site, can travel up the veins of the leg . . . to the lungs . . . to the heart . . . even the brain. Once the clot's begun traveling, she notes gravely, the danger of death is very real.

Can there be any more monsoon-like clouds on the horizon?

FINDING HOPE WHEN DOCTORS SAY THERE IS NONE

CHAPTER 44

THE MUSIC THEY PLAYED—
ANOTHER QUESTIONABLE AREA
TURNS UP ON A CT

After the third cycle of chemo, there's yet another CT to go through. Rationale for the frequency or infrequency of these scans is never spelled out. And still, no one's determined to my satisfaction what this fist-sized thing is within me. This impassioned conflict dogs me constantly.

This time for me, lying on the cold scanner table, the struggle's far more frightening, more foreboding. The days leading up to the procedure bring a series of acute physical (psychosomatic?) warnings: Penetrating pains, precisely where the 'scar tissue' now resides, begin to contract continually, pointedly. Day in and day out, inhaling and exhaling is imagined to be unnatural, more labored (Oh, please, not lung metastases!). My vision seems fuzzy at times (Brain metastases?).

You're never sure.

Are these physical manifestations genuine or just hallucinatory aches and pains my mind's evoked in justifiable fear of this all-seeing diagnostic procedure? If the CT results are favorable, even the fiercest misgivings and pains dissolve in a flash—and seem ludicrous . . . even frivolous. You smile! You laugh! You revel in chilled champagne—for a time.

With this dispiriting scan out of the way, Jane and I sit nervously in Dr. Malone's office. Predictably this small woman comes in exhibiting a certain caution, going through the nonessentials, like blood work, before getting to the CT results. Again, she reads the report while we watch, her face, her eyes, divulging nothing. Masterful at five-card draw, would she be.

"What's the word on the bowel loops or scar tissue or whatever it is?" I venture restlessly.

"It remains visualized," she replies slowly, tentatively. "However, now they're talking about a questionable area . . ." Her inflection trailing off as she continues reading. "The pleural cavity at the base of the left lung; a fluid build-up." This catchword, 'questionable,' when uttered by your oncologist, seems always to foretell of ill tidings.

Damn! Damn! *Damn!* I'm thinking, gazing out the 7th-story window at the stalled lines of chrome and color on the 101.

"What" Jane asks, coughing tightly, "does that mean, doctor?"

Not answering right away, reading further, Dr. Malone replies: "They've noted a trace of effusion—fluid—at the base of the lung. The body's response, I suspect, to the radiation. An irritation, most probably."

Having her offer this as a conceivable rationale for this new concern—the fluid accumulation—helps falsely to restore my frame of mind. "Radiation can do that?" I ask, recalling Dr. Goetz saying radiation can bring about all sorts of strange aftereffects, including the atrophy of the kidney.

"We could biopsy the fluid, but I don't think it's necessary," the doctor volunteers appeasingly. "The best thing, I think, at this point, is just to watch it."

So, instead of hearing in concrete terms what is or is not there relative to the scar tissue, via the CT results, I'm left with even more questions. Troubling mysteries nesting within me. I carry them everywhere.

"What next, doctor?" I ask, demoralized.

"Well," she replies, thumbing through my file, outwardly relieved to be moving on to a new subject, "you have, let's see, one more chemo cycle—"

"Excuse me, doctor," I interrupt, exasperated, "but I believe there are three more cycles."

"Oh, heavens, you're right," she yields unnerved, looking further into the file.

Her impreciseness is further undermining my faith, what limited faith there is. Does she or does not know what the hell she's doing?

"And the other concern—the soft-tissue thing—is still there?" I ask redundantly.

Riffling through earlier CT results, she's comparing numbers. "Actually, Mr. Scribner, it's shrunken a bit," she notes, relieved. "Was 8 cm, now they're saying it's 6."

"All right!" Jane cries, throwing her arms up. "Best news of the day!"

This marginal discovery does, in fact, help lessen the sting of this newest finding—the fluid build up. We leave Dr. Malone's with her saying that she's going to call Dr. Goetz, see what he thinks of this fluid issue in light of the radiation treatments.

All these unanswered questions surging about like so many famished piranhas. I continue working, commuting every day. Allowing the daily grind to immerse me seems to help to a degree. However, the moment the pace slackens, apocalyptic thoughts of a hideous cancer death seep in like flood water under a locked door. I feel yanked in every direction—unworkable schedule demands on the job; on-going chemo-induced listlessness; the ever-present phobia of a new blood clot; once-a-day doses of blood thinner (rat poison?); the incessant monitoring and fine-tuning of coagulation; the next CT and its inevitable mysteries . . .

God, where's it all going to end?

The freeway commute yields too much time to wallow in perpetual negatives . . . unwholesome possibilities. Time and again I find myself neck-deep in a woe-is-me pool of self-pity. Never have I been one to linger on such things, but the feeling of dying, truly leaving this life . . . seems to overwhelm me.

Enmeshed in the maudlin minutiae of my own passing, I find myself in stop-and-go traffic, living out those final moments . . . a panting, short-windedness . . . clutching at life and those about me . . . the pain-racked sorrow . . . the last rites . . . the blathering of well-wishers at a verdant, earth-smelling grave site.

These final-days images are so crushingly real, often my vision's blurry as I try concentrating on other humdrum, workaday commuters . . . applying lipstick, drinking coffee, smoking, cussing at other motorists' maneuvers. Even while caught up in this self-pity I can see the absurdity, the vainglory of it. But the mind's high-handed and has a custom of ripping itself free of your intentions and doing as it damn well pleases . . . . I hate myself, though, for this groveling, this self-pity.

FINDING HOPE WHEN DOCTORS SAY THERE IS NONE

CHAPTER 45

LET US NOT PRETEND—
HOW AM I BETTER OFF *AFTER* CHEMO?

For the next couple of months I continue the twice-a-day commute, go on taking handfuls of daily prescriptions, having a coagulation blood test every 10 days, undergoing chemo the first five days of each month.

Throughout all this lurks a disheartening specter, a sort of cryptic despondency floating above everything: What's *really* going on inside me?

If this disease was only accompanied by explicit signs—pain, some insignificant spasm—something signaling its early presence. In its budding stages, cancer ordinarily offers few if any physical warning signs. The silence that is cancer . . . is its true terror. It's this aspect of the disease—its deadly silence—that people fear most.

Statistically more Americans pass away from heart disease than cancer, yet cancer's the disease people fear most. Quite possibly this is because conventional wisdom holds that people with heart disease die quickly, often quietly in their sleep; with cancer we've been conditioned to anticipate—to accept—an agonizing, humiliating death that can take months, even years.

April 1993: Dr. Malone concludes, for whatever reason, I've had sufficient 5-FU and carboplatin. She terminates treatment at five months, not the six originally planned. She doesn't make known, even when asked, her logic. Is it the prospect of *more* blood clots? I ask. She avoids saying, moving on abruptly to a fresh subject.

More and more it appears that she has no agenda—instead has a hat somewhere she's grabbing answers out of. Nothing she does suggests methodical reasoning. Again, because of my TDKB brainwashing—and the fact the HMO makes changing oncologists near impossible—I accept her unclear decision to terminate treatment. But what had we achieved?

On one occasion at Dr. Malone's office, I unthinkingly ask my friend, the talkative lab technician, how she'd rate the doctors in this oncology group. A straightforward comeback isn't anticipated. Introspective, the light-haired technician doesn't appear as if she's going to answer. My blood specimen, with her watching it, goes on spinning.

"If I . . . were a cancer patient," she begins vaguely, almost whispering, not making eye contact, "I wouldn't come here. But, if for some reason I had to . . . I'd want your doctor."

"You actually said that?" I respond quietly, thunderstruck, feeling her candor create a bizarre cavern within me. "Wow. . . ."

Arched eyebrows, her only rejoinder.

"You're saying . . . the other oncologists are even worse?"

She nods a silent yes. Damn, I shouldn't have posed such a seemingly harmless question. Now the fallout must be dealt with. Needless to say my sense of reliance and trust in Dr. Malone takes an even steeper nosedive.

As touched upon earlier, it's been shown that the more confidence you have in your treatment team, the more likely you are to see a positive outcome from their treatment. So now, along with the myriad misgivings I harbor, I have this second-party lack of confidence to deal with. Where to go . . . what to do—if anything—with this new and disturbing discovery?

Since my chemo's now finished—but how am I better off than when I started?—I figure it's safe to begin Dr. Crandle's timetable for reducing steroid intake. Not in any real haste to let go of this stimulating drug, I begin loping off one milligram of Prednisone every two weeks. I don't bother specifying this to Dr. Malone. She'd most likely say: "That's between you and your endocrinologist."

Two months later: I'm down to four milligrams of steroid per day. Numerous undesirable changes have surfaced. In addition to sore joints and lack of stamina, my heartbeat's often erratic. Dr. Paravano puts me on a 24-hour Holter monitor. From this she concludes that my heart's indeed behaving strangely, increasing in speed just prior to sun-up. A stress-echo heart test with a cardiologist is next.

God, will this dismal parade of doctors never end? Seems everywhere I turn there's a cancer-driven medical controversy glaring me in the eye. This snowballing has a benumbing effect.

While I pass the stress-echo test with flying colors, nothing yet explains away the occasionally erratic heartbeat. My hypothesis: it's related to the Prednisone cutback. Dr. Paravano, on the other hand, thinks it's related to my caffeine consumption—ice tea. The problem does seem to taper off a bit once I discontinue caffeinated tea. But there are still too many episodes where the heart thumps unevenly for my liking.

In July, an ordinary trip to the dentist (one recommended by a neighbor) lands me back in the hospital. More doctors. At the dentist's office, a young dental technician attempts five x-rays of my painful eye-tooth root, missing the uppermost portion each time, before summoning the dentist. Once he's successfully taken the x-ray, this well-seasoned, straw-haired dentist—an individual whose breath is abominable, who has to be reminded over and again to don his surgical mask so as not to spread germs to this recent chemotherapy patient—drills the tooth, extracting the nerve, replacing it with an interim, medicated filling.   Pleasantly, the usually dreaded root-canal procedure goes painlessly well.

Three days later: The temporary filling's removed, replaced with permanent metallic material. Again, I have to prod the malodorous dentist and his assistant to don their protective masks. Chuckling, the dentist carries on about 'the old days,' when he didn't have to fret about transmittable diseases, like AIDS. Washing the exposed root canal with an antiseptic mixture, he presses the metallic material in place.

First day following the procedure: The tooth's slightly tender.

Day two: The gum bordering the tooth and that side of my face look inflamed. Returning, I lie back in the chair while the dentist checks the area, concluding a sequence of penicillin will clear up the tenderness, the inflammation. Next day, Saturday, the tooth and gum are more painful, more swollen. The prescribed penicillin hasn't had any effect. I re-contact the dentist via his emergency line.

He and a tittering teenage girl meet me after hours at his office. He's taking this opportunity to acquaint this girl—his child? a potential dental hygienist? a next-door-neighbor?—as to what's transpired, permitting her to gawk wide-eyed into my mouth—as if it were the open hood of some exotic car—while he digs out the root-canal filler. Again, I have to demand he and his 'assistant' put on surgical masks. Replacing the filler material, the dentist feels, will do the trick—knock out the infection.

The ensuing morning, Sunday: I awaken to nonstop pain, powerful swelling on the entire left side of my face. Again, I call the dentist. In an about-face, he sounds panicky, confounded. He'll call an endodontist, he volunteers gravely, to see if this root-canal expert can see me right away or suggest a quick fix.

An hour later the dentist phones back: He's conferred with an endodontist. The verdict? I should go immediately to the hospital emergency room and be seen by an MD.

FINDING HOPE WHEN DOCTORS SAY THERE IS NONE

CHAPTER 46

RENEWAL OF THE MIND—
A NEW RADIATION ONCODOC AGREES
TO REVIEW UNCERTAIN CT FILMS

One look at the massive facial swelling and discoloration and the ER doctor has me admitted right then. He directs an RN to start three distinct kinds of IV antibiotics. So here I am, back at square one . . . in the despised hospital once more.

Sadly, it seems my entire being is collapsing.

Every minor medical issue now deposits me back in this . . . pseudo nursing home. Cancer, like a soundless, ghostly specter, seems ever prowling in the wings, directing my undoing. And, this grotesque force—cancer—is, apparently, gaining ground. Each time I taste the smallest sense of victory, of moving toward health or normalcy, the disease grabs me by the scruff of the neck, yanking me back, reminding me who—or what—is in charge.

The HMO on-duty doctor, who had approved on the phone my coming here, meets up with me once I'm in a room. This HMO doctor, a fretful fellow in his late thirties, appears new at the trade, behaving excitably. Even with a trace of frenzy. Within an hour, he has an ENT specialist poring over me—ears, nose, and throat.

Both doctors seem unduly disconcerted and animated in their hushed conversation outside my room. To me, we're looking at a simple abscess. Zap it with trusty old antibiotics. No big deal. Not so simple, the ENT doctor clarifies soberly. This breed of infection, he explains, can spread quickly, even invade the brain, creating major problems.

As he speaks, an old sense of danger stirs in me: Reminiscent of the time, in the pre-dawn darkness, I was crouching at a deer stand, perfectly still, bow and arrow ready, mindful of the sudden crunch of bone-dry leaves behind me, certain a cougar was inching nearer, ready to pounce.

During these three tedious days in the hospital, my spirit's no doubt more bruised than is my physical being. The doctors, though alarmed, I'm sure will knock out this infection. I find myself yearning again and again to be that naive little kid . . . walking the Chesapeake shoreline.

Lying here quite still for hours on end, there's little more to think about than the aggressiveness of this ruthless disease, as May winds gently buffet the windows overlooking the distant Pacific. My latest reading, a religious work, has offered a secular meditation: You close your eyes, and keep repeating in your mind what's termed the Centering Prayer: "Lord, Jesus Christ, Son of God, have mercy on me." Focusing entirely on this plea affords a soothing medium for deflecting negative thoughts.

While repeating this Centering Prayer, I petition God, asking Him to radiate down upon me a healing beam of light—not unlike a stage spotlight. In specific regions of my body where I suspect cancer to be re-growing, I imagine narrower, more intense beams within the main healing beam, glowing white hot, burning away malignant cells.

 Liberated from the hospital on day three, I start a series of potent pill-form antibiotics for an additional 10 days. These drugs give me sterile bowel and other awkward intestinal issues. Once adequately cured, it's off to the endodontist to conclude the root-canal procedure. The level of professionalism—and sterility—exhibited by this doctor and his staff is exceptional. Never does anyone not wear a surgical mask or latex gloves. In defiance of the Don't-Say-Anything-Bad-About-Your-Fellow-Dentists brotherhood, this endodontist is visibly dismayed at hearing about the first dentist's manner, techniques.

 Four days after this, I undergo yet another CT of the chest, abdomen, pelvis. While I don't feel any remarkable physical symptoms, there are the predictable pre-scan abdominal spasms, throbs. We are, if nothing else, animals of habit.

 The following week: Dr. Malone tells Jane and me that the scan results are essentially unchanged. Unchanged? Is this good news or bad news? Fluid remains at the base of the left lung, and the troubling 6-cm soft-tissue mass is still there.

 I ask why, if the fluid's a response to radiation treatments, it hasn't diminished since the prior scan a couple of months ago? Dr. Malone offers no credible defense. She contends we should continue 'watching' the areas—as though this were a resolution in itself. This watch-and-see approach in cancer care can prove *extremely* perilous.

 During this period I've been deliberately cutting back my Prednisone intake, thinking, wrongly, that this, as earlier directed by Dr. Crandle, was in my best behalf. When I dutifully communicate this reduction in steroid intake to Dr. Malone, she makes no reply—as though to say, by inference, it's not her concern. The week following the CT scan, my Prednisone intake reaches zero. Almost at once I feel like a balloon without air. Zero energy. All joints, particularly the larger ones, ache brutally.

 A week later, at my next visit with Dr. Crandle, cavorting, he maintains these manifestations are universal, par for the course. He also says the achiness will abate as my remaining adrenal gland, the right one, further 'wakes up' and starts generating its full share of cortisol. "This," he assures me with a twist of sadistic glee, "could take a while."

As I re-enter my responsibilities at Rockwell, listlessness and biting joint pain persists over the next several weeks. Other signs, more troublesome, begin emerging: An utter lack of stamina, profound windedness at mounting a single flight of stairs, insomnia, a growing lack of appetite, unpredictable nausea and vomiting. Even brushing my teeth makes me gag.

Jane, noting these symptoms, becomes worried. Hey, I argue, it's to be expected—part of the withdrawal pattern Dr. Crandle predicted.

"Eric, are you relying on that weirdo's word again?" Jane inquires, appropriately piqued. "I wouldn't believe a word he says. At any rate . . . ." She stops, reflective. "Since you and he are so tight, I think it'd be a good idea to let him know what's going on, particularly the not sleeping and the vomiting part. Since all of this is his doing."

The next morning, on the phone, explaining the circumstances in some detail, fully expecting Crandle to guffaw, to tell me to quit acting like a damn baby, he comes back with: "Oow, this is not good. What I'm hearing are symptoms of acute adrenal crisis. Which means, most likely, you're not producing any cortisol at all. Do you still have some Prednisone on hand?"

I tell him I do.

"Start—right now—taking 10 milligrams. Cut back tomorrow to seven milligrams. Keep taking seven till we can set you up with a cortisol stimulation test. I'll coordinate things with your primary. In the meantime, keep taking the Prednisone."

Within 12 hours, I begin feeling relatively normal. My appetite reappears the following morning; the vomiting, which accompanied even the lightest meal, is gone. Later, when I fill Jane in on Dr. Crandle's feedback, she simply shudders: "What a loser! Why didn't he foresee any of this? He must've been one of those 'C' students in medical school."

"You know, actually, you may have a point," I say, thinking, viewing the situation more clearly in hindsight. "He should've checked my cortisol production before stopping the Prednisone. That's something he should've recognized or suspected. Everything I've read says Mitotane's capable of knocking out all adrenal function—permanently. You're absolutely right: He should've seen this coming."

Putting two and two together, I realize Crandle's been dealing with me, not as an endocrine cancer patient, but as a patient with an adrenal insufficiency problem that would right itself over time.

Three weeks later: The HMO sanctions the cortisol stimulation test. Wonderful, isn't it, how the HMO review process has slowed the pace of medicine to a crawl, to the point where it can be argued that lives are designedly lost for the sake of 'cost effectiveness.'

In the interim, I'm scheduled to have another follow-up exam with Dr. Goetz, the radiation oncologist. Having scheduled this appointment months before, I show up at the radiation center expecting to see him. I am shocked to learn he's had a medical crisis and will be out indefinitely. Signing in, I ask the girls behind the counter what happened. Unexpectedly secretive, they discreetly avoid answering. Another radiation oncologist, Dr. Trilling, they tell me, is seeing Dr. Goetz's patients.

A composed, slow-moving man, Dr. Trilling is in his late sixties, on the short side, all of five-foot-seven. Wire-framed spectacles, nicely combed gray hair. He too accounts vaguely for Dr. Goetz's indefinite absence. Again, no details. My questions are politely skirted. Letting the mystery drop for now, I delicately inquire about this new doctor's qualifications. He's the retired radiation oncology director of a distinguished cancer clinic up the coast. He's looking forward to returning to the freedom of retirement, he tells me, as I peel off my shirt.

He asks, compassionately, why I'm here; what treatments I've undergone. This is, not doctor small talk, but a framework in which to view me, a previously irradiated cancer patient. After hearing some of the procedures, some of the calamities I'd endured, Dr. Trilling nods understandingly, while continuing to palpate my bare abdomen.

"Doctor," I begin as he probes with honest, forceful fingers, "could you possibly do me a huge favor . . . and give me your opinion on my last CT films? There's some kind of fluid build-up at the base of this lung (I indicate the left) and some sort of soft-tissue mass that's appeared after my last surgery, here (I indicate the area). Nobody seems really sure what these represent."

Dr. Trilling readily agrees to re-examine the films, reminding me he's had some 30 years' seasoning in radiation oncology, x-rays, CT scans. At last, maybe I've connected with someone of wisdom who'll render a plausible opinion.

Later, shaking my hand, he says he'll take care of getting the films to review. Little do I realize this benevolent man's about to alter the entire course of my life.

Chapter 47

A New Doctor Presents the Most Impossible of Conclusions

A couple of weeks afterward, still not having started the cortisol stimulation test, I'm sitting in my office at work, in the thick of the things—executives coming and going like ants returning food to the nest—when the phone rings. The indecisive vice president is sitting across the desk in one of his focused, hands-on sessions.

Thinking this is yet another soul within the plant wanting something work-related, I cradle the phone against my ear. It's nearing 10:00 a.m. Burning stress juices are already rampaging across my chest, my gut.

"May I . . . please," a baffling male voice asks guardedly, sounding miles away, "speak with Mr. Scribner?"

"You got him," I comeback as I frequently do, still reasoning it's someone desirous of something work-related.

"Oh, good . . . Eric. This is Dr. Trilling—from the radiation center. You remember, filling in for Dr. Goetz. You asked me to take a second look at your CT films."

"Oh, yes! Dr. Trilling! I remember." Quickly, with a biting flash of apprehension, I shift gears mentally. "How'd . . . everything go?"

"Well, Eric, I've never been one to beat around the bush. It's my conclusion," the doctor's timbre falls appreciably; he clears his throat, "after considerable study, we should get that area—the effusion—biopsied. As promptly as possible."

Swallowing hard, I know exactly what he's implying: The unthinkable. All of this disease's anguish, its torment returns full force. ". . . A biopsy?" I murmur, smarting, hating the very sound of the word.

Looking up as if suddenly prodded with a hot skewer, the VP, discerning what's taking place, stands awkwardly, slinking from the office like a stray dog being yelled at for digging in the trash. Now I'm alone.

Booting the door shut: "It's . . . that big a deal, doctor?" I inquire, swallowing hard, hoping, somehow, to summon from him a reassuring Naw-Eric-It-Ain't-All-That-Bad response.

"I suggest, Eric, we do this promptly." Dr. Trilling's utilizing my name compassionately, as if he understands, cares. "My conjecture is—and I've seen a lot of these—we're looking at a new malignancy."

His words falling like lead pellets. The core of my spirit's trembling. Immediately, sweat's appeared under my arms, on my face. Oh God, no, no, no, no, no, no, no! Not again! Not this soon!

"You really think . . ." I hesitate, caught remarkably unprepared for this, not knowing what to ask or what I'm saying. "Could you . . . I mean . . . have this confused?"

"If only that were the case," he says, pausing kindly. "It's those nodules I'm most concerned with."

"I don't follow. What nodules?"

"Those your first radiologist cited. In his narrative."

I hadn't insisted on a Xerox of the CT report (which you, as a cancer patient, should always do) from Dr. Malone. So I hadn't read or seen any mention of nodules. In my recollection, Dr. Malone hadn't intimated this.

"Most likely," Dr. Trilling explains, "this condition . . . is indicative of a new metastatic finding."

All he's saying—the truth of what he's saying—is being blanked out. Always I've feared hearing that word—metastasis—used in reference to me, my condition. Now, it's surfaced. And right here—in this indifferent, corporate office.

"What . . ." I implore childishly, feeling incredibly isolated, "do you recommend . . . next?"

"I'll call Dr. Malone," he answers. "Relate to her what I've advised you. The rest . . . I'll leave to you two."

Numb, I hear myself asking what a biopsy would entail.

"The procedure itself is relatively uncomplicated," he explains, wording things now more airily as though describing something clear-cut, something he's more comfortable with. "We utilize a CT-guided needle. The whole procedure may take an hour or so. You can expect some discomfort."

Once Dr. Trilling is off the phone, I call Jane. She instantly perceives my state of mind. She doesn't seem as bummed by the news, however, for various reasons: (1) she's inclined toward screening unfavorable information more impartially, (2) she's less pessimistic in general, and (3) conceivably the biopsy could turn out negative.

Hanging up, I linger for God knows how long—maybe 10 minutes, maybe a half-hour—in my cramped office, my eyes remaining on a jagged crack in the opposite wall. My mind, in flame-bursts, is reliving the horrors of this cancer . . . as my concern for the day's business agenda, the day's activities dissolves.

My gray-haired, fifty-something aide-de-camp and reliable backer, Eleanor, taps delicately at the door. Astutely, she's perceived something's profoundly wrong.

"Oh, no, Eric—not the demon again?" she asks, sitting where the VP had.

Without looking at her, I grant: "Damn doctor just phoned . . . says he's spotted something new. Something bad."

It isn't the message that annoys me so: I'll be forever indebted to Dr. Trilling for taking the time to reread my films and calling me. But information of this nature should only be communicated face-to-face between you and your physician. Today's time-delayed HMO medicine, however, won't often allow it.

Gripping the arms of her chair, Ellie says: "No, Eric, not this soon. Is he sure? This can't be." Honest concern in her voice: She is, after all, a breast cancer survivor herself.

"One in a million, he's wrong," I concede, liking to hear myself say these encouraging words. "One can dream. But the truth is . . . this doctor seems to know more than all of my other doctors put together."

"He's not the one you've been seeing?"

"He's filling in. Doing follow-up for the radiation oncologist. Guess I should be thankful he is."

"Damn," Ellie mutters quietly, reliving the depths of my distress, as I know only she, another survivor, can. "What now?" she asks, knowing all I've been through already.

"We've got to determine what's there. Biopsy, he's saying."

"That's only a test, Eric."

At this, I grin. "Ellie, I understand what you're trying to do. But we all know better. I've had a lot of things going on lately inside me that my oncologist hasn't been able to get a handle on. If she even cares. This fellow, unfortunately, has confirmed my worst suspicions."

The sterile work place's no place to sit, to dwell on life's most heinous news. In the car, a half-hour later, these grim thoughts become more focused and are underscored by the endless freeway stripes, the lament of the car's tires on the pavement.

Once at home, I find I'm greatly angered. Calling Dr. Malone's office, I want to challenge her. She's unavailable. She'll call me back. To get things off my chest, I rant and rave to whoever's on the other end of the phone about Dr. Trilling's call, the need for a biopsy.

Dusk. A bleeding sun, out over the Pacific, is outlining a shocking pink and purple skyline. I'm gazing from the bedroom window. Lethargically I'm exercising, riding the stationary bike, my mind miles away, when Jane gets home from work. She stops, dumbfoundedly, in the bedroom doorway.

"Called your office earlier," she offers, walking by, giving me a kiss. "Whoever picked up the phone said you'd left, sounding weird. I thought if anything, you'd be meditating or involved in doing some relaxation activity. Not this."

"That's come and gone. Exercise helps displace the anxiety," I reply, actually feeling a sense of diversion from the pedaling. "Physical movement."

"So you called what's-her-name? Dr. Malone?"

"The minute I walked in."

"And her take on this?"

"She's supposed to call . . . eventually. Ain't holding my breath. She was naturally tied up."

"You short-change her, Eric, I think," Jane goes on, changing clothes. "I think she's a lot more on your side than you think."

I offer no comment, knowing to do so will only occasion a dispute.

"So, tell me, what's that little pea-brain of yours cooked up in response?" Jane jokes after a minute. "I know you've got ideas."

"I'm working on it, you're right," I respond, hearing myself say this for the first time. "Another face-to-face with the folks in Houston is a good possibility. Getting them involved. Seems they're the only ones who don't shoot from the hip."

An hour afterward: Jane's sautéing onions for spaghetti sauce. She picks up the ringing kitchen phone. Her end of the dialogue: "Oh, yes, Dr. Malone! He heard from that other doctor today—the one from the Radiation Center . . . (Pause) Um-hm, filling in for Dr. Goetz. (Pause) Dr. Trilling, I believe is his name. Apparently, he wants Eric to have some sort of biopsy . . . Sure, hold on."

Jane passes me the phone.

"Mr. Scribner," Dr. Malone begins emphatically, a detectable edge to her voice. "You spoke today with some other doctor, as I understand?"

"That's correct. Like Jane said, Dr. Trilling. He feels that due to the nodules—that appeared in my earlier CT—he'd very much like to see a biopsy . . . right away."

"That doctor, Mr. Scribner, really overstepped his bounds. You're my patient. He should've cleared all this through me before even thinking of calling you. You've been, I'm afraid, unduly alarmed."

A defensive anger sears in me. "Hold on a minute, doctor," I reply, trying to suppress my exasperation and express some of my disillusionment. "Why didn't you say anything about these nodules?"

A superficial hesitation, "I indicated we could get a biopsy," she replies defensively.

"Yes, but," I counter, "I understood you to mean that soft-tissue mass. These nodules he's talking about are apparently in the lung area."

"Perhaps," she offers, provoked, "we miscommunicated."

Doing my best to control my words: "Dr. Malone, I told you early on in our relationship I wanted to maintain the most aggressive approach possible. I relied on you for guidance. This doesn't sound like what I'm hearing. At our last couple of meetings, you said, as I recall, all you wanted to do was watch these areas."

Another pause. I visualize her mentally asking herself why she shouldn't tell this patient to go to hell. "What is it you expect of me, Mr. Scribner?"

"I want you to be up-front with me, doctor," I say determinedly. "If there's a problem, I want to know about it. So I can react. Do something." As the words come out, I recognize, at that instant, this is sort of a new beginning: I'm becoming more tenacious, less dependent on the TDKB principle. "I'm thinking of taking my films and going to Houston. See how they piece all this together."

"Can you," Dr. Malone responds brusquely, "come to the office tomorrow, Mr. Scribner?"

CHAPTER 48

MOVING ON TOWARD A BIOPSY

The next day Jane and I find ourselves sitting in one of Dr. Malone's tiny exam rooms, waiting. I'm musing on life seven stories below. Jane's thumbing through a magazine. A drizzly, silver day. Always I'm amazed at how detached from reality the cars on the freeway seem. Like some never-ending, schizophrenic snake, constantly on the move, heading everywhere... and nowhere.

"You're thinking you're through with her," Jane's saying as she tosses aside an obsolete Auto Club magazine, picking up another, "aren't you?"

Weighing this, I watch the freeway come to halt in both directions.

"Trust's a major part of this. How you see your doctor. I never really felt a whole lot of connection with this person." I stop a moment, thinking whether I want to go on, whether I want to hear myself disclose this festering wound within. Finally, I resume: "Now, I guess, I can admit that. Till now I've worked pretty hard at convincing myself she's on the right track. But I can't escape the feeling she doesn't like me. Yes, I know, I'm being paranoid. Maybe she's just frightened by men in general. *Something.*"

"Your imagination, Eric, as usual, is in outer space."

"Okay," I say, somewhat annoyed. "Take that time with the ACTH blood test. The results came back showing my level was through the roof and she was going to accept those numbers as a lab error and do nothing. I'm the one who suggested we do a re-test. Then there was the time she was thumbing through my file—you were there—and she wanted to discontinue my chemo at four months instead of the planned-on six. It's like she has no clue what's going on. And what about the fact she *did* halt my chemo at five months, instead of six. All with no justification. And now there's this situation—where she didn't tell me about these nodules. It's about time, I think, to move on."

No sooner do these words leave my mouth, when Dr. Malone marches in, the air at once seeming more fragile.

"That other radiologist, Mr. Scribner, Dr. Trilling," Dr. Malone begins in a huff, going to and leaning immediately on the counter on the opposite end of the cramped room, "should never have spoken directly with you."

This she says as if to shut all doors, satisfy all doubts. As though Dr. Trilling's violating medicine's sacred trust had neutralized his discoveries. I, however, will be infinitely indebted for his chutzpah, his 'thoughtlessness.' It's stimulating to see a physician of principle, such as him.

"That's a matter of opinion, doctor," I respond, feeling now a sense of equality brought on by my earlier-admitted disavowal of her. "As I said yesterday and many times prior to that, it's my intention to continue the most aggressive approach possible in attacking this disease. That's my position. The rest I leave to you—figuring you know what's best."

"Are you inferring something, Mr. Scribner?"

"My point is this—I'd feel more at ease getting this biopsy out of the way as soon as possible."

"That other doctor," she reiterates, tensing her lean, already folded arms, "should never have distressed you this way."

"Dr. Malone," I respond, looking her dead in the eye, "you're upset with him. I'm thinking he's a hero. He did what's right. A patient should be told what he's facing—and how to deal with it."

"Mr. Scribner, " she goes on impassively, "the manner in which we were dealing with your situation was entirely adequate."

At this, I smirk. "Doctor, adequate's not a good word. I want us in there kicking butt." Stating this, I feel suddenly uncomfortably masculine in this close-knit feminine setting.

"So be it," Dr. Malone replies, as if to cleanse her hands of the affair. "I'll prepare the paperwork for a biopsy."

"Since I'm here, doctor," I venture, "lately I've had a couple of bouts of uneven heart rhythms." I pause, watching her mouse-gray eyes watch me. "I'm a bit concerned. It's the same situation I had before my last surgery."

"In that case, Mr. Scribner," she replies mechanically, scrawling on a note pad, "I'll send a request for an echo-EKG as well. We might as well see if there's some involvement with radiation scarring and the heart muscles."

Heart and scar tissue involvement? This remark, made for whatever motive, has me instantly alarmed. Seems doctors will often use their status to get in that last dig.

"You had her pissed off," Jane complains in the car.

"Maybe that was my intent. Does it matter?" I reply. "Isn't it better to confess you have no trust in somebody and move on?"

"This is all a big misunderstanding, Eric—and you're going to regret it."

"Then why didn't you *say* something?"

"You know you don't mean that."

"Look, Jane, I know this sounds trite as hell, but fate only doles out one life per person. You know how many midnights I've laid there, deliberating. A good deal of laying awake was brought on by this doctor; how she doesn't know her ass from a hole in the ground. Or, maybe, she just doesn't care."

"Sometimes, Eric," Jane goes on, "you have a real twisted way of looking at things. She responded to your call last night, for heaven's sake."

"Jane, she was going down her damn call-back list."

"She cares. She's a dedicated physician!"

"Honey," I say, "you're still trapped in the antiquated notion that doctors are invariably right. If we don't look out for ourselves, no one will."

While I feel better about taking greater charge of my care, and recognizing the various illogical things Dr. Malone has and has not done, I harbor acute fears as well: Of instability, of being set adrift—having no one to turn to.

Three days afterward: Dr. Paravano's nurse calls, setting up the cortisol stimulation test. It's now been about a month since Dr. Crandle called Dr. Paravano launching this. The HMO has at last consented.

Now, each morning, prior to going to work, I drive 10 minutes in the opposite direction, to the HMO clinic. Day One of the cortisol stimulation test, Dr. Paravano has me substitute one tiny dexamethesone pill for my normal dosage of Prednisone. (Dr. Paravano's carrying out the test because the HMO believes it's not essential to have an endocrinologist—Dr. Crandle—do it.) I have an injection of ACTH that morning, a blood draw to observe cortisol levels the next. This routine continues for six days.

Days after the test's concluded, Dr. Paravano telephones, telling me to resume taking Prednisone at seven milligrams per day: Results of the cortisol stimulation test, she says, indicate I'm not producing any cortisol.... I'm so glad that cocky Dr. Crandle put me through that arbitrary Prednisone-reduction hell without first being aware whether my body was producing this crucial adrenal steroid.

While awaiting the HMO's consent for the biopsy and ultrasound heart test, I continue formulating an outline for one more pilgrimage to Houston.

Coincidentally, the annual M.D. Anderson Patient Network conference's scheduled for early September. I've long thought about attending one of these three-day, cancer-patient-oriented gatherings where doctors and patients come together conferring in non-medical surroundings. Now that I've resolved to take my plight to the MDA doctors, I rationalize I can kill two birds with one stone: Be present at the conference *and* see the endocrine cancer specialists.

Late August 1993. Paperwork comes through consenting to the biopsy, the heart test. I'm instructed to see a community pulmonologist, a private doctor not directly under the thumb of the HMO. This means, of course, he's more thorough, more aboveboard in his overall evaluation of the condition.

Dr. Norman's a fellow of about 40, a onetime Air Force official . . . so it says on the sleek plaques on the waiting room wall. A meager-boned guy, he's just about six foot, with smooth, camel-colored hair, an open-minded disposition.

Sitting at his desk, rather than in a lifeless exam room, we review the purpose of this visit. With me are the CT films Dr. Trilling had examined. Dr. Norman proposes we review them together.

With the individual films—perhaps seven of them—arranged on an illuminated wall, Dr. Norman slips on his reading spectacles, moving soberly from film to film.

"You understand these at all, Mr. Scribner?" he asks graciously.

Caught off guard, I respond, "Pretty much. I had some training reading industrial x-rays years ago."

He now takes me on a condensed tour of the CT procedure: "Your feet are down here," Dr. Norman explains, pointing to base of the first film. "We're looking up, toward your head. The scanner's taking 10 millimeter slices of your abdomen and chest."

He's explaining this process, evidently, so we can start on equal footing.

"The image we see here," he's pointing to a gray oval on one of the films, "is that soft-tissue mass they're talking about in the left adrenal area." He moves on, to another film, nodding, saying, "Um-hm," to himself.

"Now we're looking at your lungs," he goes on. "From the feet up again, remember. And this," he circles a crescent-shaped area with his finger, "is the fluid we're concerned with."

With his explaining the CT process, these images become recognizable. His style seems so unconfined, so leisurely I can't conceive of him giving me bad news. Entranced am I by his interpretations of the films. I'm also betraying myself.

"Do you feel anything at all—in that area?" he asks, looking at me over his half-glasses. "When you breathe deeply, or exert yourself?"

"Nothing abnormal," I reply, hoping he'll say: 'Well, in that case, the silly biopsy's not necessary—this *isn't* a malignancy. It's a such and such. I've seen hundreds of them and they're all harmless.'

Dr. Norman's kneading his smooth chin, scrutinizing once more the crescent outline in the lung area.

"Mr. Scribner, I've got to say this," he commences unemotionally. "I've never seen one of these effusive conditions, like this . . . that wasn't a malignancy. Cancer."

The office backdrop now implodes around me. An immense foreboding, an awareness of burning, encircles me. All I want to believe is true is being shattered. Once more. "But doctor," I plead, "I feel fine. No coughing, no shortness of breath —nothing!"

"Eric," Dr. Norman continues, now using my first name, "I've seen patients with three times this amount of effusion—fluid around the lungs—and still feel nothing. Not exhibit any symptoms."

An abrupt expanse appears between us. It's me, I know—I'm forcing this hopeless account through my uncooperative filters, not his.

We now proceed to an exam room. As he gives me a meticulous physical, I disclose my thoughts about going to MDA for another opinion. At this, he smiles—obviously supportive of a patient striving for the best.

He wraps the stethoscope loosely about his neck. "An excellent idea!" he offers, pausing for a second. "You see, in all honesty, we, here, don't perform these sort of biopsies all that often. But they do, the doctors at Anderson. Not that we can't do them, but if I were you, I'd want to go where they do this sort of thing on a routine basis."

My stunned psyche's immediately consoled.

"In fact, if you're serious about going there," he continues, "I'll second the motion. If that'll help."

By the time I leave his office, I believe Dr. Norman's a compatriot of sorts—at least an individual of considerable goodness, not an HMO lackey.

The ball, once again, is in my court.

FINDING HOPE WHEN DOCTORS SAY THERE IS NONE

CHAPTER 49

FLIGHT OF FANTASY—
BACK TO HOUSTON FOR REASSURANCE

September 5, 1993: The immense cloak of brownish-yellow sludge below, beneath the plane's wings, indeed as far as the eye can see, looks contemptible—like the remnants of some disturbing, self-concocted nightmare. The four-hour flight, despite the plane being chock full, seems . . . well, forsaken. From my window seat, I'm reflecting on the dreary artery-like network of dirt roads below . . . the isolated dwellings of loners . . . the far edge of this world.

"Hard to explain, babe," I say, turning slowly from the window, "but I still say it's unfair—having this friggin' disease . . . and not having any pain. Doesn't make sense."

"That's because," Jane replies, accepting a Pepsi and peanuts from a gray-haired stewardess, "you don't have the disease."

"Aren't we being charitable today," I respond, accepting a plastic glass of orange juice. "What changed Miss Pro-Malone's mind?"

"Let's leave that back home, okay?" she says good-naturedly. "You know I've always been on your team. Despite what you think."

To neutralize my frame of mind, I need a shot of booze: But I'm still not allowed alcohol because of the blood thinner. This is to be no joyous excursion, for sure. There *can* be a degree of enjoyment, nonetheless: We're planning to attend MDA's Patient Conference, possibly connecting face-to-face other ACC patients.

The HMO, remarkably—with Dr. Bristol's urging I'm sure—has agreed to pay for the needed tests and biopsy at M.D. Anderson. (No one, as yet, has told me that the HMO will also reimburse airfare and lodging expenses. If one knows how to ask for it.)

This time there's no bundle of CT scans in the overhead bins: When I spoke with my new MDA endocrinologist, he proposed I FedEx the films in advance, so he and his associates could review them. There's a peculiar, remotely violated feeling, being miles above the earth, watching kaleidoscopic patches of grassland pass below, knowing a crew of doctors in a city 2000 miles away is reviewing my CT films, pointing to shadowy images, forming opinions—all this minus the attached flesh-and-blood human being.

Thus far, the obvious watchfulness of this new MDA doctor's been remarkable. As part of his review he wants me to undergo a 24-hour urine test to identify specific excreted steroids. He has his nurse lay out details as to how to get the vessel, after hours at the clinic.

We arrive at the seven-story Rotary House Hotel at roughly 8:00 p.m. Air temperature's positively invigorating, tropical. Delightful sultriness on the bare skin—a welcome contrast from California's perpetually dry weather. Reminiscent, this feeling is, for a split second, of my fondly remembered youth on Maryland's summer beaches.

This is our initial stay at this hotel, dedicated principally to housing MDA patients and family. It's located across the boulevard from MDA's hospital and clinics. Going to and from MDA you traverse an enclosed bridgeway. On rainy or sticky days, the short bridgeway affords shelter.

At check in, the hotel clerk (the staff's been specially trained to interact with fragile-minded cancer patients) explains that my MDA agenda—list of appointments—is in our room. "Please, glance through it right away, Mr. Scribner," the young lady says cordially, "and see that, relative to scheduled times, it meets with your approval."

In the six-floor room, Jane unpacks. I'm inspecting tomorrow's timetable—a single, computer-generated sheet.

"Can you believe this place?" Jane asks, pausing, hanging up a shirt. "They even furnish a printout of what's going to happen. Pret-ty impressive, I'd say."

"Always the pushover for efficiency," I reply, stretching out on the bed. "Already, though, I feel more grounded. Like coming home." Studying the agenda, I note that I'm scheduled for blood work the following morning. Eight o'clock.

"You okay being here?" I ask Jane. "I mean you're being so . . . companionable."

"I don't really disagree with anything you do. Once you've made up your mind."

Even though the MDA clinic's technically closed at this hour—8:30 p.m.— I go over to the Endocrine Section and pick up the 24-hour urine receptacle. This drill, to my way of reasoning, will render a test of the staff's expertise: Will the container be where it's supposed to be . . . or will someone have forgotten to 'hide' it for me?

In the ghostly murkiness of the seventh-floor Endocrine Section, I go to the nurses' desk, as instructed—and, there on the carpeted floor, is a paper bag. Bold letters spell out my name.

Next morning, before eating, we traverse the bridgeway, heading for the eight o'clock blood draw. The lab area's jammed with cancer patients, of assorted ages, in different phases of therapy. I have only a brief wait.

Next destination, at 10:30, is for a CT scan. My new endocrinologist wants a up-to-date scan, generated by this facility, for correlation. He's asked for—and remarkably been given—consent by my HMO. (Dr. Bristol, I suspect, has okayed this.)

The scanning procedure here's different. Don a hospital gown and remain, waiting in an icy room, for an available scanner, with as many as 10 other patients. During the wait, three sociable RNs circulate, starting IVs to expedite the CT process. By the time the scan's completed, it's near midday. Still, I haven't eaten. We head downstairs, to the cafeteria.

The trek to the swarming cafeteria offers a fearful sense of *esprit de corps*—pale-skinned, hairless children; grown-ups in wheelchairs; others pulling small oxygen tanks; some bandaged curiously. Eating, I find myself communicating with others, with a slight nod, an inexplicable awareness of community. Reminiscent, this is, tragically, of a combat zone. This carnage, though, hasn't been perpetrated by bullets or napalm but by modern medical therapies designed to treat malfunctioning bodies.

There's now time to ease off, to relax a bit. Back in the room, with my legs propped near the massive window overlooking the grassy courtyard, I'm remotely conscious of being poised at branching roads: Where's this expedition ultimately leading me? In a best-case scenario, I'm hoping—yes, as I'm wont to do—the doctors will compare the scans, laugh quietly, slap me on the back, saying Dr. Malone's approach—watching and waiting—is justifiable, no misgivings here.

Through the window, across the boulevard, at the mouth of the imposing rose-hued MDA facade, ant-size people are coming and going, coming and going, a soul-deep fear eating at all of them.

"Did I tell you . . ." I commence, hearing myself say this aloud, "that Dr. Trilling finally told me what happened to Dr. Goetz? Why he's out on medical."

"Can't say as you did," Jane says, reclining on the bed, hands behind her head.

"Brain aneurysm. Woke up one morning and couldn't move one whole side of his body."

"You're kidding."

"Nope. That's the reason he gave."

"How old is Goetz?" she asks, looking curiously my way.

"Hell, early forties would be my guess."

"Just the other day," Jane says, "I was reading . . . where people who mess with certain drugs sometimes get brain aneurysms."

"Him, you think?"

"He's talkative as any used-car salesman, overly friendly. Maybe that's the reason."

"Now who's going overboard?" I say, recalling some of the eccentric things this doctor's said, done. "He would have access, though."

On one elbow, Jane questions: "When's he due back?"

"Trilling didn't know. Maybe . . . never."

"Poor guy. Had it so good."

Our room—perfectly equipped with large-screen TV and VCR, room-darkening drapes, a generous closet, ironing board and iron, and kitchenette with fridge, microwave, toaster, dishes, flatware, garbage disposal—is intensely silent, well shielded from the bustling world below. A benevolent dwelling for cancer patients to withdraw, observe seclusion.

1:30: Checking in at the fifth-floor nurses' station, I appreciate a sign above the nurses' desk: *If you find your wait longer than 20 minutes, please return to this desk.* This breed of patient-oriented concern I like. I'm sitting with other frightened patients who're hugging bulky medical files. Close to 20 minutes go by. A nurse calls my name. Jane and I accompany her to an examination room.

Taking my vital signs, the nurse, a tall woman with a refined but business-like attitude, says the doctor will be in momentarily. She directs me to disrobe, put on a gown.

With the nurse departed, Jane observes quietly: "Why the gown? Thought this was supposed to be a consultation. You did notice the signs as we came in."

"Dept. of Surgery? That one?"

"Are we . . . in the right place?"

"They called my name."

"Seems sort of . . . weird."

"God willing," I volunteer, cringing at the significance of being in the department of surgery, "this is where my new doctor sees his patients. Or, who knows, maybe every patient sees a surgeon; some kind of new system. Doctors here work in teams, you know." As I speak these words, they give birth to a familiar sense of premonition.

Chapter 50

As Smoke Becomes Fire—
Surgery's Scheduled . . . *Again*

Within minutes a dark-haired, athletic-looking guy in his early forties shows up. A collection of CT films, as well as a file jacket, is under his arm. He seems all business and in a hurry.

"Mr. Scribner," he says, pumping my hand, "Mrs. Scribner," he goes on, grasping Jane's. "I'm Dr. Elliot. I've studied your films, except for today's, and," he goes on, sitting on a stool, "I need to know how soon you can be ready for surgery?"

Before I can even gulp, this fellow's cut to the quick. "Whoa, doctor," I say trying to grin, to assimilate what's taken place in the last 10 seconds. "I think there's been an error. I merely came here for a biopsy, another opinion . . . now you want to open me up?"

"You have an obvious recurrent neoplasm, Mr. Scribner," Dr. Elliot proceeds, "which requires resecting. Did you not have this in mind?"

This is breaking so abruptly I have no time—like a wounded bird—to find shelter. "Well, actually, no," I say, clearing my throat. "You're catching me off guard, a little. I had hoped you'd agree with my local oncologist's view of things and I'd be on my way. It was just nine months ago I had major surgery."

Unswayed, he motions for me to stand. He examines me convincingly, with forceful surgeon-like hands. Poking here and there, checking lymph nodes, checking for anything out of the ordinary . . . digging, digging, digging. When he requires I drop my drawers, I tell Jane to step outside—not because of self-consciousness, but because the prostate exam's somewhat crude. Satisfied all's okay, the doctor opens the door, motioning for Jane's return.

"I take it you've seen these films, Mr. Scribner?" he asks, heading out the open door, beckoning us to follow. Down a short hallway, in another room with a lighted wall, Dr. Elliot sticks the films, about six of them, up for review. He slips on his tortoise-shell glasses.

"This area," he's saying, circling with his finger the familiar grayish oval shape, "is what troubles us most."

"Oh, that," I say with relief. "That's been there since my last surgery, since my radiation treatments, anyway. It's just a chunk of scar tissue." I feel exonerated announcing news that promises to relax the doctor's hard-edged approach.

"Really?" the doctor asks dramatically, a la Perry Mason. "How did you determine that?"

"Well," I begin, feeling his words now plugging into some panic circuitry in my mind, recalling nuns grilling me in grade school because I *looked* guilty, "my doctors in California say so."

Dr. Elliot nodding almost mockingly. "How did they reach this conclusion?"

"Well," I proceed uncertainly, "the mass . . . hasn't changed since I had radiation."

"Changed how?"

"Gotten bigger or smaller."

"What do your California doctors recommend you do about it?"

An opportunity to play my ace. "Nothing. We're watching it," I reply authoritatively, as if this 'oncological term' will quiet his skepticism.

Dramatically removing his glasses, Dr. Elliot looking me dead in the eye: "What are you watching it do, Mr. Scribner—kill you?"

All of my bodily functions seem to shut down instantly. I'm hollow . . . suspended in this new foreboding. . . . 'What're you watching it do, Mr. Scribner—kill you?' Searing words. Clearing my throat, I feel indeed a child in the wilderness, stammering: "Well . . ."

"This may well be scar tissue, Mr. Scribner," the doctor concedes. "But more likely it represents a recurrence. It's our educated opinion that whatever this is, it doesn't belong. Have you considered this?"

"In . . . the back of my mind, but not that I want to admit," I reply, envisioning myself again in pain, in the hospital. "I just *had* surgery, doctor."

"This, as you probably know, is an unpredictable cancer. At Anderson, we've seen cases like this where patients thought they were living with post-surgery scarring, only to discover, much later, sometimes years later, it was indeed a malignancy and now it's metastasized."

Blocking all avenues of escape—he is, after all, the expert. "You've actually . . . seen cases like this before?"

"Often enough."

As we converse, I pray there's something—anything—we could laugh about . . . something we could all summon up and chuckle about. But there's nothing. Only fright. This has become profoundly ugly business—once again.

"Looking through your file a while ago," the doctor resumes, leafing through pages, "I didn't see a copy of your surgical report—the last one. Did you happen to bring one?"

"My God," I ask, still caught off guard by this guy's doggedness, "do you really need all this at this point?"

"Before we do anything surgically, I'll will."

Fishing through my day planner, which I always have with me since it holds my computer medical record, I hand him the surgeon's business card, suggesting he have his nurse call and get a faxed copy. Dr. Elliot excuses himself briefly. Returning, he says his nurse's making the call. All of this seems too machine-like, too onerous. Like being flung before a charging locomotive.

"Actually, doctor," I presevere, "the whole purpose of this trip was to get another opinion. On this fluid." I point to the crescent-shaped area on the films. "This area. The mass—something we thought was scar tissue—didn't seem that big a deal."

"Indeed. Our next concern is that fluid," he responds matter-of-factly. "In fact, that may prove our undoing. If this effusion's malignant—which I suspect it is—surgery's out of the question."

His words cause the blood to thicken behind my eyes, a new chasm of hopelessness opens within. "Why . . ." I ask cautiously, my throat gone suddenly bone-dry, "would that be?"

"Because," Dr. Elliot says popping on his glasses once more, "if the effusion—this fluid—has within it malignant cells, there's no point in operating to remove the other. Not when there's tumor seeding in the pleural area. Do you see what I'm saying, Mr. Scribner? The malignancy may already be at the cellular level . . . in the fluid. Understand?"

Instantly, I dislike this man, his reference to 'seeding,' as though I were some scrap of indifferent, fallow ground. Asking for further clarification, I'm trying, primarily, to stave off the unavoidable.

"You see, Mr. Scribner," he goes on, striving now to blend professionalism with mercy, as if recalling some patient-doctor workshop role-playing session, "if there are any malignant cells in the fluid, this would suggest the disease could be anywhere."

"In . . . my body."

"Exactly."

A nurse taps on the door—startling me—sticking her head in, handing the doctor a fax.

"Wow, that's service," Dr. Elliot observes, smiling, as if this worldly intrusion could disrupt the tautness. "Sometimes the velocity of technology astonishes even me." He skims the two-page surgical narrative, shaking his head, uttering, "Um," thoughtfully at one point.

"What's wrong?" I ask reluctantly.

"This business with the tumor being cut into," he replies, shaking his head. "Not what we like to hear. That's most likely the reason these cells were able to migrate beneath the diaphragm."

"Creating the effusion?" I continue, the silhouette of Dr. Tzu standing over my bed in ICU, his cruel words, coming back.

"It would appear, Mr. Scribner," Dr. Elliot goes on soberly, in a canned-sermon fashion. "One word of advice: Never ever have complicated cancer surgery done by a doctor who's never been there before—or done it only sparingly. It breaks my heart seeing people come here after they have been mistreated—either with chemo or surgery—by inexpert local doctors. I tell everyone to always go to one of the major cancer centers across the country . . . for cancer treatment of any kind. This is where you're going to find state-of-the-art medicine."

"So . . . what's all this boil down to, doctor, this problem in the surgical report?"

"Basically this," Dr. Elliot explains. "We want to remove the soft-tissue mass so there's no further confusion as to what it is, but we can't—if what we're seeing here (he points to the effusion again) is malignant. That's the point."

"You're saying, then, I could be . . . inoperable?"

"A good chance." While trying to appear concerned, he's still too business-like. "From what I'm reading here."

Right away I feel angry about this man not being more aware, more conscious of patients' emotions, when we're confronted with words like inoperable. Surely he's seen what such a label can do to a patient. (In hindsight, I may've been too impassioned—but when it's your very survival, your life that's at stake . . .)

"What next?" I ask, feeling my sense of etiquette slipping away.

"We'll need a biopsy of that fluid before we can do anything. When can you be ready for surgery—if the biopsy's negative?"

In vacuum of fear, I stammer: "Well, shit, I don't know. Hadn't anticipated things coming out like this. I was looking to have maybe a simple biopsy then head home . . ." Quickly, in my head, I'm calculating my work schedule, whether the HMO will even sanction this. "Couple of weeks, maybe?"

"Sounds good." Dr. Elliot stands, offering his hand once more. Smiling cordially, he tells us his nurse will be in shortly to go over his surgery calendar.

Jane and I are now isolated in this suffocating room. An enormous vortex unexpectedly emerges, sucking away our sentiment for life. Inoperable, that dreaded utterance, now may apply to me; a death sentence, plain and simple.

Jane, too, is unmistakably stricken, sitting in a cold metal chair, her thoughts written plainly on her bloodless face. Grief on the inside's working its way to the surface. I'm hoping that she can pull off one of her, Oh-This-Is-No-Big-Deal remarks, but no. Her being, though, is refusing to react as negatively as mine.

Minutes drag by, neither of us saying a thing. Muffled air streaming through the wall vents is like thunder. Re-entering, the nurse ushers in a sense of wakefulness—of real time, of humanity. "We can schedule the surgery for the 29th," she offers. "About two weeks . . . . Does that suit you?"

FINDING HOPE WHEN DOCTORS SAY THERE IS NONE

CHAPTER 51

AND WE SHALL BE CHANGED—
MY FIRST MEETING WITH ANOTHER
ACC PATIENT

The following afternoon, after a sleepless night, I have my first face-to-face encounter with another human being fighting adrenal cortical carcinoma. Leigh's her name. We're both attending the MDA Patient Conference at a large Houston hotel. In her late thirties, very self-assured, Leigh's married and has two young boys. Speech therapy had been her vocation—her life's passion—prior to her incapacitating run-in with ACC.

Leigh's right adrenal is the one that's been affected. During a nine-plus-hour surgery at MDA, a massive adrenal tumor—nearly eight pounds—was removed together with the right kidney and a good portion of her liver.

Talking with this wonderfully up-beat lady—another being who's suffering from the identical rare disease—feels . . .well, strangely like conversing with a mirror. She, too, seems almost speechless at meeting another person who talks, who understands, the 'foreign' language of this rare endocrine cancer.

At one of the conference's breakout sessions—ironically addressing doctor-patient relationships—Leigh and I sit in adjoining plastic chairs, a soft distance apart, sensing an unspoken intimacy, as our arms, our shoulders, frequently touch; a spontaneous bonding. We share a singular, an undesirable link: a deadly disease.

Prior to the session and as it progresses, we're oblivious to the speakers. Leigh, leaning my way, whispering softly of her ill fortune with doctors—how they only begrudgingly lent an ear to her complaints of early ACC symptoms; that these same doctors began taking her complaints seriously, running hormone and adrenal-function tests. (Regrettably, this is an account heard all too often: Doctors who don't, won't listen. [See Appendix C: The Perfect Doctor].)

By then, Leigh tells me ruefully, it may already have been too late: Her condition may have been so advanced it was only manageable, and then, only for a time.

Over the next six months Leigh and I talk often on the phone, offering encouragement and comparing treatment notes, frequently running up large long-distance charges. This camaraderie provides a sense of calm: just knowing I'm not alone on earth with this disease. Always Leigh's cheerful, maintaining she's 'going to live every day till she dies.' An admirable and courageous approach to life in the shadow of an ominous cancer.

Nine months later, x-rays revealed disturbing new spots in Leigh's lungs and liver. When months of experimental chemotherapy fail, her will to 'live everyday' begins to fade and she succumbs to an embittered end. That her two boys—ages seven and nine—will never experience the uniqueness of their mother—nor she them—bothers her as much as the doctors' forsaking her.

When she doesn't respond to any of their last-ditch chemo cocktails, her doctors, saying they have no more in their arsenal, retreat, telling her brazenly she's on her own. That one human being can withdraw, telling another human being in dire need there's nothing more they can do, wounds her irreparably. I was both inspired and frightened by the intensity, by the core of desperation that propelled her final anger.

The cocky world of modern medicine—this often holier-than-thou science—deserted her . . . tossed her aside like a piece of failed machinery.

Listening to this proud, strong-willed lady struggling—just days before dying—with her physical and mental decline, her inability to walk across the living room without oxygen, I felt a shivering wave of guilt, of fear.

Leigh's passing derailed my own progress for a long while. Simply put, her death brought home the obvious: This disease *can* indeed take your life.

But I'm getting ahead of myself . . .

Later that day, after the conference, though it seems anticlimactic, there's yet another doctor appointment—a meeting with my new MDA endocrinologist. I'm dreading this since this fellow will, I know, have details of yesterday's CT scan.

Jane and I, arriving in a noticeably uncrowded, 7th floor Endocrine Station waiting area (seems there aren't too many endocrine cancer patients, comparatively speaking), take a seat. My appointment is at 3:00 p.m.

We strike up a dialogue with the lone person in the area, a thyroid cancer patient. This thirty-something woman in trim business suit, casually thumbing through a magazine, discloses blithely she's had three major surgeries and is in line for a fourth. She recounts her surgeries as though they were as unmeaningful as teeth cleanings. Dr. Elliot, the surgeon, is incredible, she tells us.

While at the MDA hospital and clinics, I'm struck with one constant: Whomever I chance upon always seems worse off than me. This judgment is, of course, from my point of view, in the scheme of things, a message.

For better than two hours we linger here, waiting.

From all opinions—this thyroid patient and others on the MDA Patient Network—this unusual doctor is well worth the wait. Once Jane and I are guided to a small office/examination room, we are welcomed warmly by a clean-shaven, balding man of perhaps 50.

Taking his chair at the built-in writing desk, Dr. Gleghorn invites me to describe my general state of health, also proposing that I interject anything of relevance as we go along. With my MDA file and my abbreviated history before him, he consciously, painstakingly, surveys my records.

His easy-going aura implies that, while he's practical and sociable, he's also remarkably focused, a veteran at this. His exactness and composure seize you, making you feel you're one of a kind, in extraordinarily skilled hands. This doctor is, in fact, world-renowned, with patients visiting from many foreign countries to gain his expertise.

Comparing yesterday's blood work with earlier blood work, he notes that a couple of my liver enzymes are running high—have been for some time, nearly two years. (Something else Dr. Malone didn't note or react to.) This, he explains, could foretell of a metastatic condition (somehow, him saying this doesn't sound as horrendous as it might have), or it could simply reflect residual damage done by Mitotane.

"Is there anyway to tell?" I ask. "Why those numbers are up?"

"My first guess would be the Mitotane. Determining the other will take time."

"Did yesterday's scan, doctor," I resume uneasily since we've covered the preliminaries, "reveal anything new?"

"You met with Dr. Elliot, I know," he acknowledges somewhat evasively, continuing to thumb the pages of my file. "And he spelled out our concerns with this effusion issue. The dilemma we're facing?"

"He did. And I've got to confess the whole thing is a surprise to me. I thought, when he first started in, he had me confused with someone else. That he'd looked at the wrong film. But . . ."

"We have reviewed yesterday's film. And our radiologists," Dr. Gleghorn deliberates a moment as if to soften what he's about to say, "after a protracted sequence of calculations, say it looks as if the mass and the fluid have grown. But we'll put those details on hold while we await the biopsy. In the interim, Mr. Scribner, I'm certainly open to discussing alternatives." (How different this is from that discussion with Dr. Drake years back where he refused to discuss any what-ifs.)

This news—the mass, the fluid increasing in size—is nothing short of suffocating. Nothing's going my way!

There is, oddly, a fragment of logic in the back of my mind, saying: You've got to get off your butt and do something on your own to ensure your state of health. But what? Diet, lifestyle changes—two of the aspects of treatment a patient can manipulate?

Dr. Gleghorn continues coming across as a very thoughtful human being. He possesses the ability to make you feel you're his sole patient. He truly sees the psychological impact of the news he's delivering.

Tossing out more nervous questions, many of them the same as I've asked other doctors, I get fresh, more decisive, more thought-out answers. He tells me, for example, about new ACC studies being conducted with exotic drugs like suramin and gossypol, how they're showing promise but aren't yet ready for use.

We also review details of my recent cortisol stimulation test, and how my local endocrinologist hadn't foreseen the negative results of my going without oral adrenal steroids. Dr. Gleghorn notes in many cases the adrenal gland, once bombed with Mitotane, never returns to normal functioning. "Doctors out in the community," he adds diplomatically, "aren't always aware of the drug's long-term effects."

Once again he reiterates that if the fluid in my pleural area contains malignant cells, surgery is not an option. A more potent chemotherapy may be my only option—my only hope. There is an ounce of encouragement here, however: At least there is an option, if surgery's not. Maybe . . . just maybe, I'll luck out.

"Is there no *good* news here?" I ask Dr. Gleghorn.

"Data from your 24-hour urine test look good; nothing to be concerned about there. Yours appears to be a nonfunctioning tumor—meaning it's not secreting any hormones. Which is in your favor."

At this, I can almost smile. I feel for split second like a shiny green sapling left standing after a forest fire.

"I see where you've already had carboplatin and 5-FU," the doctor continues, thumbing more deeply in my file. "I talked yesterday with one of my colleagues—Dr. Berger, our medical oncologist—regarding your situation. He thinks perhaps we can look at cisplatin and etopiside. Even Taxol. As alternative therapies."

While I don't like hearing any of these options, as they pertain to me, I do appreciate that he's talked with another doctor regarding my predicament. I also appreciate that there is a third alternative drug—Taxol. Recent news accounts of this chemo show it as being 'encouragingly' in treating women with ovarian cancer. But still, it's not a cure.

"You're using Taxol—with adrenocortical carcinoma patients?"

"We've had some results, in some cases," Dr. Gleghorn replies with little fervor. "Nothing's really very promising—long-term. There's not really much out there. This disease is too rare to spark an interest among the pharmaceutical folk."

CHAPTER 52

TALK NOT OF OTHERS' LIVES

In all, I spend over two absorbing hours with Dr. Gleghorn. One of the most fruitful consultations I've ever engaged in concerning ACC's available therapies. In the realm of viable treatments, we even pondered me going back on Mitotane. Dr. Gleghorn said he wasn't pushing the plan, but he absolutely wouldn't eliminate the drug from the field of future candidates.

"Not like our last trip here," Jane observes quietly as we enter the darkened hotel room.

"A far cry."

"Terrific guy," she goes on. "People like that give you faith. You noticed too, I hope, how, when he talked about bad things, you didn't feel like he was dragging you down some dead-end road?"

"This is a man who can wear the title 'doctor' with pride," I add, glad to have discovered this gracious and knowledgeable man, thinking that, Yes, he can zero in on negative topics without leaving you feeling there's no hope. "I'm sitting there, you know, hearing him talk, thinking what a waste of time it is to discuss this disease with people like Crandle and Tzu and Malone."

"That doesn't take away from the fact that these people want to do more surgery," Jane reflects solemnly. "On you."

"At least I feel more a part of things here," I respond, still dismayed with the idea. "Seeing this from maybe their point of view. This scar-tissue thing, as you know, has long bugged me. Without knowing what the hell it is, how am I—the patient—supposed to know which treatment to take? Those doctors back home, I'd say, prefer the easy way out. Doesn't matter that we're talking somebody's life."

"How're you digesting all this?" Jane asks, passing me a mug of water. "Slowly?"

"Mostly," I reply, sipping the water's coolness, wishing for something stronger, "I guess, I'm just . . . discouraged as hell."

"Could've fooled me."

"And," I volunteer after a moment's thought, "I'm getting to where I don't feel I can trust this body anymore."

"No, Eric," Jane responds quickly, alarmed. "That's no good to say. Don't say that."

"Why not, if it's true? It's like an old friend who's letting me down."

"Bodies don't let their owners down."

"Mine is."

"It's bad talking like this. Your body's you. I asked how you're holding up—because I care."

Walking to the window, I regard MDA patients coming and going from the building. "This meeting with Dr. Gleghorn helped. Talking with somebody who seems to care. Of course, I'm not looking forward to any kind of surgery, that's for sure. And from the way I see things, looks like it has to be done here, in Houston. Which introduces more problems . . . like who's going to get our big-hearted HMO to okay all this out-of-state treatment? Where am I going to stay for four to six weeks recovering? All things I don't want to think about."

"Hey," Jane offers sprightly, out of the blue, grabbing me by the arm, "why don't we—you and me—jump in our rented Buick and track down a nice Mexican café? Spicy food's just what we need for getting our minds off all this."

Buzzing like electric razors, seasonal locusts sing from nearby trees as we share a warm plate of nachos on a tree- and flower-lined verandah. The afternoon sun's low, now fallen behind tiers of old brick buildings across the way. Polite Southern breezes waft through, thick with humidity, smelling of honeysuckle. I am able, I find, off and on, to lose myself for a moment or two, becoming in that instant the cancer-free human being of old. The feeling's enjoyable, if only transient.

"What's . . ." Jane asks, scooping some guacamole, glancing quickly at a playful couple at a neighboring table, "in line for tomorrow?" Though her glance was instantaneous, Jane's feelings are obvious. At times I, too, have found myself harboring similar feelings . . . of jealousy, of fleeting ill will, at seeing an everyday couple, cavorting, sitting in animated conversation—as if death were a millions miles away.

"More vocalizing, I guess. Dr. Elliot wants to see me again. He will have seen those new films. Needless to say," I offer, sampling an icy strawberry virgin margarita, "all this panics me. What if . . . they dig up something new—something we never thought of?"

"We're going to remain determined. That's the ticket, remember?"

"Oh, of course," I reply, resenting even Jane's freedom from disease. "Talk's cheap."

That evening, drawing our room-darkening drapes tightly closed, we vow to snooze till we wake naturally. Maybe never awaken, I wish silently. Slumber, the great eraser.

One o'clock following day: Dr. Elliot seems even more rushed this time.

"So," I say resolutely, having a bit more esteem for this man after listening to the thyroid patient yesterday laud his expertise, "my new films, I'm told, show things have grown."

"There appears to be—yes—some growth."

"Radiologists back home," I offer again as mild contradiction, "said everything was unchanged—no new growth."

"We'd have to take issue with that," the dark-haired Dr. Elliot responds, looking over a two-page report. "We definitely see a change."

"That means surgery's even more certain now?" I ask dispiritedly. "If the other's okay, I mean."

"Again," Dr. Elliot continues, his dark eyes flat, indifferent, "I'm compelled to remind you, Mr. Scribner: Don't go getting your hopes up. Surgery will not be an option if the biopsy on the effusion is positive."

"I feel honored, doctor, to have all these wonderful options," I say as politely but as sarcastically as I can.

"I've got Dr. Ryman, right now, coming to take you down to radiology," Dr. Elliot goes on unfazed. "For the biopsy."

"This instant?" I ask, unexpectedly struck with the same kind of fear I've experienced when compelled to give unrehearsed presentations. "We're going to do that now? You're not going to give me any time to—"

"You'll do just fine, Mr. Scribner. Sit tight, my nurse will be in." With that he exits the exam room.

"Well, hell," I say to Jane, "it'd be nice to have a minute or two to digest all this."

"They won't operate . . ." she asks, thinking aloud, "if the fluid has cancer cells in it?"

"That's what we're hearing. There'd be no point in going through the trauma of taking out that chunk of scar tissue if the cancer's already spread beyond that point. I can't believe I'm sitting here saying this! Like I'm talking about somebody else. Times like this, I wish I was back on the Chesapeake with my crab net."

"God," Jane sighs, backsliding for a moment, "the things this disease robs you of."

"Never seems to back off, does it?" I ask, feeling slightly vindicated at her recognition of what I've been preaching for so long. "Always presenting you with new, even more unexpected snarls."

"Enough of this!" she announces, perkily, her eyes damp. "Here's our approach: Believe with all our hearts this biopsy will come out good."

"Now that sounds curative as hell," I say, chuckling uneasily.

"Hey you, you're the one always preaching belief."

"I know, I know. But that one word—'inoperable'—keeps getting in the way. You don't know how I've dreaded it—that word."

Squeezing my hand: "We'll do it."

"Damn it," I say, quaking at what the next moment holds, "they're coming to get me, like some friggin' death-row loser. Like some shabby black-and-white movie."

"C'mon, you're going to depress yourself more. Now stop."

"Anymore . . . I don't know if I care . . . . This is so much work."

"I said stop! This is just one more step in the whole process."

"But what do you do . . . when you feel all the passageways narrowing?"

"Oh," Jane replies, her eyes moist once again, "that makes *me* feel real good."

A delicate knocking on the door.

CHAPTER 53

A SHAFT OF LIGHT—
BIOPSY FIRST IMPRESSIONS LOOK GOOD

Now, all optimism, all civility's been drained from me. Playing out on a destitute stretch of my intellect—not unlike a vast dry lake—are the reasons for which I'm going to fail. Positioned in neat rows, these reasons glare back like so many shadowy gargoyles.

In the barely opened door, an affable male face appears.

"Mr. Scribner? I'm here to take you to radiology," the fair-skinned, soft-featured man says almost submissively, perceiving in a flash our gloom—as if we're clutching hand-lettered signs. "I'm Dr. Ryman." He steps inside.

Feeling set apart from humanity, I'm not in the least bit sociable. Why should I be? No smile, no hand extended in greeting. Standing indifferently, as if to underscore my mood, I bid farewell to Jane, and accompany this fellow, as if to the gallows. (Jane will be taken later by a hospital volunteer to the CT waiting area.)

Dr. Ryman tries his damnedest to make small talk as we traipse along the glossy corridors. Refusing to cooperate, I say nothing. One 10-mile-long hallway, then another, then an elevator, then another long hallway. The label inoperable floats before me . . .

Dr. Ryman's saying hello—to doctors, nurses, patients. Me, in a vacuum of self-pity—feeling nothing, save for despondency. For maybe the first time ever, I sense little or no hope: This biopsy, I'm convinced, is going to authenticate what the doctors have been alluding to.

"You local?" Dr. Ryman asks. "From Texas, I mean?"

"California," I answer sullenly. Thinking: Why should I feel coerced by decorum, gentility?

"Really? Where about? Santa Barbara was my old stomping grounds—in high school."

We pass a white-haired woman, sitting hunched over, head down, in a black-and-chrome wheelchair. She sits transfixed, as if a symbol: A failed idea left to wallow in this healing wilderness.

"Down the coast from there is where I live," I mumble, a programmed response. I want to say, 'Who gives a damn where you went to high school?' but instead, follow with, "In Ventura."

We're now entering the always cold and damp-feeling radiology area. For the first time I peek at this man's ID badge. Strange to see he's really a physician; so informal is he, so at home with this cheerless situation.

"What we're going to do," he clarifies, "is have you lie here, face down, while we move you in and out of the scanner. So we can precisely position the biopsy needle. I do this all the time so try not to worry."

These words, as meaningless as a dog's bark at 2:00 a.m., resound in thin air. Feeling a downright lassitude, I just don't care. Never before have I felt this wave of hollowness.

"Would you like something—a sedative—to soothe you?" the doctor's asking, as I put on the metal-free gown, removing my pants. "There really shouldn't be much discomfort."

Again these meaningless words trickle in. I don't respond.

"I see," Dr. Ryman resumes directly. "It's my policy—when a patient doesn't respond—to take that for a 'Yes.' I'll have my nurse administer both Demerol and valium. You've got to promise, though . . ." He pauses.

I'm looking up into his pale blue eyes. He has my attention. Maybe the drugs will realign my spirits, I'm thinking, recalling the serenity that Demerol bestowed after the last surgery.

"What's that?" I respond carelessly.

"You won't go to sleep on me, okay? During this entire procedure you can't move a muscle—not one—or we'll have to start over from scratch. You'll stay awake?"

I signal yes. With me sitting on the CT table, Dr. Ryman withdraws, retreating to a glassed-in console area, conferring with another male doctor or technician. Moments later an RN appears, starting my IV.

Within minutes, I'm being re-positioned, face down, on the concave table.

Lying there, I'm thinking how much I loathe Dr. Hubbard for cutting into the tumor . . . Dr. Malone for wanting to stand by and watch this thing kill me . . . Dr. Tzu for . . . when suddenly I'm being inundated with wave after wave of disconnectedness, of weightlessness, of warm exhilaration. My environment—the sterile radiology area—now softens, changing into something quite pleasurable. The balmy narcotics are kicking in. Big time. Now, I'm part of a new world—and want to remain permanently in it.

Instantly nothing matters. I'm now an ultra-cooperative rag doll, rolling this way, that.

A 10-inch-long, piano-wire-looking gadget—the biopsy needle—is sticking in the left-center of my back—hurting like I'm being deeply bruised—being maneuvered in, out, right, left by Dr. Ryman after each of five or six CT slices.

"No dozing now, remember?" he urges, catching my eyelids weakening.

Lying still as a corpse, I'm concentrating on the unadorned wall at the far end of the room, mindful of the scanner's continuous humming. The pale green wall melts into my vision. "No . . . problem . . . doc," I murmur, now in touch with a distant piece of myself I didn't know existed. Hell, saw off one leg, doc, I won't complain.

"We're making good progress," Dr. Ryman calls out, returning to his glassed-in nook.

This goes on now for 40 minutes or so. In the booth there are now several curious doctors peering over Dr. Ryman's shoulder. I take for granted they are doctors by their dress, their intrigue. Are they here to see me—this mutation—or, I consider more positively, to behold some radiological finding no one will believe?

"About does it," Dr. Ryman's saying next, the biopsy device now removed. "And, I've got some promising news." He's helping me to a sitting position. "The fluid we took today is not discolored. That doesn't necessarily mean you're out of the woods—don't hold me to that—but it's an excellent sign. And those nodules? As we were positioning you on your stomach, they disappeared . . . meaning they're not nodules after all, but small fluid-filled sacks."

Wandering now in a glorious desert of sun and sand—the gargoyle-plagued lake transformed—I feel myself returning to a consciousness brimming with hope. "You're not . . . putting me on?" I respond, thinking perhaps this is some drug-induced hallucination.

"Usually—and I emphasize usually—when the fluid's off-color, that's not good. Say a burgundy-red. Yours, however, was a clear, yellowish tone."

Between these implausible words and the rapture of drugs, I feel a renewal. "In other words . . . the fluid may not be malignant?"

"No guarantees, but things look good. That's all I can offer at this point. We'll have to wait and see what the pathology folks come back with."

"That'll take how long?"

"Couple of days, probably. I know you're anxious."

"The verdict won't be ready tomorrow then, before I leave?"

"Not likely. But one of your doctors will be in touch."

With me still sitting, he says, "What we need to do now is move you to the holding area. Till we're sure there's no bleeding. We'll let your wife know."

Drugs are wearing thin. This environment—this sterile world—is beginning to push through, revealing its hard-edged features once more.

"Doctor, I've got to admit: You knew what you were doing with those sedatives," I compliment him. "Any chance I could get another blast . . . for the road?"

He massages his chin, chuckling. "Well, Mr. Scribner, this is highly irregular—but, under the circumstances, maybe we could go out on a limb. Nurse," he calls out, "please give this gentleman another dose of sedatives before you pull his IV. Then see that he gets to Recovery."

With the RN inserting a needle into the transparent IV line, I bid Dr. Ryman good-bye, thanking him—appreciating now his sensibility, his ingenuity in the subtle psychology of patient care.

By the time I'm wheeled into Recovery, I'm floating again. Bliss city. This state of wellbeing seems terribly unfair, however—in light of the five or six other patients parked in wheelchairs in the waiting area, still mired in their own despair. You can see this in their dead-fish eyes. While I sense a connectedness with them, I also feel sublime, thanks to the drugs and Dr. Ryman's stay of execution.

An elderly, red-faced volunteer assists Jane to Recovery. Reaching out a colorless, bony hand, he touches me, making me feel ashamed for my poor-little-me reaction earlier. How many people had tolerated what I tolerated today and not squawked about it?

That afternoon the famed cancer surgeon and author Dr. Bernie Siegel is the keynote speaker at the MDA Patient Conference. Very much I want to hear him in person—this man whose books I'd read, tapes I'd listened to. But as luck would have it, the biopsy took too long—an hour and a half in all, with recovery. By the time Jane and I return to the hotel, wash up, and drive to the conference site, Bernie's speech is only available on tape.

Tomorrow it's back to California. With Dr. Ryman's appraisal—his rejuvenating words—coursing through me like warm soup on an icy day, I feel almost safe.

CHAPTER 54

FIGHT TILL THE LAST GASP—
A NEW SHRINK, A NEW APPROACH

Dr. Gleghorn calls the hotel the next morning prior to our leaving Houston, saying he'll follow up on the biopsy, get in touch when he's got some solid information. Still feeling pretty buoyant, I pass along Dr. Ryman's comments about the fluid color. Dr. Gleghorn, though very tentative, shares my excitement. His slight hesitation, though, sets my thoughts off in a negative direction.

"We'll have to retain ultimate judgment till we see the pathology." Plainly Dr. Gleghorn's learned cynicism won't allow him even this small morsel of hope. "You have to know," he continues, I can hear caution in his voice, "that even if the pathology shows no malignancy, the fluid could *still* prove problematic."

"Now you've got me really confused."

"Needle biopsies, Eric, are not all that accurate. Often we find them in error because so little tissue or fluid is removed for examination."

Another balloon punctured.

"They biopsied the mass too?" I ask.

"That's correct. But keep in mind there are times when tissue samples of this sort show negatively—giving false hope. Then in surgery, show the opposite."

The next Monday morning: Once again I'm in my office, back in the role of editorial ramrod. Right away I'm ass-deep in crocodiles, as they say, mired in raucous schedule and publication crises. Frenzied executives are reaching out from all sides.

Reentering a work project following a medical leave's a lot like hurling yourself back into a ragging white-water current: there's never a get-acquainted or re-education interval. You're instantly swimming for your life in a hostile, flash-flood environment.

But, in a curious manner, this is good: it keeps the gray matter from dwelling on the morose. Dr. Ryman's encouragement, though less persuasive now, continues to sustain me.

Not many of my colleagues bother asking how things went in Houston. For sure the self-centered VP doesn't concern himself. He doesn't even acknowledge that I've been gone. People, to grant humanity the benefit of doubt, are oftentimes apprehensive about asking questions for fear of what a cancer patient might tell them.

What do you come back with, for example, when someone says: 'They told me I only have six months to live?' You can't offer the pat rejoinder: 'Oh, everything's going to be okay.' The knowledge one is dying is gut-wrenching. How *do* you respond?

Then again, perhaps people are just too damn overworked or self-centered to care. Seems that way, at least, in Southern California. This could be what's plaguing our modern world: nobody feels it's necessary to make time for anyone else. It's me, me, me.

Thursday morning, five days after arriving back from Houston: I'm in my office, sipping a giant glass of ice water (coffee and tea were discontinued eons ago) when the ringing phone startles me. "Your biopsy results just came in, Eric," Dr. Gleghorn's personable voice relates without excitement. "They're saying both the fluid and the mass are negative."

"Meaning," I respond elatedly, expecting to hear real cheer in his voice, "everything's a go? We're talking good news, right, doctor?"

"We have to proceed very carefully, Eric," are his sobering words, "not jumping too far ahead. Too often these biopsies miss the mark. In fact, as I indicated before, the rate of precision's not at all what we'd like to see. For now all we can do is set up your surgery date and hope. When can you be available? Dr. Elliot did have you stop the Coumadin, right?"

"He did, yes. I can be ready . . . whenever. All I've got to do is get the go-ahead from my HMO—no easy task. Do you suppose . . . you could coordinate things with my primary doctor . . . get the ball rolling, so to speak?"

Remarkably, he says he'll be glad to.

Employing some spur-of-the-moment strategy, I give him Dr. Bristol's—rather than Dr. Paravano's—direct phone number. Even though Dr. Paravano's now my primary-care doctor, Dr. Bristol, I feel, can pull the right strings, promptly . . . if she's inclined to.

Later that day Dr. Gleghorn calls back. Dr. Bristol's approved the surgery to take place in 10 days—on September 29, in Houston. Wow, talk about expeditious! Having a doctor-friend in the world of tortoise-slow HMO deliberations pays off! But there's good news/bad news here: Good, the surgery's approved without delay; bad, that I have to recuperate in an unfamiliar city, thousands of miles from home. The scene, the logistics are daunting.

That evening, I'd scheduled an introductory appointment with a new psychologist. With all this chaos of late, an educated shoulder to cry on can't hurt. To orchestrate this meeting, I called the HMO's mental health line weeks ago to request authorization, justifying to some 18-year-old clerk why I, a 50-year-old cancer patient, needed to see a shrink. A week later the HMO girl called back, saying I could see this doctor—but only for three visits. Any visits beyond that will require an explicit written petition from the shrink himself.

Since I hadn't had the greatest luck with shrinks in the past, this one's going through a no-holds-barred, third-degree introductory interview. So inflexible am I, that I'm almost angry, resentful.

I find myself convening with this guy in a tasteful, ground-floor office, with file cabinets, oriental rug, pillowed couch, cushioned chair. The shrink—an undersized man, captivatingly proper, about my age, with thinning hair, possessing a commanding baritone voice—remains seated at his desk, his ebony high-backed leather chair swiveled my way.

This is a job interview—only I'm not being interviewed or grilled, he is. I am deliberately brittle, somewhat vague and discourteous—nothing to lose, as I see it. Ready am I to move on if his comebacks aren't on the money. Boldly, I question his education, grade-point average, where he went to grad school. No more pseudo-shrinks or divinity doctors masquerading as shrinks. Laying down the law, I tell this fellow—the TDKB syndrome losing more of its hold on me—I'll continue seeing him only if he agrees to deal with prevailing medical issues—and those alone. No rummaging in extraneous relationships, or my past.

Without objection, this small strong-voiced man agrees. Engagingly at ease, is he, disarmingly so. Once we've set the formula—all consultations are to be in the present tense—I paint a detailed picture of my medical condition, describing in particular past surgeries, radiation, chemo cycles, what heartless buffoons some of the HMO doctors could be. I also go into how I behaved intellectually and physically in these straits. Listening closely, scribbling extensively on a yellow legal pad in his lap, Dr. Nolin seems now and then shocked, throwing out pointed questions: "Well, why the hell didn't he prescribe adequate pain medication following your first surgery?"

After giving my situation some study, Dr. Nolin proposes we approach future medical treatments (he starts to say 'traumas,' but catches himself) as challenges. A modest word, an appealingly achievable plan: challenges.

"My greatest fear," I go on, weighing the flimsiness of this 'challenge' notion, "is that I'll get to Houston, they'll open me up . . . and then say I'm inoperable. The biopsy was wrong. How I'll react, I don't know. Maybe come off the table or bed or wherever, swinging, I don't know. Maybe, toss in the towel—say to hell with it. Aside from regaining consciousness in a coffin, six feet under, that's my biggest fear: 'We sewed you back up . . . there was nothing more we could do.' "

Resting snugly in a padded armchair, I'm gawking out the window, taking in the gray-violet twilight. A commiserating brook—actually a fountain and small koi pond beneath the window—sets the backdrop. Serene ambiance.

This person, this doctor, actually seems to be taking in all I say, remaining exclusively centered on my difficulties. A shame, though, I'm thinking, we have to depend on specialists like this for a sympathizing ear—we've become so insular we now have 'paid-for' confidants.

"You're a reasonably astute man," the shrink's commenting, jotting a note in his journal, "one who's clearly done a lot of homework. What I'm getting at is . . . you've proven you can handle these things. So why the doubt . . . now?"

"Things are piling up," I reply, relishing that someone's acknowledged my efforts, even if only superficially.

"With your diverse treatments. You've fared pretty well, right? Overall. Your first oncologist—admittedly a rather uncivilized soul—said (the shrink's now flipping pages, re-reading his notes) you'd only make it a year and a half. Obviously you've beaten those odds."

"Does that make me a hero or what?"

"We should see this possibility—that things may not come out so well—as a further challenge. One you'll meet and again beat."

"Sounds too . . . uncomplicated, doctor," I reply skeptically, resuming my nothing-to-lose tone.

"A lot of solutions—keys to outwardly perplexing issues—are simple."

Striving to see a grain of logic here, I mull this over. I had met innumerable challenges so far—maybe not recognizing them as such—and conquered them. Just hadn't tallied my won-lost column, I guess. "At some point, though," I offer darkly, "there's going to be a challenge I can't meet."

Studying me a moment, he nibbles the inside of his cheek: "Isn't that true—of all of us? You've done a superlative job thus far—you may not know it, but you have. Trust in yourself."

Aware the guy's stroking me, but also exposing a kernel of truth, as he sees it, I reply, "So how does one go about implementing this?"

"You rise up—as it were—and meet this thing, whatever it is, head on. You are a warrior."

"Digging pretty deep, aren't we, doc," I say laughingly.

He shrugs in appreciation.

While being a straightforward, albeit simplified solution, this challenge thing's sounding less and less like corn. Understanding if I'm to go on, I must do something to survive.

We ordinary folk, at times, need to put our objectives aside, to heed others—authority figures like doctors—offering positive courses of action in loud, unmistakable voices. The answers are always there, it's just a matter of clearing away the chaff.

I smile, feeling good . . . feeling we may've hit upon an approach—at least a workable idea—I can truly latch onto. Our first night's session—lasting well over three hours—reaches a conclusion with Dr. Nolin flipping his legal pad closed, saying, "So, what do you think, Eric—coming back for more?"

Feeling considerably more mollified, and centered: "I think you'll fill the bill. Just remember: No exhuming the past."

"No sweat."

We shake and I leave, much more outfitted for the ominous struggle ahead . . . whatever that might be.

FINDING HOPE WHEN DOCTORS SAY THERE IS NONE

CHAPTER 55

TIME: THAT ENDLESS SONG—
FINDING RELIEF IN MUSIC

The following morning, my lower left leg is aching badly, awakening me before the rattling 5:00 a.m. alarm, a painful throbbing in the calf. Immediately I'm seized with panic, with despair: A new clot! Climbing out of bed, I try the leg. Again, I limp in pain. The base of the heel, however, doesn't have that stone-bruised sensation. Good sign. If this is a new clot, I don't want it hindering the approaching surgery. Or, God forbid . . . killing me.

Is this bloodthirsty, non-stop cancer-driven invasion never going to end?

Driven by renewed fear and that hospital doctor's remark about people with malignancies being predisposed to clots—and, considering I'd just ceased taking the blood thinner—I call Dr. Paravano as soon as the HMO clinic opens. Don't want to tangle with the HMO's Urgent Care circus act at this hour.

As luck'd have it, Dr. Paravano's on holiday. Another HMO doctor, indeed the same excitable guy who filled in for her when I was hospitalized for the root-canal infection, sees me. Upon hearing the symptoms, this inexperienced, wrought-up guy seems already to have forged a theory: this isn't a new clot.

"This," the doctor informs me, "is what amounts to sympathy pains." Sometimes the leg remembers, he explains. He's compressing the calf, palming the flesh to feel its temperature, rotating the foot, watching my eyes. Measuring the diameter one calf versus the other. "We don't quite know why, but our bodies sometimes like to relive certain experiences," he offers unpersuasively. "Phantom pain, we call it."

Sure, I'm thinking, we all like reliving our most painful moments.

"Not to doubt you," I reply, seeing all this as some miserly HMO ruse, "but is there some way we can be a little more precise? A test, maybe? I just quit taking Coumadin, the drug that's supposed to prevent this. And I'm a little scared, to be truthful. In a few days I'm supposed to go to Houston for surgery—at the Anderson Cancer Center." This latter I throw in thinking it'll somehow impress this doctor, coerce him into thinking more rationally about further testing.

"I get you . . ." he offers oddly, gaping ineptly into space. "Since you've had recently a similar problem . . . with that same leg, I think I can send you over to the hospital and let them do a Doppler test . . . I shouldn't have to go through Utilization Review for this. Right?"

"You're asking me?" Ghastly images of this clot traveling to my lungs or brain and ending my life—or at a minimum canceling all hopes of going to Houston—are overshadowing my every thought.

Five hours later: "Lie back, Mr. Scribner," a thickset, heavily perfumed female technician says, running a gel-coated Doppler probe over my lower left leg.

"The old clot," she says nonchalantly after a moment, "I can still see."

"You can? It hasn't gone away?" I ask, sitting up, stretching to see the TV monitor. "Where?"

With one long orange-painted fingernail, she taps the glass screen, pointing to an insignificant, fuzzy likeness. "Probably had you on blood thinners for a while, didn't they?"

"Just recently stopped."

"And you thought that dissolved your clot, right?"

I nod yes.

"Everyone thinks that. But Coumadin doesn't work that way. Mainly it keeps new ones from forming. Sometimes the clots get dissolved, sometimes they don't. I don't see much else here. Nothing new," she says reassuringly, watching the blurry, gray screen. "Veins usually re-route themselves around the clotted ones. Nature's pretty weird, huh?"

"You're sure. . ." I persist redundantly, "you don't see anything new?"

"Tell you what," she offers, after deliberating a bit, "this is unscientific as heck . . . but I've been doing this for nearly eight years, and I've never seen a patient with a clot who could point their toes down and not have it hurt like heck. Try it."

I do; happily there's no added discomfort. "So you're saying, in your experienced Doppler opinion, this is further proof there's nothing to worry about?"

The green-eyed tech raises her eyebrows. "That's what my report's going to show."

Considering my luck of late, I'm still apprehensive. But at least for now I can go about my daily concerns with some semblance of immunity, overlooking this troublesome burning in my leg. (Later I learned from a friendly non-HMO doctor that this tech's point-your-toes-at-the-wall clot test is flawed—there *are* patients who can indeed point their toes without pain *and* have a clot.)

The following weekend Jane and I are slated to see our favorite rock group, the Moody Blues, in a sunset concert at the Hollywood Bowl. The group's lyrics are free of rhetorical clutter, like spring air, ringing of truth. Coincidentally, this melodic group recorded what we've decided is our song—'Tuesday Afternoon.' It was, after all, a Tuesday afternoon when Jane and I first met. But that's another tale.

The twilight evening is starry, summery, an open-air venue, amphitheater backdrop.

Moderately high up, we're in a rearward section—despite my calling the Hollywood Bowl months ago for 'good' tickets. We plunk down our backpack of munchies—crackers, cheese, chilled white wine, a sweet-smelling loaf of French bread. (Yes, I can now sneak a glass or two of wine inasmuch as the blood thinner's a thing of the past.)

Many other followers—an overflow crowd, it appears—share our passion for this English symphonic rock group. Rabid cheering erupts like distant fireworks with the first notes of each song. The Bowl's renowned acoustics are phenomenal, caressing the flesh in tepid waves. Neon-colored lasers are now fanning the darkening sky. Pathetically, though, the group—like many of us—is displaying signs of age. Not so much in appearance or energy, but in vocalization.

Their repertoire of tunes—scattered new ones, mostly old ones—pulls the partisan crowd in many pleasant, memory-laden directions. The faithful grow more involved, more spontaneous after each well-known piece—particularly following the group's trademark song, 'Nights in White Satin.' Out come thousands of cigarette lighters, held high to produce a sea of dancing flames.

The group's consistency isn't quite what it once was, coming tonight from these aging rock and rollers (the group's now middle-aged). This aging issue, though, seems eminently applicable in that I've been dwelling a lot lately on how humans are a frail breed, a kaleidoscopic species. Our essential being—like everything—never remains fixed, unchanged. Not from day to day, nor minute to minute. Materially you're not who you were yesterday, or the day before—billions of cells have died off, billions of new ones were created in their place.

One intriguing theory of alternative cancer treatment holds that—through meditation and other major life-style changes—we can bring into being an internal environment where the new cells don't 'remember' the harmful things the old cells were doing . . . thus denying the duplication of disease in our bodies. Fascinating belief.

Roosting here, at the Hollywood Bowl on a comfortable foam pad, under starry and soft summer sky, surrounded by raucous and care-free revelers reliving their past, the juxtaposition of me, a cancer patient, just days away from something as foreboding as major surgery and its questionable results, seems well, disturbingly surreal—ugly. In a few days doctors in Houston'll be poring over me, shaving here and there, painting me with Betadine, gearing up for extensive thoracic and abdominal surgery. Blazing, white-hot operating-room lights. Unexcitable, masked humanoids hovering over me.

As the balmy evening wears on, the group's symphonic tunes carry me back, if only for a unclouded split second . . . to a time when I was inexperienced and immune to death, to life's suffering, to being old, or sickly, or needing any kind of life-preserving surgery. The short-lived feeling's euphoric, making this whole night worthwhile.

Filing out of the Bowl, jostled by throngs of energized Moody Blues fans, my positive frame of mind's suddenly overtaken by a mawkish observation: This may be the final time I see this place . . . this group . . . a lot of everyday things.

These desolate little thoughts, like winged bats darting about the evening sky, are not worth brooding over—now get rid of them.

"Couldn't quite hold the high ones, could they?" Jane remarks dispiritedly on the brightly lit city bus on the way home.

"Um," I concede sadly, observing more bats darting erratically among my thoughts. "Were sure trying, though."

"'Least we have their tapes and CDs," she goes on wistfully, massaging my thigh soothingly, putting her head on my shoulder. "Thanks for tonight. We really needed this."

"There was something in it for me, too," I reply.

"You're worried, aren't you—about the surgery?"

"Age leaves its mark, no doubt about that."

"The surgery, I was asking about, and the leg? I saw you were limping."

"Actually, the leg's . . . almost normal. Since that Doppler technician told me not to worry. Placebo effect, you think? And yes, the surgery's sunken its teeth into me."

"Someday, babe," she says looking up at me, "we're going to live in a little house in the mountains, in the forest, with a great view of the chaotic world below, and all these bad things will be distant memories."

Now the last pre-surgery weekend's gone—digested like a prisoner's last meal. There are just a few days of routine life left till the plane touches down in Houston . . . for the inescapable.

CHAPTER 56

HOUSTON: THE FINAL TREK—
THE HARD REALITIES OF CANCER SURGERY

Blindly, like irresponsible flower children of old, Jane and I are heading out—without a place of recuperation for me. Staying at the Rotary House Hotel for a couple of weeks is a possibility. An obliging social worker, assigned to the Endocrine Section at MDA, is researching places for us to stay for the duration. Answers will come sooner or later, I trust. This is the least of my fears.

Because a close friend pulled some strings, Jane and I find ourselves on one of the better airlines, bumped up to first-class. This wearisome journey's all of a sudden become relatively pleasurable—being waited on, pampered. That I'm about to submit to an unexpected surgery in a remote city still haunts me, however.

On this opulent flight, with the great unknown awaiting me, I've chosen to throw caution to the wind—saying to hell with temperance. Swilling two full glasses of frosty champagne before the plane even leaves the ground, I'm pretty much airborne already.

With my Walkman earphones in place, I ease back in the roomy leather seats. Dr. Bernie Siegel, on one of his texts on tape, is explaining how to gear up, mentally, for the mysteries of cancer surgery. A strange mix: liquor and sobering cancer advice. One unchanging essential of the Siegel tapes is this: Those who're angered by a cancer diagnosis, those who are fighters, fair better than patients who're passive, who take the news lying down.

A pair of lively flight attendants keeps our champagne glasses all but overflowing, our bowls of heated cashews brimming. LA's jaundiced overcast—viewed through desensitizing bubbles—is without impact, does not stir any menacing mental pictures.

Two hours into the flight, in a conversation with a silver-haired flight attendant smelling vaguely of roses, Jane, loosened considerably by champagne, reveals the purpose of our journey. Visibly touched, the attendant reluctantly mentions her younger sister just died after years of treatment for breast cancer.

While preparing to land, this same rose-smelling attendant, whispering a heart-felt good luck—telling me she could get in big trouble for this—slips me a paper-wrapped, unopened bottle of Cabernet Sauvignon... saying only, "Because

I know." So astonished am I by this blatant act of kindness, this simple gesture, that I'm tongue-tied. She squeezes my hand—we exchange smiles.

Mid-morning, the following day: After a restless night at the Rotary House Hotel, I'm once more perched on an inhospitable exam table. The endocrine surgeon's prodding here and there methodically, as if looking under the hood of a car, describing the proposed procedure: "We expect this to be a two-phased surgery," he's saying. "Dr. Garret, the thoracic surgeon, will go in first, from the back side, doing a thoracoscopy. If the pleural fluid he removes is negative—not malignant—then we'll roll you over (he gestures grandly, using a twisting motion to illustrate) and I'll resect the soft-tissue mass from the adrenal bed."

"Hold on a minute," I say, swallowing stiffly, feeling as if ants had just been sprinkled on every inch of my flesh, "we already decided the fluid was okay, I thought."

"That was a preliminary biopsy, Mr. Scribner—nowhere near as complete as the thoracoscopy will be. Dr. Garret will take considerably more fluid. For a more thorough study."

"So, we could be back to square one?"

"A clear possibility," the doctor replies flatly. "At this point, we believe the fluid to be negative. If that's not the case, you understand, we stop right there. Phase two of the surgery—resecting the soft-tissue mass—is not an option."

Disoriented once again, as if reeling from a smack in the forehead with a heavy object, I ask frantically, though already well aware of the answer: "Why—why can't we go on?"

"There'd be no point," Dr. Elliot replies somewhat rankled, choosing his words too bluntly for my liking . . . as if he were discussing this situation before a class of med students. "As I implied at our first meeting, Mr. Scribner, if the fluid shows positive, that'll denote pleural seeding. In other words, there are cancer cells suspended in the fluid . . . that can't be expunged surgically."

"What if . . ." I'm now a cornered animal, stammering, seeking avenues of escape: "I gave you permission to take more? Cut out all you have to?"

"That's simply not ethical, Mr. Scribner. And not fair to you. I'd literally have to cut like this (with his finger he draws a line from my left armpit to the base of my neck, then down to my navel, then across to my left side), removing all that. And even that'd be of little value . . . the cancer could still be anywhere."

How can this be happening? I hear echoing within. I didn't do anything to deserve this!

A half-hour afterward, nerves still ajar, I'm in yet another surgical exam room. Dr. Garret, the thoracic surgeon, however, radiates a sense of empathy. He has me feeling composed in just minutes.

"Dr. Elliot, I'm certain, has gone over each step of the procedure with you, Mr. Scribner—correct?"

"Can't say as I was too thrilled, though."

"Understood," says Dr. Garret, a slow-talking man with a glistening forehead. "What I'll do is go in through here (he touches a spot midway up my left rib cage, under the arm) using a miniature fiberoptic camera device. After we deflate your lung, we'll take a good look around, gathering at the same time a quantity of fluid; hopefully, all of it for histological examination."

"There's already been a biopsy," I put in weakly, hoping this will somehow hold water, like perhaps he'll say, 'Oh, in that case, we'll skip this step.'

"Yes, I'm aware," the doctor replies.

"It said the fluid's okay."

"This time we'll be more exact. We're going to take a lot more fluid and get a more factual picture. No sense subjecting you to the trauma of major surgery if pleural seeding has begun."

Damn! That ugly term again. In me, I'm watching this bloodthirsty tug-of-war: Will I or will I not have this Godforsaken surgery?

"You're going to deflate my lung?"

"Don't sweat it," the doctor says soothingly. "Standard procedure. You won't even know it. Very little can go wrong."

Scrambling to find something positive here as one or more of my self-help books advised, I try focusing on how fortunate I am to be at this prestigious cancer center . . . to have an 'in' at the tight-fisted HMO like Dr. Bristol who'll allow me this freedom.

Next I'm in a glassed-in office enclosure, a male clerk going over insurance forms. Dr. Bristol's faxed ahead a preliminary, hand-written HMO authorization, saying the official typed version will follow presently. Seems her fax satisfies all paperwork requirements.

(I had in fact phoned Dr. Bristol the week before, boldly proposing that the HMO also approve payment for lodging and/or air fare. Piqued, she indicated I was looking a gift horse in the mouth. I remained undeterred, however. A friend of a friend gave me the phone number of a middle manager—"Who could get things done"—at the HMO's corporate office. I approached her as well about lodging and air fare reimbursement. This personable woman said the HMO would assign me a case manger and most likely would cover all reasonable air and lodging costs —since my primary-care doctor had determined I must go out of state for this specialized surgery.

Moral: When dealing with HMOs be tenacious, talk to supervisors, people with power. *Never* accept 'no' from the HMO's first-line resistance—usually poorly trained, 18-year-old, minimum-wage people answering their ballyhooed 'Help' lines.)

Finalizing his duties, the MDA insurance clerk asks that I remain seated till the anesthesiologist comes in. Peculiar place to meet another doctor, I'm thinking.

A fine-featured black woman with kind, greenish-topaz eyes, in her mid-thirties, appears minutes later—Dr. Turrell—elevating immediately my frame of mind:

"You're Mr. Scribner?" she asks exaggeratedly. "The patient? Can't be, you look too good, too healthy. Usually my patients are, well, pallid . . . delicate looking."

The thought strikes me: Yes, we're seeing again the curse of this disease: You can look healthy as hell *and* be dying at the same time.

Shaking her thin, yet forceful hand, I acknowledge: "I'm your guy—the one you folks are going to be slicing on in the morning."

We're discussing possible allergic reactions and what have you, when an unfamiliar nurse pokes her head in, asking my name. "Thank God, it's you," she breathes. "Dr. Elliot wants you to go to Admissions right after you finish here. He wants you in a room A-S-A-P."

"Me? You're talking about me?" I ask, looking at my watch, seeing it's only 11:45. "Tomorrow's when I'm supposed to check in."

"Absolutely he means you. Wants you starting the purging procedure."

Once more the unforeseen has caught me off guard. Jane and I'd planned to sneak out for a breather, a few hours of brainless sight-seeing. "Can you give me a couple hours, at least?" I implore desperately, thinking I need to buy some space, some time to get my head together.

Punching a few numbers on the phone, the nurse has her answer within seconds: "Yes, but only if you guarantee to be in Admissions by 3:00 p.m. Today."

A short time later, at lunch in the busy ground-floor cafeteria, Jane—her eyes following a sickly little girl, no more than five, lacking a single strand of hair—says: "This place . . . just bombards your spirits, doesn't it? It's awful. That poor little thing."

Staring at my toasted BLT and avocado sandwich: "Gets a person to wondering . . . about a God who'd do this."

"It makes me so sad . . ." Jane resumes quietly, watching the slow-moving child. "That could just as easily be our little girl, Eric."

"More people need to experience the ugliness of this disease firsthand. Maybe then we'd see some real cancer research funding."

"Pretty serious, they are," Jane announces perkily after a moment, bouncing back, "about things. Around here, I mean. Once they say you need surgery, they mean like yesterday."

"I'm waiting for somebody to pinch me, telling me this somebody else's bad dream," I persist. "Am I really sitting here, about to check into a major cancer hospital in a matter of hours?"

Back in the otherworldliness of our hotel room, I pitch a few things in a modest carrying case, knowing Jane can bring over whatever I need later. Reclining on the bed, I try removing myself, meditating far beyond this . . . to a place where the sunlight falls warmly on my skin . . . where small children—innocents—are never stricken with terminal illnesses.

The chiming phone awakens me, terrifying every bone.

FINDING HOPE WHEN DOCTORS SAY THERE IS NONE

CHAPTER 57

DRINK, FOR TOMORROW—
PURGING THE SYSTEM PRIOR TO SURGERY

I'm not dreaming. Admissions is on the phone. Time to check back in the dreaded hospital for yet another round of cancer surgery—another petrifying journey into the unknown. This is all breaking so swiftly. Bang, bang, bang!

Before I know it, I'm snatched off to a fifth-floor room. An engaging paleskinned black RN comes in, taking a condensed medical history, jotting commentary on a clipboard. She and I joke back and forth. Finishing up, she says I must put on a gown and get in bed.

"But—" I quip, "it's not even dusk . . . and I sure don't look sick!"

"Moreover," she continues, unmoved, on her way out, "Dr. Elliot wants you starting on Colyte. His orders, as I recall, say a gallon and a half."

Plainly I'd caught what the nurse said. But the volume of whatever she's talking about can't be correct. Nobody can consume a gallon and a half of anything. I must have misunderstood. Moments later, with gown on, I'm sitting on the bed, feeling remotely slapstick—out of place in the light of day. Returning, the nurse plunks down on a nearby table a plastic gallon bottle brimming with some cloudy solution.

"Ever had this?" she inquires, unscrewing the cap, pouring a cup. "Oh, sure, what am I saying? 'Course, you have—you've had other surgery."

"What are we—" I ask, accepting the plastic cup, "talking about here?"

"Called Colyte. Cleanses the system. We're going to need you almost sterile for surgery."

The first sampling tastes like watered-down lemonade. Not really that offensive and I am thirsty. "For my other surgeries," I explain, sipping more, "they had me on a clear-liquid diet. I've never had this."

"Better get cookin', Sugar," the nurse urges good-naturedly, nodding toward the over-sized clock on the wall. "Dr. E wants you getting all this down by six-thirty."

"Six-thirty? You're kidding," I respond, instantly angered by this constraint, glancing at the near-full gallon container. "That's just over two hours from now!"

With surgery still many hours away, why has he established this time constraint? Unless . . . this is some kind of deluded, impossible-to-achieve-challenge that control freaks, no matter where you unearth them, feel compelled to impose on inferiors. This, to let you know who's in charge, as if that's in doubt.

"I'll leave the rest for you. There's somebody I have to check on down the hall." The nurse withdraws.

"You don't really think he expects me to get all this down," I say to Jane, refilling the cup, looking for sympathy, "do you? Not by six-thirty."

"You heard the nurse," she replies unsympathetically, like this is somehow amusing. "Sounded like she said a gallon and half to me."

"That's sadistic," I complain, feeling a burst of hostile defiance. "He can't be serious . . . Nobody drinks that much of anything. In my college days, I don't recall guzzling that much beer at one sitting, for God's sake."

"Check with your nurse," Jane says, tittering, thumbing through a hospital brochure, "when she comes back."

Ten minutes later, the nurse returns.

"You weren't really. . . serious, were you," I venture, "about me getting all this awful stuff down? It started off tasting okay—like lemonade—but now that I'm getting stuffed, it tastes like, well . . ."

"Fact is, I re-checked Dr. E's orders. He does want to you drinking that gallon plus half of one more. That's a little more than usual, but he knows what he's doing."

All of a sudden, looking at the now half-full gallon jug, I feel beaten—near sickened. "This is the kind of torture," I throw out rudely, "they put people through in Vietnam. POW camps. I'm already full to the point of vomiting!"

The nurse, crouching down, is reorganizing bedding materials in one of the lower cabinets. "Don't you worry," she assures me, winking at Jane, as though this were an inside joke between the two of them. "That won't last."

At once I get her drift. I look at Jane. "Remember my mother drinking Colyte," Jane remarks, glancing up from her literature, "before her last surgery?"

Her words evoke images of her wide-eyed mother trotting miserably to and from the bathroom every few minutes.

Five-thirty: Having drained off about 90 percent of the initial gallon, and having shuffled in and out of the john a minimum of 10 times, I wave the near-empty jug at the nurse, asking if that's adequate. After some pondering, she hints it could be but, she says, she'll have to examine my next BM—prior to flushing—to more accurately judge.

This pattern—me racing for the john, her inspecting the substance—goes on for another hour or so. At one point I'm so unthinkably gorged, so obscenely full to bursting, I tell Jane—meaning every word of it—I'm backing out of the surgery. "This is patient abuse! Drinking this crap's worse than any surgery or cancer could ever be," I growl, feeling positively rebellious, like an about-to-burst-at-the-seams adolescent.

"You're being irrational," is Jane's only remark. "Think about what you're saying."

The nurse, hearing this exchange, realizing I'm nearing a breakpoint, says if the next toiletful is clear, or almost clear, she'll permit me to discontinue the Colyte. By this point, however, I've downed almost the full gallon and a half.

Seven o'clock: Dr. Elliot shows up. An End-of-Day, I'm-Going-Home mirth about him. Have I consumed all the Colyte I'm supposed to is his first concern. Obviously he doesn't want to operate unless my innards are as chaste as a soon-to-be-cooked chicken.

I give him an ear-full of Colyte horrors. Yes, I've downed the whole gallon and a half. The nurse, standing nearby, grins, not disputing this.

"In that case, all systems are go for the morning," he says, patting me freely on the shoulder, as if we're fishing buddies joining up at sunrise.

"You're in charge," I acknowledge numbly. "At least at this point."

"With things scheduled for 7:30," he goes on, "they'll come and get you around six for prep. Any final questions?"

Thinking a moment, none pop up. I glance at Jane; she shrugs.

In me, there's a resigned conviction. A naiveté I've since learned never to presuppose, take for granted: Earlier in the day, after Jane and I'd returned to the hotel room, we were considering the ins and outs of surgery and recuperating some 2000 miles from home, when I made the off-hand remark: "Well, how much worse can things get? They're already going to operate."

Fanciful last words. Stupid. Stupid. Stupid.

Hours later: The room's barren, lost. Just me, a Deepak Chopra book, my wooden rosary beads, and a Bernie Siegel tape. The time of reflection's arrived. Jane's returned to the hotel—to grab something to eat, to take a Valium, to get some slumber in preparation for tomorrow. It's expected to be a drawn-out day—for both of us. Dr. Elliot told her he'll come find her in the waiting area following the surgery. Seems all our bases are covered, excluding a place of recuperation—that's still in the works.

Being in a strange city, in a strange hospital with strange noises and odors, seems almost Twilight Zone-ish. A deep-down loneliness begins creeping in—carried on the silent, ivory-yellow light below the door—fueling my nervous jitters. Lying still, heeding the scattered midnight intonations of the hospital—voices, twittering wheels on handcarts, doctors being quietly paged—remarkably, for what reason I don't know, I begin seeing again the people I've known who've died.

Why, I don't know.

Reanimated, they're suspended over this room, viewing me. Particularly I focus on the dispirited stare of my folks. In flash, I'm their dependent child again. Blond. Dirty hands. Scabbed knees. Their somber, grave expressions convey many things. My mother in tears; father prodding me, 'Time to kick some butt, boy!' This man, you may recall, died of prostate cancer.

Once again, I recall—cowering with guilt—that I didn't attend his last hours, his burial ceremony. Does he hold this against me? Dad, I just wasn't as clear-sighted as I am today, I tell him mentally. Still, a stinging sense of guilt prevails. Because I too know what it's like—confronting the eyes of death.

Despite my nervousness I succeed in scrounging up a snippet of optimism in the face of all this—i.e., since the primary biopsy'd come back negative, the thoracoscopy would also. The biggest obstacle is going to be the physical discomfort, about this time tomorrow.

Lying awake, I'm whispering back and forth with my folks.

Unwillingly, or perhaps willingly, I am their helpless child again. The feeling, though, is rapturous, calming. Doing most of the talking, they're reminiscing and saying how they excuse me for being a jerk—'a teenage A-hole,' as my father puts it. His use of this expression has me smiling—my highly educated father, a man who never relied on fowl language of any sort. His hallmark. Speech of that variety, he maintained, was for those who had no literacy, no proper upbringing.

Now, having kids of my own, I realize, applaud what my folks forfeited for me. Alas sadly, too late. At one point, regret slithers across my cheeks. Its fine patter I hear striking the cloth of the pillow. Feels good, actually, being 'little' again.

"Are either of you scared . . ." I want to know. "About tomorrow?" Neither answers straightway.

"Whatever happens," my mother replies, her voice sincere, "happens for the best."

"Mom, that's not a real answer," I tell her. "It's weasel words."

"What she's saying," my father puts in defensively, "is however things go, you'll be up to it."

"C'mon, you guys," I complain, "drop the clichés. You're sounding like TV angels."

"Sometimes . . . " my Always-Larger-Then-Life father resumes with self-assurance, "life is a cliché, son. Think about it. Everything's been done before. What is a cliché, after all, but a life lived—a life looked back upon?"

There is a dusting of stars across the black window. Reflecting on them, I strive to resurrect other happier times when I'd glanced up, seeing these same revitalizing flickering particles of light: Like the time as kids, John and I 'camped out' in his backyard on a balmy summer night, contemplating the Milky Way's splash across the late night sky, trying to find Zeus, as we sat laughing quietly, swapping dirty stories, consuming nectarine after nectarine off his tree—till we actually became ill.

Next thing I know: White lights are stabbing my sensitive eyes. Three or so drab figures are milling about over me, rousing me from a twitchy sleep.

"Mr. Scribner," a low-pitched voice says, "it's time."

FINDING HOPE WHEN DOCTORS SAY THERE IS NONE

Chapter 58

Into The Dim Unknown—
Malignancy Halts the Second Surgery

So... the time's come. In a twinkling they have me on a gurney, plowing down lengthy corridors, one, then another, then down an elevator heading for the OR. Gazing up at the orderly's brooding upside-down face, I ask if he's ever had a flat tire on one of these things or maybe taken a patient to the wrong OR. A smirk's all I can elicit from this hollow-cheeked young fellow. Am I, in reacting to my own fear, violating some unwritten surgical code?

In the operating room, Dr. Howell, a new anesthesiologist—not the female doctor I'd met yesterday—presents himself, asking where I'm from. No other doctors are present yet.

With the oral sedative they gave me earlier now starting to blur my thoughts, I tell him where I'm from. He smiles easily, making me feel better.

"So what've got going today?" he wants to know, unwrapping a length of clear tubing. "Full oil change and lube? We going to check that rear end too?"

Lifting my head for emphasis: "You guys did talk, right?"

"Just pulling your leg, guy..." He chuckles, squeezing my shoulder. "We'll be in and out so fast you won't even know it."

"You're supposed to take some pleural fluid and check it." I say this, but omit mentioning the possibility the fluid may be bad. "Once that's okay, you're going to roll me over and take out a 6-cm mass in the left adrenal area."

Raising his eyebrows, Dr. Howell asks: "You've got both Dr. Elliot and Garret on this one?"

These are the last words I recall prior to regaining consciousness.

Later an underwater kind of murkiness fills my head. Bits and pieces of reality float by as I attempt to push through and regain consciousness. No voices, no machine-made reverberations. Total silence. No pain. Where am I? Dead?

My mental faculties, though slow and greatly fogged, perform a slow but methodical test, ticking off each area of the body—the good, the bad—searching out desirable signs of pain: in the abdomen. Midway up the left rib cage a slight stinging sensation's detected. That's all.

The absence of pain in other areas instantly registers as: I have inoperable cancer! They didn't complete the second phase of the surgery. Suddenly my mind's racing in a hundred different directions.

Hauling my head off the pillow—a near-impossible task—I try breaking completely through this oppressive fog. They didn't do it! They didn't do it! I need to talk to someone.

Could this be an evil dream—something caused by the drugs?

Feeling only a single, needlepoint of discomfort in my rib area, I look groggily about. The room seems colossal, like a gymnasium. Surrounded am I, as on a battlefield, by other corpse-like or drugged humans, as many as 10 of them, in beds.

A solitary female figure, looking like the Virgin Mary, stands over a nearby bed.

"Nurse!" I call out weakly, desperately, feeling the extreme weight of my recent discovery. "Where's my doctor? I need somebody—here! Now! To tell me what's going on!"

She signals, shushing me.

The knowledge that they didn't complete the surgery—the foreboding that carries with it—burns deeply. Why do I have to wait for someone to come and clarify things?

Maybe—just maybe—my foolhardy psyche conjures up, something else took place. Maybe . . . they were able to do both surgeries from the back side—that's why I feel only a single pain site! Or maybe they did both operations as planned but the pain medication is so effective, I can't feel the second incision.

In my soul, though, I know.

"Nurse!" I clamor irrationally. "Where the hell's my doctor?"

Fading in, fading out. Next thing I know, the nurse is standing over me. Too youthful, she seems—too dispassionate to understand this sort of life-sapping despair.

"What is it you need, sir?" she whispers firmly, but civilly.

"I want my doctor!" I demand. "I was supposed to have *two* operations. I need some answers—now!" In the next bed, maybe five feet away, a gaunt-faced man with disheveled gray hair, rouses drunkenly, as if out of a coffin, giving me a contemptible glare.

"Sir, please, you're disturbing other patients."

"I don't give a damn. I want Dr. Elliot—here, now!" My mind is raging. Nothing can tame me now. "What kind of place is this that nobody's around to fill patients in on what happened? This is *crazy*!"

A male figure—a doctor—suddenly appears through the haze, beside my bed. He's saying his name's Dr. Winters. He's a post-surgery pain specialist.

"We didn't expect you coming around so soon," he says cautiously.

"Where's Dr. Elliot?"

"He'll be along any minute. As I said, we didn't expect you regaining consciousness this quickly. I've been doing this for years and have never seen a patient come back so swiftly."

"They didn't they do it, did they, the other surgery?"

"Those particulars, Mr. Scribner, I'm not privy to," this doctor says as quietly as possible. "I wasn't there, in surgery. I expect Dr. Elliot will be along any moment."

Dr. Winters seems edgy, and keeps dwelling on the swiftness with which I broke through the heavy anesthesia, as if I qualify for some Guinness World Record.

Minutes tick by. The waiting amplifies my frantic state. This is, I know, a turning point in my life. The doctor at my side, drawing back his white sleeve, checks his watch. He doesn't say how much time's gone by since his arrival.

"Better go see what's cooking," he offers oddly, as if embarrassed. "Be right back—promise."

Again I summon the nurse, restating my desperation. She only looks on, shrugging.

By the time the pain doctor comes back, several long minutes have slipped by. Conceivably hours, I don't know.

"Found him," he tells me. "He's tied up just now, but he'll be along as soon as he can break free."

"This is really poor policy," I manage to say, still drifting in and out of a fog. "Here's somebody you guys didn't operate on—like you were supposed to—and he's left lying here . . . with nobody to fill him in!"

"Somebody should be here, you're right," Dr. Winters says finally, a look of uncertainty in his eyes. "You're well within your rights, being upset."

"Doctor," I begin, knowing in my mind this eventuality was a very real possibility, "this means, I know, I'm inoperable. I've got Stage IV cancer. I'm suddenly feeling detached . . . like everything's now been decided."

"Perfectly understandable. Be pissed off—give your doctor a little hell when he gets here."

"Don't worry," I reply.

When Dr. Elliot's face does emerge through the fog, I'm primed. Dr. Winters, without saying anything more, sort of backs away.

"Yes, Mr. Scribner," Dr. Elliot begins, guardedly. "You have some concerns, I understand."

"Answers are what I'm really looking for. I don't know what your policies are here, but in my other surgeries in California," I begin, striving to remain composed, striving not to carry on tearfully like the child I'm feeling inside, "the doctors have always had the decency to hang around, letting me know what happened. Apparently, that's not your style."

"I regret your being irritated, Mr. Scribner. But you have to understand—you came out the anesthesia much ahead of schedule."

"I need some answers, doctor."

Dr. Elliot's eyes flash, then grow narrow. Intentionally I avoid using the profanity that would satisfy my deep-seated anger, recognizing that individuals of his ilk will seize upon language like that to absolve themselves, to flee, saying, in a righteous snit, 'I don't need to listen to this!'

"Perhaps your doctors in California," Dr. Elliot replies almost sneeringly, "are better suited for this."

"That's not what I'm saying," I respond, feeling a growing indignation, a widening emptiness. "Explain what the hell happened."

"You were fairly warned, Mr. Scribner," Dr. Elliot goes on officiously, easing back on some of his apparent ire. "I told you there was a clear possibility the effusion could be malignant. That, plain and simple, was the case. We even called in our chief pathologist—who concurred."

These words shred all hope—that isolated, that forlorn was I. "Why the hell . . . did you wait so long telling me?"

"You were, Mr. Scribner, unconscious."

"This means I'm Stage IV. Do you have any idea what that means to a patient—knowing that?"

"I do have other responsibilities, Mr. Scribner."

"You don't like being bothered with this messy stuff—someone's grief, do you?"

"Look, I'm sorry about your dilemma," Dr. Elliot says indignantly, backing away, "but this has gone too far already. This is not a result of my impropriety and I don't have time to stand here any longer."

"Go ahead, just slither away . . . " I say quietly, as he disappears, "like some bloodless snake."

CHAPTER 59

LET US NOT PRETEND—
A CLERGYMAN OFFERS A SOLUTION

A cadence of nothingness is droning in my head. I don't actually recall returning to my room. Never have I felt this detached—so lacking in purpose. Empty thoughts. No expectations.

Once in bed, the nurse who'd so gregariously flooded me yesterday with Colyte steals in to check the IV. Moving quietly from place to place, she's very precise, as if she might awaken a sleeping infant, an obvious vulnerability about her—softened body language, cheerless eyes.

"I heard," she whispers with incredible poignancy, standing at the foot of the bed. "I'm so sorry."

While I want to yell at her, at everyone, I can't help but acknowledge her warmth. Her recognition, though, only furthers my sense of failure. Nodding in appreciation, I work at smiling.

Within minutes Jane is bedside. "You don't need to say anything," she says, kissing me, pressing her wet cheek to mine. "I saw the doctor. He told me everything."

Sitting on the bed, she's watching me, pitifully, as I stare into space. For several long minutes we say nothing, communicating silently as long-time companions do.

"Didn't work, babe," I offer feebly, holding in my grief.

"Wasn't you."

"Who then?"

"It was way beyond you."

"Worthless friggin' doctor. Didn't seem all that disturbed. When he finally got there to see me."

"Eric, it wasn't his fault. Don't go pointing fingers—please."

"Well, somebody has to be responsible. I'm tired of blaming me."

"Didn't Dr. Nolin, your new psychologist, say to see this—if it happened—as a challenge?"

"Easy to say, hard to do," I respond testily. "I just learned—in so many words—this cancer's getting the upper hand."

"You've got to look around . . . see other things. I'm here, with you."

"Why should I do anything? What've I got to care about anymore—the good will of some blasé doctor?"

"What did happen—there in Recovery? Dr. Elliot says you said some things."

"I was feeling pissed—like never before. Maybe betrayed is a better word." Somehow, possessing and recognizing this deep-seated rage feels good—a revitalization, a deliverance. "And don't go looking for me to express any regret."

"We're all disappointed."

An hour later, with Jane back at the hotel, Dr. Winters, the pain doctor comes in. With him, a much younger doctor, also a member of the 'pain team.' "Mr. Scribner, are you comfortable at this moment?" this youthful assistant, Dr. Ruell, asks machine-like, easing me to the side, inspecting my epidural.

"There's little *physical* pain," I reply.

"You're upset, I know," Dr. Winters interjects, maintaining a cautious distance to the rear of this other doctor. "Would you like someone to talk with?"

"Someone? You have someone who can change events?"

"One of our staff psychologists, I meant. Somebody from Patient Affairs?"

I shake my head, thinking: What's to be gained?

Late afternoon: Another unfamiliar doctor enters from the department of thoracic surgery—not Dr. Garret, but a representative. He fingers the transparent line running from the wound site, pulls away the cumbersome surgical dressing, looking closely at the inch-long thoracoscopy incision.

Summoning a nurse, he informs her the dressing and adhesive are to be replaced every few hours—or whenever it becomes saturated with the lemon-colored goo that's oozing out of me.

"We removed quite a bit of fluid, Mr. Scribner," this doctor explains, pointing out at the same time that he'd assisted in the surgery. "We looked very closely—did a lot of digging—and didn't find any nodules. The images we picked up on your scans—the nodules—were apparently produced by the fluid. Encouraging news."

"How's that?" I ask passively, figuring he's heard this Scribner guy's a jerk and he wants only to get in and out of this room without a confrontation.

"It means we didn't find any obvious seeding. Meaning, usually, that whatever they use on you next will have a greater chance of being effective."

"What're you saying," I ask, this remark nabbing my waning attention, "use on me next?"

"I'm not aware of what's planned from here on out. That's up to you and your oncologist, Dr. Berger."

After he leaves, every few hours a nurse inspects and replaces my dressing. This process grows incredibly excruciating—like splashing hot sauce across a naked abrasion. I dread anyone saying the adhesive has to come off.

After dinner, Dr. Garret shows up. He too reviews the surgical site, the leakage. A humane man, he restates what his assistant had: After collapsing my lung, they extracted all the fluid they could—and didn't see any nodules.

"From what the other doctor said," I tell him, feeling slightly less hostile, but no less despondent, "that's supposed to good news. If there is such a thing."

"I really got in there," he goes on emphatically, talking like a little boy swaggering before Mom, "and poked around, searching."

Staring at him, I'm thinking: Still, this doesn't undo the fact that you guys didn't do the second surgery.

"If it's any consolation," he says, "things could've been worse."

"That's one of those rubber-stamp statements you doctors like. Like when you're talking about dying, how you tell us we could step off a curb and get hit by a truck."

"We can safely say, I think," he goes on, contorting his mouth, "that someone's always worse off."

"Another rubber-stamp response," I volunteer, veering into self thought.

"Mr. Scribner, don't get so down on yourself," Dr. Garret says, looking me dead in the eye.

Dr. Elliot never makes an appearance that night. Conceivably, inasmuch as he didn't do his portion of the surgery, he's finished with the matter. At any rate, I'm not exceedingly eager to see him, either.

Before long a black-garbed clergyman appears in the doorway, a Catholic priest about 40 years old, with thick brownish hair, graying at the temples. Father Enright, an MDA chaplain—one of many. Seems every denomination's represented here.

"Things didn't go so well for you, I hear," he begins, moving cautiously toward my bed, as if advancing on a frenzied dog.

Not really too sure how to react, or if to bother reacting at all, I say: "Seems that way. Why are you here?"

"To offer consolation." He's now picked up a metal chair and is moving it near the bed. "To sit and talk. To allow you to vent."

"What if I don't want any of that?"

"Then perhaps . . . we can pray."

"And if I don't want that either?"

"I will . . . then . . . excuse myself. If that's your wish."

Saying nothing for a minute or two, I just stare at him.

"I will though," the priest resumes, standing humbly, turning to depart, "include you in tomorrow's mass."

"Hold it a minute," I hear myself saying as he nears the door, "maybe . . . we can go over a few things. I do have some conflicts that need airing."

Beaming, the priest returns, sitting in the chair, crossing his legs. The rattling of rosary beads emanates from his pants pocket.

"Like," I open slowly, trying to awaken my mind to form a cogent thought pattern, "why is it the Church turns a blind eye to certain issues?"

"Certain issues?"

"Messy things," I go on, reminding myself to be frank, to deal with this as if nothing mattered . . . and in fact nothing does. "Like divorce situations. Not long ago I returned to the Church—after being away for a number of years. And because I got a divorce a while back, I'm denied the right to go to Communion. To be a complete Catholic."

The priest, following me with his eyes says: "I'm listening."

"Because the Church sees divorce only one way: As sin. The only way to resolve that sin is to have the former marriage annulled. *Annulled!* I looked into the process. Essentially it takes an edict from the Pope! You have to petition some mysterious jury—can you say Inquisition?—and then get your friends to sign sworn declarations saying your marriage was a farce from the beginning. I went over all this with the parish deacon in detail. The process can take up to two years! I won't be around in two years!"

Father Enright doesn't say anything. It's apparent he's aware of the spiritual corner I'm backed into.

"And the deacon," I resume, "when he spelled out all this rigmarole—all the steps involved—seemed to delight in telling me that if the committee finds against me . . . that's it. I'm out of luck—there's no appeal. *I'd never get to receive communion!* I'd forever be on the outside looking in. The guy, I think, had a little of the sadist in him—knowing good and well it's virtually impossible to complete the process."

"Unfortunately, what you say is true," the priest confesses, looking down at his delicate, colorless hands. "In many ways the Church's behind the times. For some reason I knew you were going to bring this issue up. We've eased up on meat on Friday, women on the altar, some Communion standards . . . the mass we now say in English. But on other issues . . . like past marriages—divorce—I'm afraid . . . we're stuck in the Dark Ages."

"Let me put it this way," I interrupt, feeling invigorated. "In the world at large today there's something like a 50 percent divorce rate—okay? That means every week, as you stand there giving out Communion, you're giving it to people who are sinners. People who refuse to acknowledge the Church's position on this issue. They go right on receiving Communion. I was raised Catholic, in Catholic schools, so I've had it beaten into me—divorce is a sin.

"I can't knowingly add to that sin by receiving Communion while already being in a state of sin. My point is this: Why don't you, when you're delivering your sermon, just once in a while, remind your congregation it's a sin to receive

Communion once you've been divorced—unless you've been absolved by going through the Church's years-long annulment process?"

A troubled look twists Father Enright's face.

"I'll tell you why," I resume once more, "because if you did you wouldn't have anyone at the Communion railing! The church would be nearly empty. So, why can't the Church admit this hypocrisy?"

Stating this, I feel myself growing more acrimonious, more desperate: There are tears in my eyes. I want that badly to win this fight, to return to the roots of my religion. I want to be Catholic again. "Father," I resume impatiently, "I'm most likely not . . . going to be around in a year. I just want to have a proper bond . . . with God. That's all."

Touching my hand, he says, "I wish it were up to me. But the annulment process is still, unfortunately, the lone, recognized course of resolution. No deviations."

"Even when a person's dying?"

"In cases of death, Mr. Scribner, as you're aware, you can be absolved through the Last Rites."

"And what if there's no time—no priest around?" I respond. Here I sit, propped up in a lumpy bed, in a flimsy hospital gown, IVs dripping into me, a yellowish muck dripping out of me, alone, with this man of the cloth.

"You do, Mr. Scribner," he says quietly, "present an unusual case."

"The Church knows there are people receiving Communion who shouldn't be—you know there are people receiving Communion who shouldn't be—and yet no one does anything about it. The purest form of hypocrisy . . . when here I sit, a cancer patient, truly in need of a spiritual crutch, and I'm offered nothing. What about all this forgiveness we Catholics are so famous for?"

Again, Father Enright sits, watching me, as if grasping at something, or drafting a strategy.

"Father," I go on after a moment, "I'm seriously considering changing religions. To one—and there are many—who'll accept me as is, without some archaic ceremony. If I go through the Catholic process, and if they were to annul my former marriage of 19 years, my two kids—who I love—would be illegitimate . . . *bastards!*"

"There are ways around that, Mr. Scribner," the priest concedes.

I've now let go uncontrollably, and, being this grief-stricken, am not really listening. "You don't have any idea what it's like, Father," tears forcing themselves to the surface, so powerful is this and other issues bottled within me, "to have them tell you your condition is inoperable—when you've always seen that word as a synonym for death."

"Mr. Scribner . . . I'm not a neophyte. I spend everyday with dying patients."

"But you don't really know what it's like—*being* one."

This gives the priest pause. "You're correct. I'm sorry. I spoke too hastily. Witnessing a thing and experiencing it are two separate issues."

"I never thought facing death . . . would be this hard. Would affect my outlook this way. I thought I'd be tough, you know, like in the movies. But it isn't that simple . . . I admit, I'm scared as hell. And that fear never goes away. Do you understand what it's like to wake up in the morning knowing you're still in the same diseased body? Knowing nothing's changed? Except maybe you're a day closer."

"Dying, for all of us," the priest begins soberly, "is a time of reckoning . . . of facing something we never wanted to face. It's inexplicable—in many ways cruel—how life allows us to go along knowing we're going to die, but never being overwhelmed by that knowledge. Until we near the end."

For several long moments neither of us speaks. In the noiseless room, suspended like a whirling swarm of summertime gnats, are all the words we've uttered over the last hour. It appears I've touched something within this man—something deeper than priestliness. Just saying all this aloud has been, for me, an extraordinary release.

"Truly, Mr. Scribner, I'm troubled by this," Father Enright offers after a period, his voice cracking slightly. "I can feel your plea . . . your wanting to return to our Lord. I'm only sorry I can't offer a final solution . . . ." Clearing his throat, he pauses as if asking a private mentor if it's okay to proceed. "Other than this: When you return home, call upon your pastor. Tell him, exactly like you told me, what you're facing. I think he may, under the circumstances, confer authorization to receive Communion. If you were my parishioner, I know I would."

"That's . . . an actual possibility, Father?" I ask, feeling an awkward sense of enthusiasm.

"Again, under the circumstances, if it were up to me, I'd say yes. Your pastor's his own man. You, unquestionably, fall in a special category."

"Thanks, Father . . . for understanding. It's been helpful."

"Did you, Mr. Scribner, remarry?" he asks, standing to leave, moving the chair back in place.

"Yes. My wife's across the street sleeping at the hotel. She's worn pretty thin."

"Oh!" he says, pausing in the doorway. "Were you aware cancer patients have their own patron saint?"

"I suppose," I reply, feeling myself smile. "Isn't there a patron saint for everything?"

"In case you're interested, you might direct a few prayers St. Peregrine's way."

"Saint who?" I ask, startled, feeling a sudden shiver.

"Peregrine—you know, like the bird. He was born in Forli, Italy, somewhere in the twelve-hundreds, if I recall. Dedicated himself to helping the sick and the poor."

"Too weird."

"Why do you say that?"

"Just . . . thinking. Odd coincidence, maybe."

That night as I lay in the eerie darkness, recalling the falcon who'd watched me each day as I drove to the radiation treatments, I feel a renewed flicker of hope—perhaps, just maybe, my pastor will grant me permission to rejoin the church, to receive Communion. And, as one of the doctors tonight alluded to, maybe there is a chemo regimen out there for me.

But still, I can't get away from the ugly confines of this body: a body that's unknowingly embraced this disease—this inoperable cancer—that I must deal with, live with, every waking minute.

Even sleep, as I told Father Enright, can't eradicate that. Each morning, there it is—like some loathsome Halloween mask: the same disease to deal with, unchanged, yet again. It's not like a hangover or some other transient ailment that'll 'go away.' No, this disease sinks its teeth in, sucking the life from you slowly, fiercely.

FINDING HOPE WHEN DOCTORS SAY THERE IS NONE

CHAPTER 60

STRANGE ENCOUNTERS—
THE DISAPPEARING OLD MAN
AND THE BLUNT ONCOLOGIST

At daybreak, with the earliest traces of sunlight streaking through the window, I'm lying there like cold meat, looking at the ceiling, trying not to think, when an orderly with a patch over one eye appears, saying he's got orders to 'carry' me to x-ray. When I ask what for, he says he doesn't know—his duty is only to transport.

He helps me out of bed, into the wheelchair. I'm hanging on to and controlling the chrome IV pole as we roll toward x-ray, down several floors. A heavy-set guy in his mid-twenties, with puffy trousers and unsanitary high-top tennis shoes, the gnomish orderly isn't terribly sociable. Nor am I. Twin uglies at large in the deserted, early morning halls.

I'd spent most of the sleeping hours, dozing on and off. My current—and chilling—forecast consuming the darkness. The new day has brought no new hope.

The orderly abandons me in an empty x-ray waiting area streaked with peculiar shadows. The small enclosure's chilly, smelling of film processing chemicals. I'm the only human in sight. To say my intellectual state is a wasteland is putting it lightly. I don't feel as if I can communicate with anyone: Why should I, I rationalize, I'm going to be nothing but a memory in a matter of months. Put more plainly: In the light of this yet uncontaminated day, I don't give a damn about anything.

An unbustling, early morning feel to the hospital as I sit there, alone.

Without warning, in the unfilled space next to me, as if out of nowhere, a hospital bed appears, occupied by a lean antique of a man. To this day I can't say how he got there. His bed, for whatever reason, is cranked up high off the floor. Girdling it are a swarm of chrome IV poles, still-swaying IV bottles. Chemo overkill. Out the corner of my eye I can see this laid-up old guy's bony face, his ashen-gray crewcut.

For many tedious minutes, I sense his eyes on me. My resentment's germinating. He hasn't mouthed a word—yet. Clearing his windpipe, the elderly guy croaks weakly: "You're new."

I don't respond, or even look up.

"Wouldn't give me time to shave," he goes on, "before they drug me down here."

Glancing up, I note his silvery cheek whiskers in the pale light. Just as quickly I restore my gaze to the ashy green wall before me, my solitude.

"Why are you here?" he pursues after a minute.

"Because," I snap irritably, still not locking eyes with the man, "I have cancer."

"Um," he retorts pensively, unmoved. "Same here. See all these dang bottles? I believe these folks think I'm one of their white rats. Me being one of the first folks in Texas—maybe all the world—getting this new stuff pumped straight into his liver. Cuz you see," he pauses, not for effect but to snatch a breath, "got me a real nasty case of liver cancer."

Inexplicably, this revelation finds a receptive spot within me. We are comrades. And he has, without knowing it, trumped my misery: Liver cancer's generally understood to be one of the more virulent forms of the disease. Perhaps, I find myself thinking I've discovered, face to face, the proverbial soul who's worse off than me.

Feeling a stab of compassion for the old guy, I divulge tamely, "Mine's adrenal cancer . . . inoperable." The word 'inoperable,' I'm thinking, might cut some ice with him—bring us to an even par. Our eyes finally meet. In a flash, I'm struck with a commanding energy, a mysterious sense of connectedness. The faded blue of this man's eyes . . . is not unlike an Alaskan Husky's stare.

"How old are you, son?" he goes on.

I almost answer contemptuously, 'None of your business,' but say instead, "Fifty-one."

"Just a kid, still. Ask about me—how old I am."

When I do, he says: "Be 85 this Sunday. Big, big family get-together planned. We're really going to whoop it up. But I'll tell you something," his tone more serious now, "ain't nobody ever seen me with no long face . . . not like you got. Uh-uh."

Even as I'm speaking this following sentence, I realize how petty it sounds: "Maybe you don't understand what 'inoperable' means."

This amuses him. "You have any idea who I am?"

"Am I supposed to?"

The old guy chuckles effortlessly. "You believe in the Lord?"

Reluctantly, seeing again flashes of my catharsis with last night's priest, I nod insecurely. "I'm not so sure anymore. He sure as hell isn't looking after me now."

"In that case, here's a little story for you . . ." The old man takes a moment gathering his thoughts, as if bagging bits of pollen drifting on a spring breeze.

"There was this fella—we'll call him Clay—bought a ranch up in the Panhandle. From photos he seen in a newspaper. Real proud, this fella was, too . . . till he went up there and laid eyes on the place. Then he realized he'd been bamboozled—the ranch and that picture were two different things.

"This Godforsaken ranch was going to take a heap of fixing. A whole heap. Rail fences was rotting and lying over. Pastures all untamed. Rickety old house had half the windows busted out, holes all ate in the roofing, the walls. Old Clay, he just parked his rear-end on his tote bag, a-looking and a-looking. After a fashion—once he got over the disappointment of it all—he rolled back his sleeves and got to moving."

The old-timer rests, grabbing a breath. Only half-heartedly am I heeding this silly yarn.

"This here's a good story, now, son, you trail along . . . Clay got to slaving away, hard as the dickens for better than two years, a-sweating and a-excavating and a-hammering, a-refinishing and a-polishing the whole shebang. Mended everything in sight, sweating dawn till dark.

"One day Clay's brother, Orville, calls from Houston. Old Orville, he wants to come see his brother's fancy spread. Arriving at the gate a couple days later, Orville's standing there, taking in all the eye-pleasing sights—freshly turned bottomland showing good Texas soil, reconstructed fences, chickens pecking in the yard. Good country fragrance in the air. Regarding the just-painted ranch house, Orville says to himself: 'Boy, old Clay sure lucked-out when he bought this place.' "

Once more the old guy halts, waiting, looking at me for some reaction. An extraordinary sort of alertness—like this man's not even ailing—is emanating from those uncanny pale blue eyes. More than slightly uncomfortable am I in his gaze.

"Well, while these boys was a-shaking hands, ol' Orville blurts out, 'Clay, I envy you—you sure got yourself one hell of a spread here. The Lord surely can cause wonders when He's inclined to!' Hearing this, Clay lets out a little laugh, tossing his arm around his brother as they head toward the house.

" 'Since you brung it up, Orville, I gotta tell you something,' " Clay says to him, " 'it wasn't all that simple. You should'a been here and seen how ratty this old place was *before* . . . when the Lord had it by himself.' "

Completing the story, the old man delays long, contemplating me. He's in fact grinning as if having a terminal illness is the most distant thing from his mind. How can a man—I'm thinking—who's surely in misery, with hardly any time to live, who's getting life-or-death chemo pumped directly into his liver, smile?

"You get the point of this here story, son?"

Seeing more deeply into the old man's perplexing eyes, I feel a wave of wonderment, of humility. I don't grasp why and I don't answer for some time. Jacked-up bed, a perimeter of IV bottles, tubing going everywhere—it's now that

I observe the room's warmer, the air smelling sweet . . . of baking bread. Something of that nature.

Here he is . . . this old coot confined to a bed, me in a measly stinking wheelchair. In contrast, I'm thinking . . . how luckless can I be?

"Yeah," I contribute, listlessly, "I catch your drift."

"I'm not so sure you do."

"Hey," I retort, my hostility still not too far beneath the surface, "I said I did."

"You see, son," the old man resumes, "the Lord, He can do a lot. But you gotta bear in mind, He *ain't* gonna do it all himself. You gotta pitch in too—do your share."

At this juncture, someone from x-ray snatches my wheelchair, whisking me off to get a shot of my chest: They want to check for fluid build up, make sure the left lung's still inflated properly. Possibly 10 minutes slip by. I'm wheeled back, deposited in the same obscure waiting area. The x-ray tech, taking a phone off the wall, summons an orderly. The area's deserted.

"What happened to that old guy?" I ask the x-ray tech. "The one who was here. In that high bed."

"Old guy?" the x-ray tech responds, looking around exaggeratedly.

"The one who was here, in that jacked-up bed, with all the IV bottles. You saw him."

"How long since your surgery, sir?"

"Yesterday morning."

"That's probably it, then. Those drugs can make things seem, well, a little funky. There was no one here before. I know. I'm here this morning by myself."

This shadowy incident leaves me with a peculiar feeling, yet a new sense of level-headedness. But at this point in the day, with a multitude of doctors and more bad news ahead of me, it's not something I give emphasis to. In my memory it becomes just another encounter with a cancer patient.

Some time after lunch: Dr. Berger, my MDA oncologist, shows up in my room. A guy I'd never seen before, eyeball to eyeball. Gray-haired, sporting an ornate silk bow tie (a little weird on a grown man), he takes a chair, consciously positioning it far from my bed. Like he's a cat wanting to bask in the sun by the window. In conversation, he makes regular eye contact with his audience: Jane, myself. An indefinable pomposity, insolence about him.

"You're at a place right now, Mr. Scribner, where chemotherapy's your last hope," he's explaining in a very hygienic, business-like manner. "We have, in the past, used the drugs cisplatin and VP-16 with some success in some cases like yours. However," he's speaking more sternly now, "you should understand that if these drugs do achieve a response, it's only seen in about 40 percent of the cases.

In those cases, that response lasts about a year, maximum. Then we're looking at a recurrence."

He's just said, in effect, that even if all goes well, I have only about a year to live. "So 60 percent of the time, these drugs *don't* work?"

"That's been our experience."

"These drugs you describe, doctor," I ask, finding it a little difficult to remain sociable in light of his stark approach, but at the same time relishing his being here, "are they my only option?"

"Essentially. We have others in the pipeline—Taxol, for one, but it's far from proven. This is a very troublesome cancer to treat, Mr. Scribner."

"As you may know, doctor," I go on, seeing in my mind, for some odd reason, the dilapidated ranch house in the old man's story, "I've had carboplatin and 5-FU already."

"That's discussed in your file."

"Back home, my doctor weighed using cisplatin, but she decided against it, saying it was too toxic for the kidneys . . . since I'd had radiation to that area."

"We're looking at a situation here, Mr. Scribner," Dr. Berger says impassively, scratching his neck, "where impairment of the kidneys is the least of your concerns. Your life on dialysis is preferable to no life at all." He's now smiling thinly, as if wrapping up a sales pitch. "Agreed?"

How can he introduce this monstrous alternative and smile? Not an uplifting, consoling component to this consultation—apart from the fact there may be further treatment for me, a treatment that's only good 40 percent of the time.

Dr. Berger stands to depart, smoothing his trousers.

"Will I have to remain in Houston? For treatment?" I ask in haste, wanting to detain him—this cancer authority—feeling desperately he's my last hope, my last respite till I face this new, more potent chemotherapy.

"Shouldn't be necessary," he responds. "This isn't an unusual protocol—except in the case of adrenal cancer. Your oncologist in California can handle it, I'm sure."

"My doctor in California . . ." I recite vaguely, wondering just who the hell my doctor will be. Not Dr. Malone, she's been shelved. "Could you, Dr. Berger . . . do me a huge favor? Would you please put what we've talked about here in writing and forward it to my doctor? It's a whole lot easier dealing with an HMO when you have things in black and white . . . from a man of your stature."

He nods in agreement. I give him Dr. Bristol's address, reckoning when she—rather than my primary-care physician—sees this doctor's letter, I'll have a greater chance of seeing things put into immediate action.

"Cisplatin's the drug," I ask inanely, as a farewell comment, not knowing how else to conclude this, "where people get violently sick, right?"

With an aloof smile, Dr. Berger: "Again, that's the least of your worries, Mr. Scribner." He shakes my hand, then leaves.

"I bet that guy loved pulling the wings off of butterflies when he was a kid," I say to Jane, mustering all the sarcasm I can. "Leaves you with the feeling you're about to step aboard the *Titanic*."

CHAPTER 61

PROGENY OF LIGHT—
THE IDENTITY OF THE OLD MAN
BEGINS TO EMERGE

The following dawn the same one-eyed aide arrives, dragging me off to x-ray. Today, though, the seasoned old man makes no appearance. The waiting, the x-rays are routine. Later, when the orderly wheels me back to my room, a professionally attired woman with a short, precise haircut is awaiting my arrival.

"Mr. Scribner!" She's standing now, offering her hand. "I'm Barbara Schafer, from the vice president's office. You had some, I understand, difficulty with one of our doctors."

"Difficulty?" I respond, settling into bed. Jane, too, is in the room. She's inexplicably giddy—as if she's already conscious of good tidings.

"In Recovery, day before yesterday?"

"O-k-a-y," I reply cautiously, feeling perhaps this incident's mushroomed out of control. I'm not fond, either, of being a cause celebre.

"Would you concisely, or not so concisely," the woman says, browsing through notes in a leather-bound day planner, "relate what took place? How you came to be so distraught."

The recovery-room incident, as I hear myself retelling it, begins sounding picayunish—like I'd been a self-centered pantywaist, over-reacting.

"For your being left in Recovery without adequate follow-up, I apologize. Considering your state of mind," Barbara, a person who seems very sure of herself, says, "that was inexcusable. Though I doubt Dr. Elliot planned it that way. Would you like an apology . . . from the doctor?"

"Apology?"

"In writing or verbally. We can facilitate either."

Taken unawares, I am. First by her very presence—had word of my 'difficulty' spread that far?—and second, by this unexpected overture. "That seems a bit severe," I return, having thawed considerably since the recovery-room impasse. "You're right: Dr. Elliot most likely didn't intend it to happen. No need compounding the issue by forcing an apology."

"You're comfortable . . . leaving it at that?"

"I'm not by nature a malicious person," I explain, feeling as if someone had called my hand. "I might occasionally go off the deep end (Jane's grinning, eyebrows raised), but I get over it."

With an observable sense of relief about her, Barbara, a very clean-looking woman in her mid-forties, gathers her hands together on her knees. "I also understand," she says, beginning anew, "your next alternative's going to be chemotherapy? Most likely cisplatin and VP-16."

"That's what I hear. It's one of the few things they haven't already thrown at me." As I speak, I'm once more impressed by her investigative work. "Going to have to sink my heart and soul into this one, I think," I add.

"As I was telling your wife while you were down in x-ray," Barbara goes on, winking at Jane, "I was treated with the identical drugs. Seven years ago. For advanced ovarian cancer."

An icy chill zips across my abdomen—because, unexpectedly, she's a fellow patient—and, it's my perception that advanced ovarian cancer, like ACC, is fiercely resistant to treatment. Yet here she sits. Hearing her say this, for lack of a more suitable metaphor, is like tossing an open can of spinach to a besieged Popeye. Encouragement personified. "And you're obviously still with us today," I observe superfluously.

"And feeling better than I did in high school," Barbara says, amused, patting her cheeks for emphasis. "Putting in five days a week—sometimes more—doing what I'm doing right here."

"You . . . went through the whole business? Hair gone, everything?"

"Couldn't tell me from your standard bowling ball. And there was many a time when my rib cage ached from vomiting. But that was ages ago. Patients today are much more fortunate—queasiness is not nearly the problem it was, with all the new anti-nausea drugs."

"This all seems so . . . strange. Your being here," I find myself muttering, wonderstruck. "But here you sit. Someone who knows the ins and outs."

"See?" Jane puts in heartily. "People do make it through this stuff. Barbara's had everything—surgery, radiation, chemotherapy. And look at her—you'd never know."

"Eric," Barbara says importantly, using my first name, "so long as there's the slightest flicker of life burning in you, there's hope. We patients can't ever forget that. And don't ever let anyone—not doctors, not anyone—tell you differently. The human body's an astonishing creation. The miraculous things it can do—when it wants to—are only partially understood."

Chancing upon another everyday human being, one who's successfully exchanged blows with cancer, is an immensely fortifying experience for us—we cancer patients. For if they've made it through the highs and lows, why not us?

"Down in x-ray yesterday," I tell her, sitting up now, feeling suddenly conversational, feeling a camaraderie, "I ran into one of your more unusual patients. Tough old fellow, getting some sort of chemo pumped directly into his liver. According to him, he's the first to undergo this new treatment."

Sitting quietly for a moment, Barbara looks mystified. "Strange you mention this. We're about to start a clinical trial with direct infusion for primary liver cancer," she says, as if graciously questioning what I'd said, "but . . . we haven't yet."

"This old guy and I talked for a good 20 minutes. This Sunday, he said, he's going to be 85. Even went into this elaborate story about two Texas brothers and some ranch one of them bought and brought up to working condition."

"You didn't dream this?" she asks, smiling.

"Not at all."

"Well, that trial, I can assure you, hasn't begun yet. We're in the final paperwork stages. So, who this was . . . "

"A real flesh and blood guy, I can tell you."

"Did he offer a name?"

"Now that you mention it, no."

"Eric," Barbara says, shrugging, "I'm . . . at a loss what to say. We definitely haven't launched that infusion trial yet. But you encountered someone. At any rate, let me know if we can make your stay any more pleasant."

"Is she remarkable or what?" Jane asks once Barbara's gone. "Your exact kind of chemo she went through."

"Was nice hearing her," I admit, feeling more buoyant than I had earlier or the previous day.

" . . .That old person you guys were talking about," Jane asks, "what was all that?"

"Now I'm not sure," I tell her, going on to describe my exchange with the old man.

"But Barbara said . . . that was impossible. That he couldn't exist."

"Yes, I understand what she said. But I was there."

"He was old," Jane asks slowly, thinking, "but his eyes seemed real peppy?"

"Like they belonged to someone much younger, someone who wasn't even sick."

"I'm wondering . . ." Jane says after a long pause, her voice withering, a mysterious look in her eyes.

"What're *we* wondering now?"

"Maybe . . . I know who it was."

"You mean you'd like to offer a wild guess?"

"Eric, think about it."

"I have, and people tell me I'm seeing things."

"That's just it. This old silver-haired man. Who else could he be—but an angel!"

"And they said the drugs were affecting *me*. Jane, this was just some picturesque old man."

"I don't buy it. Not with all that stuff he told you—the brothers, the ranch. No way. This was some kind of messenger. You heard Barbara: they haven't even enrolled people in that trial yet. Even the x-ray tech couldn't explain away this fellow. But you saw him—his pale eyes."

"Hey, girl," I hear myself saying, "this certainly isn't the cynical old Jane that I remember."

"Even though I never said much, I've always believed in angels."

Despite watching her excitement, I find it hard getting worked up over an encounter with a doting old man. "Okay, you're right," I concede, to mollify her. "That's what he was."

"You're laughing now, but he was a messenger. That's a wonderful sign. Tells us that your treatment's going to work."

"Wow, are we jumping ahead, or what?"

Friday morning, two days after surgery: I'm being discharged. Monday morning I'll have to return for a final check by the thoracic doctors to be sure I'm well enough to travel on a plane.

As he's signing my release papers, Dr. Garret proposes I get some exercise—a good, extended walk would be perfect, he says, to keep the lungs clear, functioning properly. For curiosity's sake, I ask if he's aware of a clinical trial involving direct infusion of chemo into the liver. Sure, he tells me, but it's still months away.

After Jane peels off and changes my oozing dressing, we take a drive, then we go for a trek through the humid Houston bayou country. Transcendental walk-hike—it is, at that. Here I am, in effect stooped over, barely hours from being in bed at a major cancer hospital, now afoot in a lushly wooded region outside Houston, coming eyeball to eyeball with all sorts of sovereign critters—wary-eyed deer, loitering armadillos, quick-limbed lizards, sunbathing snakes, dog-paddling turtles.

Everything . . . the very soil, the grotesque tree trunks, the silently moving bayou, the overhead blue sky . . . all seem to have become something else, to have adopted virgin identities.

Catching a breather in the tall grass at the water's edge, I watch as enormous thunderheads collect in the distance. Reluctantly I tell Jane what Dr. Garret said about the liver infusion trial.

"So," she responds righteously, "you're coming around now? I hope."

"I'm afraid I still need just a shade more convincing," I reply.

As we're exiting the wooded area, a scant black and white sign fastened to a tree trunk captures my eye: *TAKE ONLY MEMORIES, LEAVE ONLY FOOTPRINTS*. While this may be a trite caveat to those who frequent this particular pathway, it's new and awe-inspiring to me—a concept I can take with me and apply to many parts of my life.

That evening, after a subdued dinner in the hotel restaurant, after changing my still-oozing dressing a third and fourth time, we go to bed, choosing to be isolated for the balance of the weekend. We've decided to close the room-darkening curtains, snooze till our eyes open naturally. We're going to do everything possible to purge our souls of the past days' misery.

Or so we thought.

FINDING HOPE WHEN DOCTORS SAY THERE IS NONE

CHAPTER 62

THE GOOD, THE BAD, AND HMOS

I'm dreaming I'm careening down a long dimly lit corridor, going where I don't know, when the hollow ringing of the phone jolts me awake, scaring the hell out of me. Fumbling to get the receiver to my ear, I'm disoriented, wondering who could be calling on Saturday morning. The hotel room's dark, shadowy. A knife-blade of daylight is slicing through a gap in the curtains.

"H-e-l-l-o?" I say, clearing my throat.

"Eric?" a courteous masculine voice on the other end asks. "Mr. Scribner?"

"Um-hm."

He pushes on: "This Dr. Gleghorn, Eric. I want to let you know how sorry I am about missing you before you were discharged. Did I wake you? In any event, I was wondering if we could get together for a few minutes."

"Sure . . . yeah . . . of course . . ." I stammer. "What did you have in mind?" I ask, attempting to focus my thoughts. Jane, now astir, has one eye open, whispering, "Who is it?" My palm over the phone, I tell her.

"Just some points I'd like to go over," the doctor says, "prior to your heading home. How about if I come over there . . . to your hotel?"

"You want to come here?" I respond. Here's an eminent physician asking me if it's okay to get together and talk! "S-u-r-e. What time is it?"

"Just after nine."

Is he proposing this—I'm wondering, as one of many thoughts rocketing through my head—because of guilt? Surely, he too is aware of 'the Recovery room incident' by now. "How about if we . . . come to you?" I tack on hastily.

"I'd prefer to do this at your hotel. Invariably it's too raucous here."

"How about having lunch then?" I ask, feeling, for some strange reason, as if I don't want 'royalty' seeing how us 'commoners' live. "At the hotel café, here. We'll pick up the tab, of course."

"Most likely," he resumes, "I can't make lunch. I can, however, convene with you in the hotel's library area for a bit, on the second floor. We can chat comfortably there. Does eleven sound okay?"

Am I fantasizing?

Clock radio's glowing a blood red. Jane clicks on a small light. "Sure, we can be ready then." He seems delighted in saying good-bye.

"This is too . . . farfetched," I say dumbfoundedly once the phone's back in its cradle, looking at Jane. "He wants to get together—and talk. About what, I don't know."

"I don't have the foggiest," Jane comments sluggishly.

As we go about showering and getting ready and all this sinks in a little more, Jane says: "Seems kind of like we're hallucinating. You don't suppose . . . somebody's playing a joke, do you?"

The pipe-dreamer side of me is hoping Dr. Gleghorn's found some new treatment—that's what he wants to talk about. "I'm baffled too," I concede. "He's sorry, he said, he was unable to come by at the hospital to see me. Sure *sounded* like him."

Two hours later: Jane and I are occupying a small, highly burnished mahogany table in the hotel's subdued library area. A light drizzle is trickling down the large windows overlooking a grassy area. With us, sporting a multicolored Hawaiian shirt and casual slacks, is a particularly tranquil Dr. Gleghorn. Bear in mind this gentleman is the chief of a major section at MDA—he is, as they say, head honcho. His time, I surmise, is valued at hundreds per hour. With us now he's displaying that same You're-My-Only-Patient rapport he had on prior occasions.

"I feel as if I've slighted my patients," he's saying, "when I haven't sat with them prior to their being sent home."

Alas, he hasn't come to furnish information on some just-discovered wonder treatment. But he's here—and fair game for questions. As always, I have plenty. "Goes without saying, doctor, you're a hardworking guy."

"That's not justification, though. Were you left with any unanswered questions?"

"Maybe a couple." I now proceed to unload on him—gently, of course—every unanswered question I can think of, particularly those that might elicit positive responses. In doing so, we discuss at length other unnamed ACC patients who've gone through the chemo regimen I'm facing. Several have done quite well, he says. Not pressing him for what 'quite well' means, I opt instead to see these patients as being cancer-free for a very long time—years.

He goes on, explaining this chemo will produce a pronounced lack of vigor, potentially severe and prolonged nausea. He reminds me to double up on steroids under stressful circumstances—and yes, being pounded with a course of chemo is deemed stressful.

"You're a fortunate fellow," he observes. "From my recollections of your file—your history—yours is a very indolent cancer. Some patients, like you, go many years without seeing a recurrence. Some, not so lucky."

Hearing my cancer is presumably slow-growing is an odd mix of good news/bad news. "Seems like it comes back about every two years," I note, wondering: Should I smile, should I take exception to this negative prediction?

"That's a pattern we see evolve quite often. Let's hope not in your case."

For perhaps an hour and a half we talk, and talk—about only me. Astonishing this man, this renown physician, has taken time to sit one-on-one with Jane and me—to see that I, an ordinary patient, am adequately enlightened before leaving Houston.

His very presence, this in-depth concern for his patients, goes a long way toward restoring my ebbing opinion of the medical world. To say I'll forever be beholding to this extraordinary man for conferring so generously of his precious time is an obvious understatement. As Jane observed at one of our earlier meetings with Dr. Gleghorn, while he doesn't offer groundless hope—he doesn't crush what hope you have, either.

"Once I get home," I tell him, catching a flash of sheet lightning in the window, "I don't think I can go back to my current oncologist—the one who suggested we watch this fluid and tumor."

Nodding understandingly, Dr. Gleghorn says nothing—as medical mores decree.

"I've basically lost confidence in her. 'Course," I admit, going on, "I had reservations before all this. It's scary to think, but if I hadn't come here—even though things didn't come out as I'd hoped—I most likely wouldn't be around too much longer."

Again, a diplomatic nod in agreement.

"What I'm thinking of doing is having an oncologist at UCLA (since the UCLA medical school isn't far from home) oversee my care from here on out. My chemo, the works."

"Sounds like a smart move," Dr. Gleghorn volunteers, moving his glasses back on his nose. "In fact, I have several colleagues at UCLA and I'll be glad to orchestrate things. I'll cooperate however I can—a directive to your local doctors if you wish, clarifying this."

As he departs, I find I'm imbued with a rush of optimism, a real pound-the-chest, can-do spirit. But the biting question is: Can I maintain this motivation?

Sitting elbow-to-elbow on the overcrowded airplane (no first-class seating this time because of the change in return date), I still find within me a deep vein of depression, an immeasurable abyss. This do-or-die chemo could be my swan song. This formidable task—remaining motivated—is uniquely mine . . . as Clay, the Texas rancher learned.

There is still a messy ooze leaking from the surgical opening in my rib-cage area. In the cramped coach seating, the pain seems magnified. Sitting there, with my knees up to my chest, I watch the silent yellow-green grasslands slip by, trying to reflect on the good things of the last few days . . . the homespun account of the naive ranch buyer and his side-by-side work with God (was the old guy *really* an angel?) . . . the real-life cancer experience Barbara, from the vice president's office, offered coincidentally . . . the wondrous hope I derived from just sitting with Dr. Gleghorn. And then, too, there's the very real prospect that my parish priest will grant permission to receive Communion without the time-consuming annulment.

Everything . . . is up to me.

The morning after we arrive home: Calling UCLA, I speak with the chief oncologist's office, tentatively setting up an arrangement to go there for chemo treatments, follow-up. I am resolved to stay in the hands of a physician who practices and understands state-of-the-art medicine.

Having laid this preliminary groundwork, I telephone Dr. Bristol, explaining I'll no longer agree to see the HMO's oncologist, Dr. Malone, for obvious reasons.

"I want everything handled through UCLA from now on—my chemo, the whole bit," I tell her, without bad-mouthing Dr. Malone, anticipating she'll say, 'Well, sure, Eric, yours is a rare condition, requiring unique care. I thoroughly agree we should maintain the level of care you received at Anderson.'

Pulling no punches, she instead says: "We can't sanction that, Eric. Things here have changed in the past few weeks—new people at the top, new policies. I just can't push things through Utilization Review anymore. The insurance bunch wants everything accounted for and documented. Nothing impromptu flies anymore."

"Dr. Gleghorn, the chief endocrinologist at Anderson," I go on, feeling instantly deflated and angered, but hoping Dr. Gleghorn's name and influence will pull some weight, "says he'll do whatever he can to move this along."

"It's just not going to happen, Eric, is what I'm saying. I don't care who advocates differently. We're seeing too much opposition from the number crunchers. They've really taken over. We're being told to hold down expenditures on everything, everywhere. They had an absolute fit when they saw you'd been approved to go to Houston."

"But . . ." I resume, frantically, striving to influence this person who I'd considered a mentor of sorts, "I've just now spoken with Dr. Grossman at UCLA. He agrees with this whole idea."

"Well, naturally, Eric," she proceeds tersely. "Medicine is a business. He's looking for new customers. He'll tell you whatever you want to hear. We tried last week sending a breast cancer patient to UCLA for treatment. The HMO's new administrators say that patients get lost—become numbers—at facilities like UCLA. Everything there, they claim, is too impersonal. Patients end up being discouraged. What they will agree to, I know, is you switching to another oncologist—locally."

Feeling totally inept, even humiliated, I say nothing for a moment. A mature adult—*with insurance*—being told that he cannot have the level of care he requires. I'd presupposed Dr. Bristol would see things my way, agreeing with the UCLA approach. Then we'd move forward, like in the old pre-HMO days, when patients themselves chose the most appropriate place for their medical care.

"Doctor," I resume futilely, feeling like a floundering adolescent trying to piece together a battle plan to offer a rankled parent, "most authorities agree—cancer patients who have confidence and trust in their medical team have better odds of beating the disease."

"After you've been with another local oncologist for a cycle or two of chemo, then we might be able to get the number crunchers to review your status. And yes, I received Dr. Berger's summary from Houston. I understand your frustration, Eric," Dr. Bristol says curtly, contentiously. "There are two other oncologists locally. Dr. Sloan and Dr. Hamersky. UCLA, at this point, is out of the question."

Feeling a burning anger course through me, I say little more, hanging up to further hone my strategy. . . . How can someone who pays for medical insurance *not* have the right to use that insurance where he or she chooses?

Going to UCLA for treatment by a physician acquainted with rare cancers and protocols isn't an excessive desire—particularly in light of the inferior quality of care I'd seen from the HMO's local oncologists. After seething a good while, I telephone Dr. Bristol again. I allude this time to a letter I'm writing to the HMO's corporate appeals board. This procedure, if I undertake it, can take months. But it appears to be my only recourse.

Seeing this as a thinly veiled threat, Dr. Bristol counters: "Eric, you do what you have to. I've told you what the group's decision would be."

In this barbaric, keep-the-patient-from-his-desired-medical-treatment chess game, I have one closing compromise move: "In that case, Dr. Bristol," I go on, "Dr. Berger in Houston—and I hope he put this in his letter—offered that if I didn't respond to the first chemo regimen he's recommending, then he'd advise moving on to Taxol. (HMO policies, I already know, consider this drug only for use with ovarian cancer; consequently it is considered experimental and not paid for when used against unapproved types of cancer.) If I agree to see someone else—another local oncologist—would you authorize payment for that, Taxol in the future, if the need arises?"

"I know Taxol is not routinely used in cases such as yours, Eric," Dr. Bristol says, "but yes, if you see a local oncologist, like we think you should, I will approve that drug, later, if need be."

While seeing this as an ugly victory, I unenthusiastically—having her word on this Taxol issue and knowing an appeal would take months and I could be dead by then—concede to seeing a local oncologist. Selecting one of the two doctors offered, I call, make an appointment. This doctor, too, is going to experience that same job-interview-type grilling the shrink underwent.

Let's get this scary chemo business rolling—start kicking butt.

(If HMOs could defend their heartless denial of medical benefits because the money saved was being used to care for other more seriously ill patients, or for research, that *might* be defensible. But in reality, HMOs deny benefits under the guise of 'holding down costs'—a euphemistic way of saying they have to do this to maintain their obscene profits, so their CEOs can remain among America's highest paid executives. An HMO's denial of adequate health care is driven solely by the desire to build the amount of money going into that insurance company's coffers. It has absolutely nothing to do with improved patient care.)

CHAPTER 63

IN GIVING, WE RECEIVE—
THE NEW ONCODOC AND I HIT IT OFF

In the next few days, while awaiting the appointment with the new oncologist, I take several long meditative walks on the foggy October beach. I am more accepting now—realizing I don't have months to challenge the HMO through the appeals process over this UCLA denial.

Getting on with this chemo is priority number one.

While still somewhat rankled, I recognize there's but a small window during which to successfully attack this disease. Time, as the cliché so aptly warns, is of the essence. (Every day you delay starting your treatment is one more day your cancer can further entrench itself.)

To say I'm not owning up to a good deal of fear would be an enormous untruth: I am now a Stage IV cancer patient and the disease is advancing unchecked.

Physically, though, I'm feeling fairly healthy. When the body's intact—not feeling overburdened or burned-out from chemo or surgery—that's the best time to really get in there and fight. With this being my 'last stand,' so to speak, I'm going to make it a good last stand . . . Everything I can do, I'm going to do—to make this work.

Somewhere along here, on one of these solitary beach walks where it's just me and the soothing sound of the surf in the misty morning air, I resolve to radically reform my diet. This, for most of us, is all but an impossible undertaking. High cholesterol, high-fat meals—that's all we've ever known . . . and loved. Giving them up is almost unthinkable.

Food, though, is going to become my on-going 'chemotherapy.'

Having seen a lot of anecdotal reports on the favorable results of a low-fat and no-meat diet (no fish, no chicken, no red meat), I know consuming the right foods does have a decided effect on cancer. (The National Cancer Institute has recently acknowledged that as many as 70% of all cancers are diet-related. Think about that. This means that at last, medical scholars are agreeing with what a lot of us have known for years—what you put in your body, the foods you eat, or *don't* eat, have a profound effect on your health! See Appendix D.) This change in diet, to me, is the first real step I'm making toward my own renewal.

Is this what the old man at MDA was alluding to?

Dr. Sloan's office, in a modest farming community, is about 30 miles away. Roadsides on the way are teeming with verdant, shiny-leafed citrus groves, and salad-smelling green onion fields—mile after mile of them. The dawn-tinted Topa Topa Mountains rise high in the distance to the left.

"You've heard good things," Jane asks as we breeze along, "about this doctor?"

"Can't remember where exactly, but yeah, other patients have said they like him." I too, want stubbornly to like this doctor, with time being so precious.

In need of dire modernization, his waiting area's anything but regal. To put it graciously—new paint and new carpeting would go a long way toward a more professional look. The small area's almost over-crowded with uncomfortable metal chairs. A bank of semi-opaque windows hides three elderly receptionists.

A short, dark-haired nurse calls my name after a brief wait. We're ushered to the doctor's office, not an exam room. (It's always best discussing major issues with any doctor with your clothes *on*. It's far less intimidating. Keeps you on an equal footing.)

Jane and I suspensefully wait in two lightly padded chairs in a pint-sized office—which seems all the more cramped because of an overabundance of aquatic knickknacks and souvenirs. These trinkets are displayed everywhere. Enlarged colored photos of surfers riding monster waves adorn the walls. Small-scale figurines of dolphins, whales and assorted leaping fish, pieces of multi-hued coral appear randomly all over the place . . . on the desk . . . on bookshelves . . . the window ledge. Not unlike a kid's messy bedroom.

Everything in sight has a nautical theme. Because of this clutter, there's literally no space on the doctor's desk, save for the blotter square. This gives the office a sloppy, unhygienic look, not exactly conducive to instilling credibility. Looking about, I'm thinking: This isn't going to work—this doctor's going to be worse than Dr. Malone.

But I really want to like him. Because of my aggressive approach, I want this chemo to commence quickly, to prevail.

Seconds later: The oncologist—darkly tanned, sun-streaked auburn hair, forty-ish—comes breezing in (are doctors ever not in a flutter?), smiling, introducing himself, shaking hands. Taking a seat behind his desk, he invites me to explain why I'm here.

Opening with details of my recent trek to MD Anderson, I also tell him of my predilection for being treated at UCLA. This, to catch his response to something he may not agree with. He remains poker-faced. For a good 10 minutes, I go on, reciting my case history.

"Okay, now you're here, with me . . ." he says, trailing off. "Where are we headed next?"

Touching briefly on my recent exchange with Dr. Bristol and the HMO's denial of my UCLA treatment idea—chiefly to introduce that Dr. Bristol had already okayed Taxol for later use if needed—I say: "What I'd like to do, is get started as swiftly as possible with the new chemo. Can we do it this week?" I want to get things rolling so if this doesn't work—I don't respond to the drugs—I can still, hopefully, move on to Taxol—or to UCLA.

Dr. Sloan's browsing the pages of my one-and-a-half-inch-thick file. He lingers over Dr. Berger's letter—the one saying this chemo elicits a response in only 40 percent of the patients treated, and this response will last only a year, at most. In toting my file from place to place, I'd read the entire dismal verbiage of Dr. Berger's letter. It's disquieting to see, in black and white, what a renowned oncologist's saying about your probability of dying.

"We'll get things moving as quickly as we can, Mr. Scribner," Dr. Sloan says, not objecting to or questioning Dr. Berger's written battle plan. "But starting this week's a bit optimistic. In the old days we could send you over for a baseline CT tomorrow, then start your treatment the next day . . . Now we have to bow to the gods of whichever HMO's calling the shots. Everything nowadays is manipulated by someone tapping numbers into a calculator."

"Common ground."

"Hm?" he responds with raised eyebrows.

"HMOs. Sounds like we agree on disliking them. It's scary what they're doing to medicine," I comment. "We now have to beg for care that we already pay for."

"Very daunting, as a doctor," he says pensively, as if I'd touched a nerve. "If one's unlucky enough to find himself working for an HMO clinic. They fire physicians left and right. For giving patients the care they deserve: It's not cost effective, they say. How this dollars-and-cents policy is not seen by our lawmakers as a blatant conflict of interest for doctors is beyond me. I treat my patients as patients—that's why I went to medical school," he goes on with emphatic candor, "and I very much resent having invisible, non-medical bureaucrats sticking their nose in, telling me how to do things.

"I don't really work for an HMO, but I'm indirectly under contract with some of them. All of this is very complicated. You either collaborate or they starve you out. It's getting worse by the day. Saddest of all—they've even taken some of my patients and sent them back to their primary-care doctors for treatment, saying these patients don't need an oncologist. I've written letters. I've called, protesting. Nothing seems to get through to these people. I had one HMO recently take away a breast cancer patient—with existing metastases to her lungs—saying her internist could handle her care. Nine months after that she passed away. Thirty-six years old, this lady was. Just a shame."

At once it's apparent this doctor, unlike Dr. Malone, will do battle for his patients—despite HMO coercion. I'm beginning to loosen up, breathing easier, embracing Dr. Sloan as a fellow battler.

"Do you, doctor, have any objections to working with the doctors at M.D. Anderson?" I ask pointedly, having learned that many physicians see themselves as superior—not needing help from anyone. "Consultations when necessary? By phone, or whatever."

"No objections here. In fact, I think it's a good idea," he responds, seeming very much at ease. "Those fellows are on the edge everyday—they're the experts."

"Why all the ocean-oriented stuff, doctor?" I inquire as he's leading me out of his office to an exam room.

"We all have our ways of unwinding, Mr. Scribner," he says. "Mine's the water. I hit the waves every day. Before settling in here. My patients, for the most part, brought in everything you see. Hop up, please."

"You surf?"

"Never miss a day."

"Even in winter?"

"This profession takes a lot out of you," he says, passing my next test—palpating my stomach deeply, with good forceful fingers. He checks my ankles, the lymph nodes in my neck, armpits. Doesn't appear to be in some kind of mad rush, either. "I see a lot of very sick people. Once that sun cracks the skyline, I'm out there. My hideaway. Just being there, floating on the waves, waiting for the right one, seems to refresh the world."

"What got you started," I ask, lying back on the table, "doing that?"

"So what we need to do," he says, not responding to my question, "is to get a baseline CT. See what we're working with. I realize you recently had one at Anderson, but we need this so we can check the state of that effusion. And follow your response to the new chemo."

Then he volunteers, in the process of helping me to a sitting position: "In my 18 years at this . . . I've treated two other patients like you—with adrenocortical carcinoma."

"Here—in this small community?" I ask, astonished, thinking maybe this disease isn't so uncommon after all. But I make it a point not to ask how these others are doing or how they did.

"Mitotane—which you know all about—was the only known therapy at the time," he goes on, listening to my heart. "So this new regimen will be an education for me as well."

Hearing a doctor divulge he's in the process of learning anything is truly . . . rejuvenating. Perhaps I have, of late, struck a mother lode of compassionate doctors. Maybe I'd just had a run of inferior ones before.

"So we'll have you get that CT this week," Dr. Sloan's saying, "if the HMO gods consent. Then initiate chemo next week. That's about the best I can offer."

"I think I can live with that," I respond, applauding this doctor's integrity. "How'll this chemo be given? I mean, are you going to stick me in some big room with 50 other people—one of those chemo infusion centers or what?"

"Cisplatin's tough on the kidneys, calling for extensive hydration. I'll be putting you in the hospital overnight," he explains, draping his stethoscope around his neck. "The month-to-month details will be the same: You'll check in at the hospital around 10:00 on Monday morning. Once you're in a room, the nurses will start an IV, then begin giving you an anti-inflammatory and lots of fluids to be sure you're sufficiently hydrated well in advance of the cisplatin.

"Around mid-afternoon, they'll start the VP-16 after a good dose of Zofran, an anti-nausea medication. Then we'll give you something orally to relax before dinner. After dinner most patients feel pretty groggy, falling asleep around eight or so. During the night, the nurses will start the cisplatin. In the morning, if all goes according to plan, you'll wake up, feeling pretty good, not knowing anything happened, eat a good breakfast and go home. I find most patients have heard bad things about cisplatin—vomiting and so forth. So, I've found, psychologically, if they don't see it going in, they're less likely to get ill. You'll have to come back here, after your release from the hospital, for two additional doses of out-patient VP-16.

"We'll carry through with this identical schedule over the next eight months. Treatments will come three to four weeks apart, depending how well your white count behaves. . . . Sound like something you can live with?"

"I have to say, doctor, I'm pleasantly surprised. Really," I say, looking at Jane. She nods in harmony. "Sounds like a satisfactory strategy to me."

"Some people—a few," he explains, "are able to keep on working during this therapy, most are not."

"I've decided to take a medical leave," I tell him. "I want to devote my undivided attention to beating this disease. Rockwell, my employer for better than 20 years, has been, so far, extremely understanding."

"It's decided then," he says grinning, reaching for the door. "I'd most likely do the same, if my employer concurred. I'd like to compliment your enthusiasm, Mr. Scribner—about licking this disease. Attitude's a big part of the process."

"So . . ." I ask, self-consciously tugging at my hair, "I'll be without this shortly?"

"Never let that be a deterrent. Think, instead, of the alternative."

As Jane and I motor home, rolling across the long valley floor, past miles of shiny-leafed orange groves beneath a clear October sky, she says, "Seems like a really decent guy."

"He and I certainly see eye to eye on HMOs."

"So," Jane asks after a mile or two in silence, "you still think I'm full of it?"

"Full of . . . what?"

"That old man at Anderson . . . that he was an angel?" she goes on, an air of I-told-you-so. "Ever since he popped up, things have taken a definite turn for the better."

"It's not that I'm not a believer, you know that," I remark, thinking: Perhaps there *is* something to this angel business. "I just can't imagine an angel squandering time on me."

"Maybe—did you ever consider?—they have a plan for you? Something you're supposed to do with your life."

"You're saying—" I respond, seeing in my mind that mysterious peregrine on the power pole—the way his eyes followed me, "I've been, maybe, singled out?"

"Think about it."

CHAPTER 64

A DAY IN THE LIFE

In the days following my first visit with Dr. Sloan, I read another self-help manual—Michio Kushi's *The Macrobiotic Approach to Cancer: Towards Preventing and Controlling Cancer With Diet and Lifestyle*. Though I am looking for a new diet, this one seems a bit severe for right now. Maybe later, if I need it.

Along with detailing the fine points of this austere diet, Kushi, in a Zen-like manner, for the sake of health and connectedness, introduces the belief that we humans should strive to have physical contact with the earth every day—feeling her textures with the soles of our feet: sand, silt, grass.

Crucial this is if we're to stay in synch with our environment. We are, after all, an integral part of a universal oneness. Learning to ground ourselves in the here and now, so that our existence—each minute—can be genuinely appreciated, is one of the book's goals.

At first this seems trite and stale. But not when you truly think about it.

How often you go about your every day life—daily routine—not really participating in it? We often move from place to place like robots: Our minds being somewhere else, enmeshed in worries of years ago, of tomorrow. This sort of thinking taints the present. Today, right now, should be appreciated in a way the future or the past can never be.

Several days after meeting Dr. Sloan, a sense of relief, of hope has settled in. Despite being forced by an HMO denial into this doctor-patient relationship, I'm anxious to get on with this new chemo. Alone, at home, I'm gazing out the bedroom window, regarding the fogged-drenched beach, thinking about the hair loss, the involuntary vomiting this potent chemotherapy will induce. I decide to take my rosary beads and go for a walk—to reconnect with Nature, as Kushi suggests.

Sandals, walking shorts, a heavy sweatshirt, that's my uniform. Once on the misty beach, I kick off the sandals, something I've rarely done. Now, for the first time, I truly feel the tranquil sand against the bare soles of my feet, the bite of icy water against my naked legs. With every slow, purposeful step, I'm trying to savor my kinship with the earth.

For some reason, I've always been mesmerized by gloomy mornings—drizzle, fog, coolness, low-hanging clouds—making the distant world seem nearer at hand. It is, conceivably, my DNA asserting itself. Irish heritage. The friendly sound of the surf off to the right . . . two-story beach homes off to the left, barely visible in the drab mist.

I find a wondrous feeling of solitude—not another soul in sight.

Used to be, I did this very thing on the Chesapeake as a boy—a thousand years ago in the Forties. Each morning my ever-excited Collie and I roamed the shoreline, stalking Maryland blue crabs, gold doubloons left behind by the buccaneers of old, mysterious artifacts cast ashore in the night by passing Naval vessels. Walking now on this slightly chilly Pacific beach, I'm struck with how extraordinary it is, some four decades later, to be once again roaming a shoreline.

This time, though, I'm *seeking* innocence.

A sense of unshakable doom, however, lingers within. Insignificant bits of debris appear on the sand—twisted, foot-high mounds of eel-looking kelp, time-polished rocks, a scrap of Styrofoam cup, bits of colorful beach glass, pieces of shells, a shard of a rose-colored birthday balloon—materialize like signal flares, somehow underscoring this negative feeling.

In the drizzly air, an insight appears. A sudden recognition of my own unimportance, my irrelevance in the design of things. An idyllic feeling. As I walk, I feel drawn ever nearer to a God I've never known. He and I commune. There is, on my part, a good deal of remorse. There on the beach, free of all humanity, I stand, bawling like a wee lad.

As I resume walking, a huge line of jagged rocks emerges from the fog. Mounting these reef-like boulders—actually the marina's jetty—I sit for several minutes, the waves below surging to and fro—as though the ocean were breathing amid these rocks. Dancing through my head, a poem-like series of words. Though I don't have any way to jot it down now, it's still with me when I get home.

> gray-white clouds
> I wore a crown
> this beach morning
>
> peaceful waves, my soul companions,
> spoke of being
> and not being, of living
> and of dying

Walking again, once more I'm verbalizing with God. One to one. Moving along, I'm trying to ingest all that is about me. When I feel my mind rambling, I lure it back to the here, to the now. Pausing a moment, looking about, feeling a wash of cold water on my naked feet, I try utilizing the five senses—sight, sound, taste, touch, smell—riveting myself to this moment.

Still no one else is around. Not even footprints. The beach is mine, for this mind-clearing walk. Heading back, I begin my Hail Marys, aloud, fingering the wooden rosary beads that belonged to my father. Praying, walking in the chilly mist feels especially invigorating. Yet there remains that core of despair . . . but not quite as real as when I began this walk.

Will He listen? Will He intercede?

This isn't going to be a one-sided cancer struggle: Me lying back, counting on God's benevolence. No, this is going to be a good old-fashioned cooperative fight, I affirm loudly. God and me, arm in arm, trudging foreword. The strange episode with the old man at MDA comes drifting back. I smile, wondering if the old fellow really was some kind of messenger.

"If you really are an angel," I say aloud, in jest, "do something right now."

FINDING HOPE WHEN DOCTORS SAY THERE IS NONE

CHAPTER 65

TWISTED NEWS—
GOOD CT RESULTS, POOR BLOOD WORK

October 1993 . . . I've been battling cancer now for better than three years—a year and a half longer than Dr. Drake said I'd be alive.

While waiting to hear about the baseline CT, I resume my weekly consultations with Dr. Nolin, the shrink. His clear-headed approach has helped. When I recount for him 'the recovery room incident,' Dr. Nolin, usually professionally somber, appears delighted that I'd risen up, not accepting my predicament as inescapable.

"So, how are you coping," he asks, "being a confirmed Stage IV?"

"That's part of why I want to keep coming here," I respond, watching him make a notation in my file. "It feels good, opening up. With an uninvolved third party." Going on, I quote Dr. Berger's statistics for the planned treatment. The shrink wants to know how I'm dealing with these pessimistic numbers.

"First of all," I explain, hearing myself say this aloud for the first time, "I plan to take my usual aggressive approach: Putting myself in that 40 percentile group that *does* respond. From there, I'm going to try to hold onto that response for as long as I can."

"But," Dr. Nolin says, grinning, "you'll skew their stats."

"Numbers on paper," I respond disdainfully. "They're nothing more."

"I'm not questioning your intent," he goes on openly. "You've done marvelously up this point. Are there additional treatments—beyond? Or is this it?"

"Pretty much, this is it," I answer, uncomfortable at revealing this. "Taxol—that breast cancer drug—is a slight possibility. Hope things don't go that far, though. And, I'm determined to get more involved. For starters, I've decided to become a full-time vegetarian. That's probably the biggest jump I'm making. Totally altering the way I eat."

"One sure way to put some good statistics on your side," Dr. Nolin, a vegan vegetarian for some 20 years, observes. "It's pretty well understood vegetarians don't get cancer anywhere as often as the other guys. How's your wife with this? This no-meat thing is obviously easier to live with if your spouse is on board."

"She likes the idea that I'm doing something for myself. One more thing I'm doing is getting more involved in spirituality. (This word, 'spirituality,' is actually cop-out of sorts on my part—saying 'God' seems so to-the-point, so Bible Beltish.) Right now I go to church—as you know—but I'm going to dig deeper," I go on, not really having a 'spirituality plan,' per se, but liking to hear myself commit to one. This leads to my recounting the x-ray waiting area episode with the old man at MDA.

"Sounds like," the shrink observes, amused, as I finish, "you ran into one of those down-home psychologists."

"My wife thinks he was an angel," I offer, mainly to see how a veteran psychotherapist interprets this. "Sent here to put me on the right path."

"Who's to say she's wrong?"

"You're saying she could be right?"

"What do you make of it? No one else except you saw this guy, apparently."

"Well," I admit, a bit unnerved, "he certainly had strange eyes. Kind of—well—emotionally charged, for lack of a better way to say it." Further piquing the shrink's interest, I go on, telling him of the grayish falcon on the power pole as I traveled to radiation treatments . . . and how the bird has never reappeared since.

As a clinical psychologist he appears uneasy dabbling in the supernatural. But at the same time, his scholarly curiosity is getting the best of him, given my sincerity, my honesty. "Eric," he offers tentatively, "people have been known to see inexplicable things. Particularly in times of duress."

"Then there was the priest. At Anderson," I go on. "He told me about St. Peregrine and how he was the patron saint of cancer patients. Tell me that's not a weird coincidence."

"I know what you're thinking—too many things to be random. A lot goes on in the mind and out there," Dr. Nolin concedes, "that we're just now touching upon. Telepathy, for instance. Renowned physicists will confess it's verifiable—that atomic particles in different parts of the world communicate with one another—but they won't call this telepathy. For fear of being labeled kooks."

"I just never considered my connection with God," I conclude, pausing, "to be this complex."

"Okay, so what else are you planning to do? To increase your participation in a cure?"

Clearing my throat: "I haven't come up with a whole lot more."

"Might I suggest you try removing as much stress as possible from your life?"

"Like that's easy."

"We talked before about how cancer patients sometimes have to change their entire lifestyle if they hope to survive. Have you considered quitting your job?"

"Quitting?"

"Yes, you know, retiring. You're what—51?"

I had in fact toyed with this idea. "Big, big step, doctor."

"You do want to maximize your ability to fight this disease, don't you? Or is making money more important?"

"Okay, no need to rub it in."

"It's not unrealistic—retiring. You'd undoubtedly remove 90 percent of your daily stress; things that are suppressing your immune system. At the same time, you could devote more muscle to your fight."

"I'll give it some thought," I respond, pausing a moment to reflect on this. "Dr. Sloan would have to be a central figure, signing the necessary paperwork."

"If you want to keep coming here weekly—I believe it's a good idea—we need to start the begging process. Get your HMO going . . . on extending the approval." Angst in the shrink's usually placid voice. He, too, has locked horns with managed-care MBA's, their farcical 'cost-saving' maneuvers.

At the close of that week: The baseline CT and blood work are out of the way. With any CT, there's that all-consuming anxiety, that dread: You never know what's going to turn up. The soft-tissue mass in the left adrenal bed's there again, unchanged. The effusion, in that the thoracic surgeon in Houston siphoned most of it off, is, in the radiologist's report, 'all but nonexistent.'

No telling how many malignant cells, though, escaped to microscopically 'seed' in the lower left lung area. Blood test results also offer cause for concern: Dr. Sloan, skimming the numbers, reopens my file, running his finger down earlier columns.

"Something wrong, doctor?" I ask.

"Your . . . liver enzyme numbers," he replies, cryptically. "A couple of them look elevated." He resumes thumbing through my file. On his tanned, youthful face, the expression's not heartening. "I'm looking at what they were in the past."

"Is this, " Jane asks quietly, "a big deal?"

"Possibly," the doctor concedes, still reading. "If just one number's high, we don't get too excited. But when two get up there . . . most likely that's an indicator."

An indicator. Instantly I recognize what he's alluding to: Metastases to the liver. My insides immediately feel a biting acid.

"One of the enzymes," Dr. Sloan continues, "has been running high for some time."

I interject what Dr. Gleghorn said about Mitotane: When used over a period of time, that drug can boost the enzyme GGTP, and that, solely, is not cause for worry.

"Agreed," Dr. Sloan resumes congenially, apparently trying to soften the impact of this news, "but you see, there's now a second elevated number, your alkaline phosphatase, and it's up quite a bit. Looks to have been climbing for some time."

I feel my earlier enthusiasm draining away. "What would you say this means?"

"The cancer's gone to your liver?" Dr. Sloan responds questioningly, as if talking to himself. "Possible. If that's the case, it probably won't respond too well to cisplatin. That's been my experience."

"But," Jane puts in, intervening, "nothing was picked up on the CT, right? In the liver, I mean?"

Dr. Sloan, returning once more to the CT report: "No, you're right. But it's still probably too small to manifest itself."

Desensitizing words. "Is this like . . . handwriting on the wall, doctor?"

"Don't lose heart, Mr. Scribner," he offers, with an encouraging smile, closing the file on his finger. "Now's the best time to strike. If we're going to get ahead of this stuff."

That weekend: Jane's been after me to replace an overflowing potted lilac bush on our front veranda. It's not producing flowers, she maintains. I'd tried fertilizing and spraying the bush—without payoff. While not offering a rationale, I insist on replacing the lilac with a young, robust ficus, maybe two feet tall.

This will be, I decide, my comrade in arms. Not to sound too hokey, but in desperation—looking for any living thing I can bond with—I make a tacit covenant with this ficus, while tamping the soil around its roots. I'm going to take good care of this fragile little bush and, in due course, it'll flourish . . . just as I, the cancer patient, will flourish under the new drugs.

Cisplatin/VP-16 Day One: This hospital setting's anything but a distinguished teaching institution like MDA. If anything, it may be the antithesis. A one-story, antiquated facility, residing on a picturesque bluff overlooking the small town below.

My lifeless cubbyhole (room?) is surprisingly small, stark—not unlike a jail cell you'd see in a black-and-white Fellini film: bare concrete floor, undraped picture window, institutional semi-gloss green walls, a tiny private bathroom set apart by a fabric accordion door, an archaic metal hospital bunk. From the windows the sunny Topa Topa high country's visible in the distance.

In stark contrast, though, the nurses are attentive, cheery. Hand-picked are these chemo RNs, by Dr. Sloan.

Those of us receiving chemo—there are several side-by-side private rooms housing Dr. Sloan's patients—are ministered to by the RNs with true understanding and feeling. Chemotherapy here's anything but out-patient, indifferent, automated In-Your-Face doling of drugs like I'd seen with Dr. Malone. These RNs see us, the patients, as the crème de le crème—we've already earned our stripes, with all we've been through thus far in the cancer fight.

"This your first treatment?" Ellen, a fine-featured, prematurely silver-haired nurse asks, running through a unwritten litany of things (side effects) that I'll be experiencing.

In a hospital gown, I'm sitting on the bed. "First of this type," I reply.

"I can usually tell," she goes on amiably. "Try not to agonize about what you've heard. The new anti-nausea meds are great. Patients barely have any discomfort anymore. And if you do, Dr. Sloan's always close at hand. Comes by twice a day."

As I look about, everything relating to this hospital—save for the attentive care—seems contradictory and outdated: the rusty IV pole looks like it's seen numerous monsoons . . . the unrepaired spider-web cracking in the mirror over the washbasin. Where is Fellini? This below-par backdrop would be most disturbing . . . were it not for the attentive nurses and Dr. Sloan's apparent confidence in the place.

"You've had others?" Ellen inquires, suspending a pouch of crystal-clear liquid on the corroded IV rod. "Chemos?"

I relate my adventures with Mitotane, 5-FU and carboplatin.

"Not exactly a newcomer then, are you?" she says, trying to start the IV in my right arm. "As I can see from your veins."

"Damages them, chemo does, I've been told," I put in, watching her, feeling a sharp jab in my forearm.

"Yours aren't that bad," she volunteers. "There we go. Some patients are all but impossible to start. That's why we have Mary from ICU—'the IV Queen'—in reserve."

Once Ellen's gone, Jane collects my things—billfold, rings and watch—saying adieu, to return to work. I'm alone now, in the company of my latest book (*You Can't Afford the Luxury of a Negative Thought*), and my trusty Walkman. This hospital time I propose to use advantageously.

Negative Thoughts—a book I'm enthralled with. Seems authored just for me, or someone with a life-threatening condition like mine. It's every bit as good as having a paid shrink sitting at your side. Hostility, resentment, guilt, forgiveness, and other emotions . . . methodically, the authors—John-Roger and Peter McWilliams—go through every facet of personality, of temperament, as these relate to negative views in our daily lives and how these thoughts suppress our ability to combat, to recover from disease. Tools for repairing your life-outlook are clearly provided.

Another subdivision deals with the fallacy of statistics and you. I catch myself highlighting meaningful sections on how we shouldn't think positively, but instead we should *focus* positively—we shouldn't hope needlessly for things unattainable. Many paragraphs I re-read, then entire sections, then the whole book. Easy to see why it was a best seller.

Eventually, as the afternoon wears on, I pop on my Walkman earphones, listening to Dr. Carl Simonton's mediation tapes. These, too, I'd chosen for their positiveness, their point-by-point instruction on getting well, on perceiving your chemotherapy as an ally—not as a poison. How can we expect to get well if we see our remedy as a poison?

Lying there, I reflect on just what chemotherapy is: the utilization of chemicals to treat disease, any disease. We've all used chemotherapy in one form or another. Aspirin's chemotherapy . . . antibiotics are chemotherapy. (I'm attempting here to disarm the fearful word *chemotherapy*. I've even come to regard diet as a type of chemotherapy.)

At the core of any medical treatment is this: If you truly believe that a treatment will work, you will be more likely to garner its benefits. This is the most important message in this book: *Belief is at the very nucleus of healing.* You must believe you can get well . . . and you must believe your treatment will take you there.

Some doctors may attribute a cure—or remission—to the placebo effect. The placebo effect (one's inherent ability to make oneself well) is the unlisted 'medical' component that doctors and medicine men have relied on for centuries. The placebo effect is simply the body's own healing mechanism coming to the fore.

This is not to say chemotherapy's an elixir. It is not. Your contribution to the battle is your belief.

Little wiggly droplets are now trickling into my forearm. It's just a matter of time till the real thing—cisplatin and VP-16—start dripping in as well. (A little-know fact: Close to 100,000 cancer patients are effectively treated with chemotherapy each year—a remarkable statistic. This is a number we *don't* hear enough about. The press, it seems, would rather dwell on negative issues—people who're treated with chemotherapy and die despite the treatment. But as a cancer patient, you can take heart: Chemotherapy can, for legions of us, work miracles. Remember: *Belief is the key.*)

CHAPTER 66

LET THE DANCE BEGIN—
THE FIRST CHEMO SESSION GOES SMOOTHLY

Multiple eyeballs, noses, mouths. These images reflect back at me in the cracked mirror over the washbasin like a Picasso portrait. Seeing my own face spilt in a dozen kaleidoscopic pieces, I'm wondering, dismally—Can this be me? Am I really a middle-aged Stage IV cancer patient . . . being doctored to in this Twilight Zone hospital in the middle of nowhere? Is this really *my* life?

As the afternoon wears on I occasionally pace about the room, looking out the window, seeing the peaceful Topa Topa Muntains, the red-roofed township below . . . and, in my mind, my own life in simpler times.

Silver-haired Ellen comes in, attaching more sacks of fluids on the IV pole. She's setting up the Zofran (anti-nausea medication) and Decadron (an anti-inflammatory drug). She gives me an Ativan—to 'soften' things. Close to four, she returns, initiating the VP-16.

Here we go. I'm feeling that same anxiety you experience sitting—for the first time—in the seat of an about-to-start carnival ride. Chemo horror stories do take their toll. With visions of me pitching my guts—yes, I am overreacting—I focus on the first few droplets as they head toward me.

Will there be an immediate queasiness?

But there's no sensation at all. An hour passes . . . Have I made it over the hump? All of this, though, I'm reasoning, should've been predictable: Dr. Sloan, in his exactness, looks to have this chemo method down to an art form.

About five, he shows up. I welcome his interest in how things are going. Examining the IV site, he asks if I'm drowsy. I admit I am. He looks satisfied. For a moment I consider asking why he's working in this raggedy little hospital. I decide it's one of those topics best left unaddressed, like when you mention that someone's little sister ain't exactly the belle of the ball.

Jane returns around six-thirty, ladened with bags of aromatic Mexican food—cheese enchiladas, rice, beans—from my favorite restaurant. The spicy food tastes incredibly good. She and I work at playing a game of chess—a tedious contest with me battling to maintain an open eye. The chessmen grow ever fuzzy. Like a kid trying to fight off going to bed, I'm striving to concentrate on my next move. The Ativan is pulling me deeper, deeper toward slumber.

"Sure is good seeing you so unruffled, sweetheart," Jane says, smiling. "And doing so well." Her warm hand caresses mine. "Looks like this might not be so bad after all. I tell you what—why don't we let you get some sleep and me go home. I'll be back in the morning. Promise. I'll leave work the minute you call."

Daybreak: A good, strong beam of sunlight is bursting through the undraped window, creating a square-cut diamond effect on the green wall. The last of the cisplatin is still dripping in. The room's feeling slightly chilly. Running an impromptu mental and physical check, I detect that everything feels okay: no weird pangs or spasms anywhere . . . no vomiting. For several minutes I lie there, watching the clear drops silently cascading into my arm. Slipping on my earphones, I return to Dr. Simonton—he's reminding me how I have to see this chemotherapy as an ally.

Eight-thirty: The morning nurse, Belinda, disconnects the empty cisplatin bag, telling a red-cheeked candy stripper to bring in a breakfast tray. An enjoyable breakfast—toast, tea, oatmeal, poached eggs. My inaugural chemo day/night . . . seems, well, too tame. Do I at last merit something going this smoothly?

Roughly 9:30: Dr. Sloan reappears. "So, did we live up to our billing?" he asks, looking freshly showered, shaved.

"I was out cold," I respond, feeling quite fortunate: I now have a doctor I can communicate with, put faith in. The world, at least for now, is a sunny place. "Didn't feel a thing."

"Used to be . . ." Dr. Sloan's saying, checking the IV site, "when I walked in here in the morning, I had to be ready to duck. Patients literally flung things at me. They got that sick. One woman nearly bounced a metal bed pan off my head. This was prior to Zofran, though. It sure makes my job easier. And it allows us to administer higher doses of chemo, improving patients' chances of knocking out this disease.

"For the rest of today," he advises, "go home and do what you please, but take it easy. Then, day after tomorrow, come to my office and we'll give you the second dose of VP-16. Then come in again the following day for the last dose."

"When do me and this hair part ways?"

"Certainly not overnight. You that anxious?"

"I am looking forward to it—you probably think I'm nuts."

"Not really. A lot of patients think that if they haven't lost their hair the drugs aren't working."

"You hit the nail on the head."

"Well, don't worry—they're working. And before I forget," he goes on, reaching in his shirt pocket, "let me give you this prescription for Zofran. I want you taking one pill every eight hours until they're gone. Even if you don't feel queasy."

Later, when I go to pick up the prescription at the pharmacy, the druggist hands me a small pill bottle, saying, "That'll be $120.00, Mr. Scribner."

"My insurance covers it," I explain calmly, as if he'd misunderstood the billing. "Should be only a $3.00 co-pay."

"Your HMO is saying this drug's not on their formulary," the balding pharmacist explains sympathetically. "Their approved drug list."

"How can that be?" I ask, aware this issue didn't originate with him. "I have to have this medicine. My oncologist prescribed it."

"What you need to do, Mr. Scribner, is have your doctor call the HMO and tell them that. It's bothersome, I know. Fifty percent of my time every day is wasted dealing with these HMO know-nothings and their unrealistic formularies."

Realizing I have to have the Zofran to stave off nausea, I write the pharmacist a check for four pills—$24.00—far short of the original prescription amount, but enough to hold me for a day.

"I'll set this aside," the druggist says kindly, waving the check, "till your doctor straightens things out."

Dr. Sloan's nurse, when I call his office, says she'll have the doctor try to untangle this mess as quickly as possible. Several hours later, the pharmacist calls to say the HMO has decided to allow the Zofran. I can pick up the balance of the prescription, tomorrow—along with my $24.00 check.

With this time-wasting caper out of the way, I try sitting quietly, watching some afternoon TV. But I can't sit still, and I'm not queasy . . . What's taken hold of me?

Out of the blue, my wandering mind decides I should undertake a task I'd meant to carry out months ago: Video taping the house's entire contents. In case of a fire or earthquake or whatever, we'd have proof, for the insurance company, of our possessions.

So wired am I that I create an hour-long video—and ad-lib a humorous dialogue to go with it. The tape ends up being more a distorted parody—which only my charitable sister-in-law applauds—than a household-contents video.

Two days later: Feeling truly lousy—like a 200-pound anchor is lying on my chest—I'm sitting before Dr. Sloan in his tiny chemo room. "Weirdest thing happened when I got home," I'm explaining as he inserts a needle in the back of my hand.

"Oh, really?" he says, stone-faced, "What's that?"

"My mind was clicking along at a hundred miles an hour," I continue. "I tried everything to relax, but couldn't. I ended up videotaping everything in sight, all the furniture in the house and then some. I'd been meaning to do that—but not then."

"You can't imagine how often I've heard this," Dr. Sloan remarks, chuckling. "Women, as a rule, clean their closets. Men reorganize the garage. It's the Decadron. You got a sizable blast—roughly 10 times the steroid dose you're used to. That's the reason you could take on the world."

"I anticipated being sick, if anything."

"In the old days, yes—before these new anti-emetics. Chemotherapy's a far cry from what it used to be."

After the chemo, at home, a barefoot walk on the beach sounds appealing. But, once out on the sand, I find I can only trudge for a hundred yards or so. Depleted of all energy, I feel like I'm going to keel over. Backing away from the ankle-deep foam, I plop down in the cool, dry sand.

After a period of rest, I struggle back to my starting point, slumping in an aluminum chair, not moving for several long minutes. (This becomes my post-chemo routine: one day of exhilarating steroid-driven energy, a 24-hour sense of light nausea, then weeks of oppressive fatigue.)

Watching the waves come and go, I catch my breath, while trying to focus on my current good fortune. . . . This heinous cancer business began in 1989. It's now 1993. How much more savvy a patient I've become by reading, keeping my ears and eyes open, becoming involved . . . seeing doctors as less than gods.

Doctors will, one minute, quote statistics, then minutes later—when talking about expected chemo responses, say we're all different—and admit that statistics may or may not apply. *Huh?* Realistically, statistics are, at best, a tool used for *estimating* the outcome of your particular disease. Statistics are most appropriately used for researching which treatment holds the best chance for you.

Sitting here on the beach, contemplating the crashing waves becomes, in time, a post-chemo ritual. During the following months of this, a collection of portentous wonders presents themselves. All of them I see as a harbinger of good tidings.

One day, for example, a cluster of dark dorsal fins appears in the waves. Surfacing between me and the horizon, these bottle-nose dolphins, as many as 20 of them—some quite small, others fully grown—zip through the translucent surf, riding the crests as body-surfers would, then whipping back, launching themselves, spinning in the air. Eerily entertained, I glance about . . . to see who else is enjoying this. But no one's in sight.

When Jane comes home for lunch that day, I tell her about these childlike creatures, their command performance. Sliding a tomato sandwich toward me, she has that, 'Yeah, sure,' expression.

"Really, it happened. I'm not pulling your leg. Maybe . . . it was one of those angel-inspired things again," I say in jest.

This causes her to pause. "Could be you're right. Why else would they pick you—or that exact spot on the beach? To put on their show?"

Little did I know the near future held more mysterious encounters—one of them truly profound and unexplainable in everyday earthly terms.

CHAPTER 67

WHEN WEAKNESS BECOMES STRENGTH—
WORKING THROUGH THE CHEMO FATIGUE

In the days following the first chemo treatment, a crippling tiredness, and a sense of background nausea have me feeling as if I'm forcibly dragging this body, like a stagnant mass, from place to place. This is extraordinary . . . in light of that first post-treatment day, when the Decadron transformed me into a human buzz saw.

In the weeks following, there are few times when I feel really good. But, after enduring a year and 10 months in the grip of oral Mitotane . . . five months of IV carboplatin and 5-FU . . . eight bone-weary weeks of once-a-day radiation, and three debilitating surgeries, I'm not sure what 'feeling good' means anymore.

My daily routine now involves dragging myself out of bed around eight-thirty, fixing an immune-system-enhancing breakfast. Time and again accounts have popped up of folks triumphing over malignancies with the proper nutrition. At a cancer survivors' lecture one evening I cornered a naturopathic physician.

"I can't tell you how many people I've seen literally cured of cancer, through diet, in my 25 years at this," this enthusiastic fellow confesses. "But in America we aren't ready to recognize food for its curative powers, so I can't openly advertise this fact. People—the medical establishment—would rebel, calling me a quack. But they're coming around, slowly. Won't be long, though, before food is seen as a cancer treatment." (The National Institutes of Health currently have several food-based clinical trials underway.)

Each and every cell in your body's produced—and nurtured—from the foods you select and eat. Think how incredibly important this is. Food—especially vegetables, fruits and grains—is the fuel your body utilizes to build the mechanisms it calls on to fight malignancies, cells gone crazy.

As a non-meat eater you can dine in any café or restaurant—Jane and I do all the time—and have a satisfying meal. Nearly all restaurants nowadays offer vegetarian specials or stock items like pasta, egg dishes, bean-and-cheese burritos, salad bars with everything under the sun, and no-meat 'garden- or veggie-burgers,' to identify just a few. Or you can order a menu item, instructing the waiter or waitress to hold the meat.

Eating healthy is simple—and easy.

In any case, each day I have a filling breakfast—hot oatmeal or a 10-grain cereal. Then down go a handful of medications and vitamin supplements—these are best taken with meals, unless otherwise specified. Then, plopping down in Jane's grandmother's antique rocker, I meditate or listen to Dr. Simonton's visualization tapes for 20 minutes or so. This relaxation interval, though bothersome at first—sitting, accomplishing 'nothing' for so long, seemed tedious—I find to be thoroughly restful, cleansing.

After the daily mediation, if feeling well enough, I struggle over to the beach. Cool sea air caressing the skin's wonderful for bringing life into focus. These walks along the water's edge, over the course of my treatment, become sort of a gauge: the further a treatment's behind me, the further can I trudge without feeling utterly drained.

Most days I can walk only a half-mile or so. Fatigue's that debilitating. Then, returning to the aluminum chair, I catch my breath, reading a chapter or two of a plain-English Bible—as part of my spirituality program, I've decided to read this from cover to cover—before my eyes grow weary or the gusting breezes threaten to tear the fragile pages.

Emotionally, I'm in limbo. Between treatments, CT scans.

I'm putting all my faith—as best I can—in the chemo's efficacy. As Norman Cousins contends in *Anatomy of an Illness*, there are enormous curative powers in positiveness—or positive focusing, as the authors of *Negative Thoughts* put it. Believing you'll get well and focusing on this sends a powerful regenerative message to the body.

But still, with human nature being as it is . . . there's a deep-down fear: Will this last-ditch effort work? Or will the doctor ultimately say: 'Sorry, Eric, it didn't work. There's nothing more.'

Day 14, following the first chemo: I'm sitting with Dr. Sloan again. Each of the four exam room walls is adorned with hand-painted ocean scenes—watercolors presented to the doctor by young cancer patients. Going over me with good, athletic hands, digging deeply here and there, he asks how things are going.

"Other than feeling like I've just been through the first week of football training, you mean?" I ask.

"Tired, you're saying?" he replies hesitantly, scratching a note in my file.

"And my sense of taste—that's gone south. A lot food-smells make me queasy."

"Pretty much par for the course," he acknowledges, listening to my lungs. "Probably it'll get worse before it improves."

"And I'm still concerned about this hair," I go on, noting the doctor's thick, sun-streaked auburn mane. "It was supposed to be gone by now, I thought."

"That's still troubling you?"

"Well, yes . . . because . . . it must mean the chemo's not working."

"Eric, it's just not time yet," he says, now recalling my earlier concern, "for the hair to go."

"Time?"

"Yes. Day 21," he goes on, clicking his pen shut, folding his arms. "If it doesn't start happening by then, I'll be surprised."

"You can calculate it . . . to the day?"

"Most patients start seeing the hair come out on or about then. Most of them, though, aren't real excited about it."

"You're being serious?"

"Absolutely."

"Okay," I respond acceptingly. "Something else I want to tell you—since honesty's part of this relationship. I'm changing my diet. No more meat." (Your oncologist should be aware of any and all complementary therapies you're involved with—even though he'll most likely downplay their value.)

"Red meat, you're saying?"

"No. All kinds—fish, chicken, beef."

"You are an extremist, aren't you?" he says indifferently, tucking my file beneath his arm. "Kelly, my nurse, has been eating like a rabbit for several years. Doesn't seem any worse for the wear."

"No objections then? You don't think it's going overboard?"

"So long as it doesn't interfere with what we're doing. But promise me—if you start feeling more wilted you'll go back to meat. At least till we finish your chemo."

Nodding in agreement, I ask: "How about if we move the date for the next chemo up? Or maybe do the treatments more often? I'm thinking I can handle it."

"Your attitude's a real plus, Eric," Dr. Sloan asserts, patting me on the shoulder. "But things don't work that way. Your white count's got to bounce back before we can resume. Otherwise, you risk getting an infection, setting back your treatment for weeks . . . months, even. We don't just pluck dates out of the air—there is a rationale. Your fighting spirit, though . . . is what we see in patients who walk away from this."

Grinning, I relish a doctor's endorsement.

"So—we'll get some blood work, alright?" he goes on. "A couple days before. Then we'll move on to cycle two." Handing me a scribbled-on piece of paper to give the HMO clinic—so they'll sanction the required blood work—he winks, walking out.

Even the tiniest medical procedure by either patient or doctor, it seems, is scrutinized in detail by the overly-vigilant HMO . . . as if they were our newest appointed Big Brother.

With Day 21 comes the shock of lifetime.

FINDING HOPE WHEN DOCTORS SAY THERE IS NONE

CHAPTER 68

THIS... COULDN'T BE—
MY HAIR'S FALLING OUT!

Saturday. A windswept, sunless day at the oceanfront. Jane and I, wearing sweat clothes, have been over by the water, walking, then doing a little reading. Cycle two of the chemo is still a week away. At home, I hop in the shower. Pouring out a handful of shampoo, I first give the old scalp a good lathering.

As I'm washing away the shampoo, I catch a quick, blurry glimpse of something dark, something murky swirling about my feet and the shower drain. Images of the Psycho shower scene zoom through my mind—the dark swirls on the floor are blood! Somehow this chemotherapy is making me bleed from my pores!

As my eyes clear up, the makeup of the swirls on the shower floor becomes instantly clear: It's globs of hair! My hair! Mixed senses of fright—and repugnance—hit me. One minute I'm innocently showering, next my hair's falling out in thick gobs, swirling down the drain.

Despite my wanting this to happen, it's not easy to take. Watching your hair disappear, vanish down the drain, almost at once, is—well—unnerving, to say the least. Thick strands cling to the towel as I dry off.

"You were saying how ready you were," Jane reminds me, trailing me into the bedroom. "Looks like somebody cast an evil spell over you."

"He said around day 21. I just didn't expect this to happen all at once!" I respond, leaning forward, studying the half-dollar-sized sections of freshly exposed scalp. "This makes me look a lot sicker than I actually feel."

"What's your choice," an unmoved Jane asks, "the clippers?"

"Let me think about it."

Sunday, the next morning: Loose hair, great swirls of it, are strewn across my pillow like patches of seaweed on the beach. Looking in the mirror, I'm trying to envision how I'll look as a chrome-dome.

"Guess it's the clippers—or this mange look," I tell Jane. "Friggin' hair's coming out everywhere—in my food, on the pages of the whatever I'm reading, the shoulders of my shirt . . . like it was never attached. Remember those chemo patients? The ones at Anderson? How sad—and truly ill—some of them looked with patches of hair missing?"

"So," Jane wants to know, "you've decided on the polished look?"

Minutes later, I'm slick, smooth. The scalp feels like a warm bowling ball. This sudden, naked, no-hair look is startling, but unquestionably a more acceptable look, in a Yul Brenner way.

"Happier now, Slick?" Jane jests, dropping the clippers, the scissors back in the drawer. "You're the one who told Dr. Sloan you were looking forward to this."

A bittersweet sense of contentedness.

Jane, running her hand over my glassy head: "How weird."

"How's it look, though?" I ask, feeling aberrant ... as if I'd just dropped my pants before a crowd.

"Oh, better, yes, much nicer than that sickly, patchy look. In the mirror now, it'll be a healthier-looking you. That mangy unevenness was awful. . . . Say," she goes on, "you know who you remind me of?"

"This ought to be good."

"*Peanuts*," she says, laughing heartlessly. "You know, that cartoon kid."

"Thanks, Lucy. I needed that."

Instantly my head's chilly. Remarkable how much warmth hair provides. Now, whenever I go out in public, I sport a hat—for a time I'm sensitive to people's gawking. Or what I perceive as gawking. The chemo, without doubt, is doing its job. But this chrome-dome look generates a whole new sense of misgiving: Like the pain of seeing myself, *after*—if this chemo proves unsuccessful—lying inelegantly in a casket, mourners passing by, muttering under their breath how ghastly a bald Eric looks.

Days later, my son and grandson are supposed to drop by. I've told Marc not to tell my six-year-old grandson about my new baldness. I want the boy's unbiased initial reaction. Entering the living room, my grandson at first dashes toward me—then slows dramatically as if suddenly confronted with a freakish animal.

"Hey, big guy," I ask, reaching out, "what's up?"

He stops dead in his tracks, holding his ground. Eyes narrowed, not saying a word.

"It's me, Conor," I go on, having tormented the boy enough. "Your Grampa. Can't you tell?"

"Oooow, Grap-pa," the youngster begins slowly, deliberately, his head moving side to side as if this will reveal the identity of this stranger, *"you . . . got old!"*

Chuckling, but feeling strangely hollow at the same time, I explain the reason for the hair loss.

"How come . . ." the boy asks astutely, frowning in disbelief, "when I get sick . . . my medicine doesn't make my hair come out?"

Looking into the child's unspoiled eyes, I wonder: How do you explain the inhumanity of a life-sapping disease like cancer to an innocent child?

The week prior to going in the hospital for cycle two, I undergo the necessary blood test. The report's forwarded to Dr. Sloan. This succeeding chemo cycle goes precisely like the first. Dr. Sloan, on his chemo rounds, comes by in the afternoon. He doesn't bat an eye seeing my slick pate. When I call his attention to it, he jests about the convenience of not shampooing. I want to ask—but don't—if he ever feels any guilt at being the force behind a patient losing his hair.

He's more in a hurry today, saying he wants me to have a follow-up CT at the end of the month. Standard practice, he explains, to evaluate the chemo's response.

"We can see something that soon?" I ask.

"Generally," he says, "one way or the other."

At home the following day: That same explosion of steroid-driven exuberance energizes me. I walk several miles along the breezy beach, easily. Day two, though, the desolation sets back in . . . a two-ton cloak of inertia.

But this month I have a mission. I'm going to see the local parish priest, requesting his permission to return to Communion—without the rigmarole of a lengthy inquiry. Admittedly, I hadn't arranged this rendezvous till now, till my hair has fallen out, knowing my story'll have that much more impact, hairless.

Alas, all of life, it seems, is a chess match.

On my initial call I'm given a next-day appointment to see the pastor, a fine-boned man who I'd only seen at a distance, offering Mass.

A windy November afternoon at the turn-of-the-century rectory, I'm ushered into his unpretentious private study by a sour-milk-smelling elderly woman in a faded dress. When the pastor appears in the doorway, he hesitates, as if startled. Very frail—with perhaps a touch of palsy—having sparse silvery hair, pink-white hands, Father Melchur seems disconcerted, at once uneasy with my harsh appearance.

Though cordial, he maintains that man-in-charge demeanor as I take 10 minutes spelling out my dilemma, and the recommendations of the priest in Houston. The pastor, I fully expect, will smirk, pointing out how far-fetched this request is.

"Taking into account the possibility of your early . . . *demise*," Father Melchur offers quietly, with near motionless lips, "I don't see how it would be of any significance . . . whether you did or did not receive the Council's blessing."

"You're saying then . . ." I respond, stunned by the immediate ease of this, "that . . . I *can* receive Communion? Now . . . without the Council's approval?"

"I am not, of course, the ultimate authority," the priest concedes, seeming outwardly moved by my narrative, my appearance. "But I think He will understand . . . in that you may not be with us next year."

FINDING HOPE WHEN DOCTORS SAY THERE IS NONE

A dead weight has been stripped from the soul. In a matter of minutes—without any sort of haggling, as I'd expected—I'm a full-blown Catholic again.

"But Father," I ask, delighted, but quickly gathering my thoughts so as not to cause him to change his mind, "what about when I go to confession? That first time? When I tell the priest—as I'll have to—that I terminated my marriage. Won't he be required to stop right there, saying he can't absolve that sin?"

"Despite what may appear to be the case, Mr. Scribner, priests in this parish are fair-minded—quite modern," the pastor affirms, seeming satisfied with this achievement. "Tell him of our dialogue—my decision. That should resolve any inconsistencies. And," he prompts, as if calling to mind something almost overlooked, "I think you should consider receiving the healing oils."

A quick sense of fear grips me—do I look that wretched? "Healing oils? You mean like . . . for people who aren't going to be around long?"

"Not at all. Sadly, within the church we do a poor job of instructing parishioners about healing oils." The old man's stare is punctuated now by a grandfatherly grin, a moving blade of flesh from chin to Adam's apple. "The oils are utilized in cases where a person's ill—very ill—but not necessarily near death."

Father Melchur advises I make an appointment to see his assistant, Father Esperanza, and have him administer the sacrament, as well as hear my confession.

Two days later: It's sundown as I again enter the yellow, two-story rectory. Father Esperanza, a threadlike black beard framing his jaw, coming up to form a thin, sinister-looking mustache, lets me in. The floorboards creak eerily in the dim corridor in a way I hadn't noticed previously as I accompany the stoop-shouldered priest to his office.

"Please, Mr. Scribner," Father Esperanza, a man in his mid-fifties says graciously in an obscure Mexican cadence, "be seated."

His quarters are tinier, more packed with storage boxes than the pastor's. Sitting in a straight-back wooden chair adjacent to his cluttered, dark-wood desk, I've folded my hands submissively in my lap. A single desk lamp poorly illuminates the room, casting odd shadows. Ventilation carries with it a mixture of distinct odors—decaying books, stale incense, oiled wood.

"Father Melchur tells me," he begins with considerable distress, as if I were a blood relative, "you are . . . ill."

Again I recount my cancer history.

"This cancer, Mr. Scribner," the priest asks, "is where?"

"Father, I know this is matter of words—but I don't like thinking of myself as *having* cancer, or that it's anywhere in my body at the moment. But it was right here." I touch the region beneath my left ribs. "It was a very rare cancer, Father," I add needlessly, "only about one out of every two million people get it."

"Indeed, a mortifying disease," he observes gravely, gathering up a tattered black prayer book, a pint-size glass-topped flask of oil. Positioning a length of purple vestment around his neck, he opens the prayer book. Fingers of ebony hair lay across his shinning scalp. "Numerous acquaintances have I lost to this terrible plague," he goes on. "My sympathy is with you."

There is a palpable electricity in the air—as if all who'd sat in this chair before me are nearby, listening. Through the slightly distorted window glass, in the dim garden light outside, a chipped and weather-worn Virgin Mary stands, making eye contact, hands held imploringly. "It's been pretty tough, Father," I admit. "A lot of times . . . just me . . . and the guy up there."

"This cancer," Father Esperanza's been reading softly to himself for a moment, "is elsewhere?"

"Just here," I reply, my eyes suddenly drawn to a brown-bodied spider making its way across the dusty windowsill.

"Please, if you would be so kind . . . raise your shirt. I will be placing the oils directly on the skin."

Feeling a comfortable sense of neutrality, much like I've adopted with male or female doctors, I raise the shirt. As I do it occurs to me that this man, being from an isolated village in the mountains of Mexico, may be more acutely attuned—and accepting—of all things mystical.

"Father," I ask, "did you ever have an angel . . . come to you?"

FINDING HOPE WHEN DOCTORS SAY THERE IS NONE

CHAPTER 69

TILL THOU RETURN UNTO THE GROUND— BECOMING A CATHOLIC AGAIN

"I am a holy man, Mr. Scribner. You are asking me this?"

"Yes, because . . . I may've encountered one—an angel or something at the cancer center. In Houston," I volunteer, going on, telling him of the old man with the mesmerizing blue eyes . . . and his story of the rancher.

"And still you are skeptical?"

"Could this be, is all I'm asking."

"It is said that each of us has a spirit nearby, Mr. Scribner. When truly needed, they appear, giving us a message . . . sometimes a mission."

"Message . . . okay."

"Often this message is unclear," the priest explains in a near whisper. "Left for us to decipher."

"Many meaningful things, Father," I continue, opening up, feeling the pieces fall into place, "seem to have gotten better . . . since he appeared."

"Aiyee!" Father Esperanza utters this one-word response in an odd, old-world voice, his dark eyes gleaming, as if this will clarify everything.

With the glass stopper moistened with healing oil, he leans forward, touching it several times to the battlefield of my cancer, praying softly. He asks permission to lay his palm directly on the area. With consent given, he places his relaxed, warmish hand flat on the area of the incisions, murmuring trance-like in Latin, looking imploringly beyond me.

I'm trying humbly to show a synergy, seeing this sacred rite as one that'll go a long way toward fulfilling my spiritual plan. The olive-skinned priest—absorbed in reflection—begins reading from the frayed prayer book. When it's my turn to respond, he recites the phrase then looks to me. This laying-on-of-hands takes perhaps 20 minutes.

"Would you care, Mr. Scribner, to make your confession now?" Father Esperanza asks, removing the purple vestment from around his neck, as would a physician with a stethoscope.

Caught off guard, not expecting this all-in-one package, I consent, accompanying him as quietly as possible into the breezy night, to the barely illuminated red brick chapel next door. It's been—what—20 some years since my last confession. This, then, I calculate will take some time.

Sitting face to face in a 'modern' confessional—unlike the confessionals of old where the priest remained behind a barrier—Father Esperanza coaches me. Upon hearing the elapsed time since my last confession, he proposes I lump my transgressions in broad categories. When I get to the divorce, he says he's exchanged thoughts with Father Melchur about this and, in light of my situation, this issue is not an obstacle.

Thus the confession takes a matter of minutes, not hours.

When I finish, Father Esperanza catches me unaware a second time asking if I want to receive communion—right now. "We can do that right now?" I ask spontaneously, never having received the sacrament outside of Mass.

"Of course," he says, beckoning heartily, shepherding me from the confessional to the midpoint of the withered, baroque altar. The shadowy chapel, with its mute statues, its unoccupied rows of pine pews, possesses an omnipotent silence. The altar—garish, Spanish-influenced, conceivably a leftover from the Missionary days—exudes a wondrous feel, an inviting quality, as if beckoning me nearer.

"I will leave for a few minutes while you say your penance," the priest says, departing in the shadows.

Though I'd been an acolyte 40 years earlier, being this near the tabernacle once more has me—well, nervous. I find myself flashing back to . . . the sweet smell of incense . . . the metallic clanging of the incense burner chain as the priest is swinging it . . . the vile looks the priest shoots my way when I misstate my Latin.

Several minutes later, approaching the gold tabernacle, Father Esperanza reaches in, removing a lone wafer. All of this seems jarringly impromptu. A warmth instantly rushes through my body as the small disk is laid upon my tongue. Heeding my tears, Father Esperanza reaches out, clasping both shoulders, bowing insightfully.

Driving home, I feel ebullient—whole again. No longer a vast spiritual divide within me. No longer will I see myself on the outside looking in—a miscreant. This spiritual interlude: a necessary step forward in my struggle with this disease. The shrewdness of the chaplain in Houston has proven prophetic.

Jane, using the remote to mute the ten o'clock news, asks how things went—with the ceremony, the priest. Knowing she doesn't share my excitement about things spiritual, I offer only a brief summary. "Well, you certainly look euphoric," she comments, to all appearances tickled things had gone so well. She asks no more.

I truly am exhilarated—and can now concentrate on the worldly matters of subduing this disease.

FINDING HOPE WHEN DOCTORS SAY THERE IS NONE

Frequently, when not sitting at the seashore trying to digest the Bible, I'm preoccupied with some just-out manual on fighting cancer. I'm trying to read everything at the community library, at regional bookstores. Deepak Chopra, Dr. Siegel, Dr. Simonton, esoteric medical texts, you name it. The more I read, the more an overriding argument crops up: To change the course of this disease, to survive, one has to make meaningful changes in his or her life. (This, of course, is in addition to standard medical treatment.)

Simply put: You must change the life that created the cancer if you hope to put the disease behind you.

Even if this transition is interpreted as changing your employment, your marriage, your relationship with a particular individual, your living conditions . . . if you hope to defeat this disease, you *must* change that negative environment. In my case, I know without hesitation the incompatible environment: my employment. While the job compensates me well, it doesn't give me anything to be joyful about. Its nonstop stresses I've long suspected are promoting my condition—destroying me.

Just after the second chemo cycle I realize—or begin owning up to—that to truly get well I have to change occupations, or, not work at all—retire. Both options seem viable, in that my abiding goal's to stay alive, period. Dr. Nolin, the shrink, had pounded this issue home time and again.

"I was concerned, frankly," he submits, at our next session, "that you were going to side-step the issue."

"There's so much involved, doctor," I respond. "It's not like society's out there saying, 'Hey, you're real sick, and in order to get well, you need to quit work . . . we'll take care of you.' Far from it. Seems like all of society, as we know it, is geared toward getting you back to work—no matter what that's doing to you, physically or emotionally."

"Our Protestant work ethic again."

"So," I resume with the shrink lending an ear, taking notes, "I've decided to apply for Social Security Disability and my company's long-term disability."

"You are going forward with this?"

"I'm at least going to see what happens."

"How old are you again?"

"Fifty-one last July."

"You can go into this—and not go batty? Silly question," he says at once, answering his own question. "I should know that by now."

"Whatever it takes, I'm willing to do—to get well. Getting away from an ugly experience, my job, seems like one of the best tools. All the folks who write get-well cancer books—doctors and former patients—agree."

"And I'm with them. But, understand, it's a major step—one that will transform the rest of your life. Can you handle it . . . monetarily?"

"A step down, certainly," I admit. "No more condo at the beach. But . . . I'll live."

"How's the chemo going? You able to get through a regular day?"

"If I stay focused on this stuff, not too bad. But if I go off on the negatives, then everything closes in—the nausea, that morbid exhaustion."

"To occupy those down times," the shrink begins, looking over his tortoise shell half-glasses, "have you thought about getting an animal—a pet?"

"Hey, I just got re-accepted by my church . . . now you're telling me I need a pet?"

"For company. An important piece in the recovery puzzle."

"Yeah, yeah, I know—the how-to books are always saying pets are a good idea. And I have given it some thought. But just the idea of scooping up puppy shit turns my stomach—and definitely sounds unhealthy."

"That's why a cat's the perfect pet. Now let me finish . . . (the shrink's holding up his hand). They're low maintenance—virtually no cleanup—and yet they provide another consciousness, another set of eyes to communicate with. At those moments when you're feeling isolated."

"Man, I hate cats. They're so . . . distant," I say, listening for a moment to the soothing trickle of the fountain beneath the window.

"Precisely. That's why it should be a cat. They require you to come to them, not the other way around. They draw you out. That's what you need."

Seeing cats as an unmanly pet, I say, "I'll look into it."

"You are one determined individual, Eric."

"Have to be, doctor. You have to always be on guard, reading, listening, and arming yourself. This disease doesn't take a break, neither should I . . . " I offer, then: "Can I count on your help? You do agree with the plan, right? The retirement idea."

"I've documented everything we've covered since that first day. So, sure, I think you've got a case. An excellent one."

"Actually, I haven't made up my mind one way or the other . . . with respect to ending my career. This is essentially a hearing-out session. I want to hear myself saying the words while getting some well-informed feedback. This plan . . . I haven't even revealed to my wife. It's still just a sprout in a vast grassland of ideas."

"I not only think it's a good choice," Dr. Nolin says, making note of something. "I think it's the *only* choice."

"I got a call the other day," I say, going on. "From the woman who took over my duties while I'm gone. She's an MBA, mind you, and actually one of the sharpest people I've ever known. She told me she's already getting an ulcer. Her stomach aches all night. She wants to know how to deal with the vultures—the executives—hovering around my office all day."

"And you told her?"

"Jokingly, to stock up on Maalox and Valium."

"Sounds like another vote for not going back."

"It sounds odd saying this, I know," I continue, veering off the beaten path, "but there are good things about this disease. If nothing else, it gets your head out of the clouds, brings your merry ass down to terra firma. Sounds cliché, I know, but you see things like never before. Like this job thing, and changing your life—to make it better. I like to think I participate in living much more now. Mundane things. Like listening to a mountain stream or picking up a leaf and identifying with its uniqueness, its intricate vein pattern . . . understanding my infinitesimal place in this universe. Oh, never mind," I tell Dr. Nolin, "I'm just venting."

"No, no, this is what we need. Go on."

"Oh, and while I'm thinking of it . . . the damn HMO, three months after the aborted surgery in Houston, still isn't paying. So I'm getting all these calls from Anderson asking what's going on. Like I need more to worry about."

"Have you touched base with your friend, the doctor at the HMO?"

"She says she doesn't get involved in billing problems. Call the accounting department."

"Medicine's got to get back to medicine," the shrink observes, "and soon, before we all perish."

"That pretty much sums things up, doctor," I say, concluding. "The disease can end up teaching you good things . . . like how to prioritize your life. What is and is not important."

"Hard, very hard, for the uninitiated to grasp this," Dr. Nolin concedes, closing his note pad. "How an unpredictable condition—cancer, for God's sake—something capable of killing you, can make your world better."

FINDING HOPE WHEN DOCTORS SAY THERE IS NONE

Chapter 70

Betrayed—
The Things Cancer Does to Your Psyche

As a cancer patient, there are times when your eyes open in the morning and, for a split second, you forget the disease has invaded your body and is now dictating your every thought. You forget the body you've known all these years has betrayed you. In that one split second there is enormous solace.

But you know as you lie there, in bed, in peace—doing nothing—this silent disease could be spreading. It has wrapped itself around your mind, your every outlook and reshaped them. A painful hollowness accompanies this recognition. And there's an awareness of being alone: No one can step into your body and wage this war—it is yours. Feeling trapped, you can't go anywhere, do anything to escape.

Cancer has forever altered your life . . . your outlook. What was taken for granted—getting dressed in the morning, warm sunshine on your bare arm, the indifference you feel watching a mindless TV program—now takes on an ominous sense of now, of presence.

This never-ending sense of strife, this 24-hour-a-day vigilance, is exhausting—a psychological debilitation. Any sudden ache or pain . . . in your chest . . . a discomfort inside . . . a simple stomach ache . . . run-of-the-mill feelings that a few years ago wouldn't have caused you a second thought, now taunt your sanity.

Then there are times when the enormity of having cancer drags you down . . . having it redirect your life, having to deal with the ugly medical procedures it throws at you—all the time.

Physically, though, you feel almost as if you can handle anything—then your mind gets involved.

At times dark mental sessions spring forth, dragging you under. For example, you're involved in some ordinary activity—say brushing your teeth, not really thinking about anything in particular—and a wave of fatalism surfaces, out of the blue, instantly engulfing you. You're suddenly questioning your goals: 'Why am I doing this . . . carrying on this hopeless battle? The cancer's going to win—you know it is.'

Lingering negative thoughts add heavily to your sense of foreboding, of doom. And maintaining the mental armor is tough. With me, my dogged determination stands fast, built upon solid reasons for survival: a cherished alliance with Jane; a devoted son and grandson who love and care about my well-being; other inexperienced cancer patients who need tutoring; a new understanding of the pleasures of life; a renewed kinship with God.

The large body of positive wisdom . . . about diet and its impact on cancer, the benefits of exercise, changes in lifestyle, spirituality, prayer, meditation and imagery . . . attitude . . . all of this I use to overwhelm the negativism.

Quitting—you must remember—is always the coward's way out.

Late in chemo month 2: Getting a follow-up CT isn't easy, logistically. I have to see Dr. Paravano—my primary-care physician—then relate to her that Dr. Sloan wants a CT. (His office can't simply call her office and request this as in the old days.) She then seeks approval for the procedure through the HMO's Utilization Review process. To keep their CEOs' wallets fat, HMOs force their patients to jump through countless hoops.

Once the CT is authorized, it's then my responsibility to arrange with a separate diagnostic facility to get the procedure scheduled, and physically deliver to them the HMO's payment authorization. In the unfeeling world of HMO medicine, you are your own advocate—you look out for you. No one else does.

Aged and infirm patients, those who usually don't have the fighting spirit, and those who still believe in TDKB, I especially pity. They comprise a large body of submissive patients which the HMOs have factored into their actuarial tables as being their on-going profit base—i.e., those compliant patients who won't argue a decision . . . and will quietly go off and die.

(HMOs *despise* fighters . . . . Years after this, following my appeal of an HMO decision denying me the right to see an oncologist for follow-up cancer care, my new primary-care doctor decided to dispose of me as a patient, saying we'd 'lost trust in one another.' Finally a Medicare review of my HMO appeal sided with me, forcing the HMO to refer me to an oncologist, *not* allowing an internist to do the follow-up care as the HMO had wanted. But that's another story.)

This follow-up CT, because of its pivotal nature, has me rattled. Essentially this report will determine whether I continue chemotherapy . . . or there's no hope. The CT procedure itself, as I've alluded to before, isn't all that panic-inducing. In fact, it's almost old-hat by now. The killer part's the waiting—for the radiologist's findings.

Nothing tears at a cancer patient's nerves like this.

While awaiting the CT results, I find my thoughts drifting . . . seeing a faceless human, a radiologist, in a murky cubbyhole somewhere, poring over the shadowy images that appear in my films—my very future before him.

(Customarily, a radiologist remains an invisible face. But he or she needn't be. You can make an appointment to meet with them to discuss your CT results, if you wish. I frequently do . . . and find it quite beneficial. Often your oncologist might overlook parenthetical comments made by a radiologist within a CT report, recommending further testing to verify some indefinite image. So get a copy of your CT reports and *read* them carefully, looking for comments or questions raised by the radiologist. Talk directly with the radiologist, if necessary.)

The evening before this appointment with Dr. Sloan, my mind's slinking about like a neurotic cat, seeking a quiet place of solitude. While I feel and look good today, tomorrow's report can—in an instant—reverse that. A negative report can redirect your life, making you feel utterly betrayed.

Your body's done it once again—defied you. Without warning.

On this peculiar evening, Jane and I struggle at bonding, making love for some unspoken, compelling reason. Admittedly, it's an odd time for passion. Maybe—I know we're both morbidly thinking—this will be our last opportunity, ever. Neither of us, though, utters this blasphemy aloud, but the thought's there. Our sense of enthusiasm's unquestionably dulled.

As this affected, lethargic lovemaking session concludes . . . Jane and I, looking silently into each other's eyes, see only unspoken doubt. Will that piece of paper tomorrow reverse our lives *again?* If it does, can we rise up and survive yet another setback?

You quickly learn, you cannot predict what this loathsome business of cancer will next inflict.

As the decisive hour approaches—facing Dr. Sloan and the news—my sense of panic swells a thousand-fold. Never have I met a patient who takes this process lightly. If you possess a piece of lucky clothing, you wear it. If you sometimes rely on Valium or the like to cope (I do), you indulge in that as well. You reach out everywhere, with a magician's hands, for support.

By this time you've prayed and prayed. . . till each prayer's a rerun.

Sitting in the silence of the tiny exam room, I'm staring at a child's painting of a blunt-nosed whale beneath a multi-colored ocean, when a tan-faced Dr. Sloan opens the door, report in hand. Without hesitation, he gives me one thumb up, a quick wink.

"Meaning," I ask, swallowing hard, my heart still running in high gear, "the scan was okay?"

"I'm thrilled, I must say," Dr. Sloan replies, insisting we shake hands. "I probably feel better about this than you do."

This incredibly good news doesn't register all at once, like you might think. For days now I've been numb. Part of me, though, wants to leap up and shout for joy; another part needs further convincing. Waiting has taken its toll.

"I'm just glad I've got *you* . . ." are the only words I can muster.

"Doctor what's his name," Dr. Sloan's scanning the report for the radiologist's name, "Dr. Wright—says here, and I'm quoting: 'The effusion has not reappeared or increased . . . left adrenal mass remains unchanged.' Outstanding news, in light of what you dealt with in Houston."

"The drugs . . ." I ask incredulously, still not believing my ears, flashing back on Dr. Malone, her unnatural manner, "are working, then?"

"We're at least holding our own."

"And . . . what about the blood work?"

"It's looking slightly better," Dr. Sloan replies, flipping to second sheet. "Liver enzymes are down—a shade. Still on the high side, though."

"But down, right?"

"We discussed this whole issue earlier, remember, Eric? Cisplatin and elevated liver enzymes. I've never, honestly, seen that much impact."

"I'm better off than then when I started, right?" I offer, thinking: Let's climb one mountain at a time.

"Goes without saying."

"So . . . we're moving forward," I go on superfluously, like a child granted a Christmas wish, "with the chemo?"

He nods a brisk yes. "In two months we'll get another CT. Till then . . . keep doing whatever you're doing."

"Doctor," I volunteer with a sense of self-satisfaction, "I guess my liver likes fruit and vegetables . . . more than it likes animal flesh."

"You just might end up," Dr. Sloan says proudly, shaking my hand as he departs, "as the ACC poster boy."

Chemo cycle three: Except for some unusual bleeding that occurs when Mary, the 'IV Queen,' can't get my IV started, this cycle goes, mechanically, as the first two had. But this time there's a greater element of hope.

Once at home, I'm wired for a day, then fall into a pattern of being nearly comatose most others, with a growing sense of queasiness, particularly following meals—or smelling certain foods cooking. After a single sip of beer one evening, I discover I can't tolerate alcohol—it tastes the way lighter fluid smells.

During this third month: Two mysterious and inexplicable events surface, further revealing this chemo business is working (my interpretation). These bizarre incidents, because of their improbability, their freakishness, or whatever, I've never disclosed in great detail to anyone.

The first incident, as it unfolds, is eerily frightening.

CHAPTER 71

IS LIFE AN ILLUSION?

It rained yesterday, all afternoon, cats and dogs. Today is fairly cool, 55 or 60 degrees. This morning, when I opened my eyes, I had no idea this'd be one of the strangest days—ever. Eating my typical breakfast, I decide to head over to the waterfront to do a little reading, a little bonding with the cosmos, and some meditation . . . instead of meditating in the bedroom on the rocker.

Setting up my aluminum chair on the sand, I kick off my sandals and labor through a brief walk along the water's edge. No one is within eyeshot. Ten o'clock. A feeble breeze is moving across the water, definitely sweatshirt weather.

A quarter-mile down the shoreline, pausing to recuperate, I hunker down observing a flock of wiry-legged, long-beaked birds scooting in unison along the spongy sand, methodically running inches behind the receding wave foam, snatching pea-size sand crabs with their beaks before these spidery little critters can re-bury themselves.

Curiously, it seems these usually wary birds—maybe 12 of them—are, at the moment, accepting of my nearness. Usually I'm only allowed no nearer than 20 yards. Now, however, they're advancing surprisingly close. Perhaps we've achieved some sort of primitive bond—them having a sixth sense, grasping that I'm unwell. Squatting here, I watch their exploits for many long minutes, marveling at their ability to stab the precise spot in the glistening sand where their writhing little prey lie hidden.

Once one of my feathered friends bags a crab, other birds, usually gluttonous seagulls—screeching obnoxiously—pursue him till he's gobbled down or dropped his catch. This ritual is repeated each time a sandpiper snags a sand crab—eat-and-run, in reverse.

A while later: Back at the beach chair, puffing heavily, I'm awaiting my stamina's return. Being here, on the beach, alone, I love. A wonderfully unblemished day . . . the sand near and far—not just along the surf's edge—is dark and damp from yesterday's downpour. Gentle breakers, knee-high, possess a rolling nature, as if maybe the ocean had just awakened and is yawning. I'm hoping that perhaps my extravagant guests, the bottlenose dolphins, will make an encore presentation. They like tranquil days, it seems, with this slow, rolling surf. But there's no trace of them.

There is, however, an inexplicable feeling of nothingness all about.

Taking out my hefty wooden rosary beads, I launch into my prayers, mindful of the close-by, gray horizon. Praying the rosary often seems a monotonous recitation. But there's a deeper explanation: The same prayers, recited over and over, become a sort of religious mediation, a holy mantra.

The rosary takes a half-hour or so. Dropping the beads in my pocket, I sit quietly, hands folded, toes wriggled beneath the rain-wet sand, consciously utilizing all five senses, one then another, striving to ground myself, to take in the Here-I-am physical state of this free-and-easy morning. My exposed flesh feasts on the cool sea breeze, my ears on the feathery, rolling surf, my lips and nose savor the briny air, my eyes take in the gray morning atmosphere, its shallow cloud layer. Each of these observations I try to home in on—for an instant, at least—in order to absorb its spirit. Delightfully transfixed, I sit doing this.

Once relaxed, I slip on the Walkman earphones, punching the tape button. The calming voice of Dr. Simonton's leading me through another guided imagery. Having sampled many visualization tapes—his are my favorite.

On this particular tape he starts by having you breathe, then relax, then breathe, then relax and so forth. While bathing yourself in thoughts of safety, comfort, and protection, you go through each area of your body and attempt to relax each—neck, scalp, chest, heart, stomach and so forth, till everything's at rest. During this process, you attempt to descend to a point where an uninterrupted visualization's possible.

Now, with you 'floating in a state of relaxation,' Simonton speaks of appreciating the wisdom (Godliness to me) that dwells naturally within us. Our inner 'wisdom'—what the Chinese refer to as Yin and Yang—wants us to be well, wants us to be in a natural state of harmony or balance, the way we were before the onset of disease. Homeostasis, it's called in American medical terms. Simonton prods us to recognize the wisdom of universe. The inherent order of things, he says, the beauty of this world, is not accidental.

At this point, he suggests, that we, in the quiet of our minds, address the wisdom that resides within and allow that wisdom to manifest itself—in our minds—in any guise it adopts, no matter what form or shape that may be.

Though I've listened to this tape many times, I've never before tried participating to the point where I call forth any sort of 'inner wisdom,' thinking it was, well, sort of frivolous. But today, I've decided, I'm going to participate in each step and see what comes of it. So, after faithfully following each relaxation segment, I try, in the quiet of my mind, allowing whatever form of wisdom I possess to come forth, to reveal itself in some way. Secretly I'm thinking: 'This is just so much wasted energy.'

Here I sit, eyes closed, on a quiet beach, relaxing, heeding the pleasant lap of the waves, feeling the coddling breeze, trying to purge my mind of all thought, giving my gray matter free reign, allowing only the image that it generates—without my influence—to emerge.

Now . . . comes the really baffling part.

Most people, under these circumstances, would no doubt conjure a gentle-hearted image—an angel, a compassionate soft-eyed animal, a merciful source of light—as their wisdom signpost. Not me.

Something totally unforeseen appears in my mind.

My eyes still closed . . . the mental picture that emerges is of me, standing on the ground, adjacent to the front landing gear of an idle World War II bomber—a B-25.

. . . This is *my* image of wisdom? How is this relevant?

I have, of course, never flown one of these bombers, but have seen them in photos and close up as a child when I accompanied my father to military bases in the '40s. And I have seen them in flight. Still adhering to Simonton's ritual, my eyes remain closed as I watch myself standing disinterestedly on the ground, near the plane's nose gear, looking up at an open, but empty cockpit window. No one—pilot or otherwise—returns my gaze.

Nothing is happening in this lifeless representation.

I'm alone there, as I am on this beach. No other images emerge—no humans, no more planes, no runway, no nothing. The bomber just sits there. Simonton says we should let what happens happen—so, with my eyes still shut, I play along, not in any way undertaking to tamper with this vision.

Partaking in this seemingly inane exercise but a few more minutes, I open my eyes. The universe looks just as it had—the sky overhead, the ocean, the wintry sand beneath my bare feet . . . nothing has changed.

Well, that was a waste of time. How silly, sitting here, calling forth a source of wisdom from within. And I get a damn lifeless WW II bomber.

Concluding I'd put enough effort into this exercise, I pick up my Bible, and take to reading. As I read, chapter after chapter, the tide comes in a bit, the breeze picks up a little, the air gets a shade colder, the clouds thicken.

An hour or so goes by.

With my eyes needing a rest, I sit back, clasping my chilled hands behind my bald head (I'm wearing a white baseball cap), stretching, yawning, gazing haphazardly at the hazy horizon.

Several restful more minutes drift by. A orderly row of brown pelicans drifts by, gliding just inches above the waves. A faint, distant droning sound only slightly catches my ear.

Paying this little heed, I go on idly exploring the dividing line between the sky, the sea . . . pondering why being near a large body of water bestows a sense of well, deliverance, on most people. The droning is now coming nearer. Suddenly, emerging through the low clouds directly before me—is a single, silver B-25!

'Ho-ly smokes!' I mutter aloud, understanding instantly something of major significance taking place here. 'This. . . can't be! It's got to be a hallucination!'

As the bulky plane lumbers across the late-morning sky, now directly overhead, I can feel the powerful resonance of its engines. A thousand recollections from my boyhood days zip through me—the muggy Maryland air, the distinct scent of my father as he carried me asleep from the car, the invulnerability I felt in my parents' presence—the way memories bombard your senses when you catch a sudden whiff of some unforgettable scent from your past.

Sitting bolt upright, I jerk left, then right, to see who's devised this impossible prank. But no one's in sight.

Keep in mind: An hour beforehand I was sitting here, innocently trying to call up 'my wisdom'—and a motionless, unoccupied B-25 popped into my head. Now, this!

My eyes continue tracking the ancient bomber as it dissolves into a far off cloud, its convincing engines still droning powerfully . . . 'Ho-ly shit,' is all I can murmur, feeling goose bumps an inch high everywhere, 'what *is* this?'

Frenzied, I think: 'Who's going to believe this?'

Everyone will see this vision—if they're not too busy laughing, calling me wacko—as an amazing fluke. Hollywood, they'll say, was filming a WW II movie. Even if that is true, seeing this exact plane, at this exact time, after calling forth this exact mental image, would be a trillion-to-one sighting. This is 1993, for God's sake—B-25s haven't flown in 40 years!

A vexing chill flows through me. I am now very cold. Cautiously, as my thoughts merge, I quickly come to understand I've experienced some profound riddle—some grand gesture . . . but by whom . . . and for what purpose? Goose bumps still all over me. A muddled voice within whispers: Now, *use* this . . .

But how? What do I do—if anything?

CHAPTER 72

ECSTASY IN SUCH AS ME—
A MYSTERIOUS BLUE LIGHT IN THE NIGHT

A couple days later, after endless pondering on this baffling vision, I'm sitting with Dr. Nolin. Having just told him of the incident—my inner vision, then the bomber's actual appearance—I ask what he makes of it. He seems very uneasy with the whole episode. His eyes ask, 'Are you sure of this?' He doesn't openly ask this, I think, because he knows: I have no reason for making up such a story.

"So what do you make of it, doctor?" I persist.

"Truthfully, I'm at a loss."

"Okay," I persist, "considering it really happened—which it did—what would you say was behind it? Some zillion-to-one random event? I checked and there was no air show that day. No one was making a movie—I checked on that as well."

Looking over his tortoise-shell half-glasses: "Definitely, you're sure you saw something?"

A compact man, Dr. Nolin is sitting in a grand, throne-like black leather chair, turned toward me, at his desk. I'm sitting—almost sprawling—on a six-foot, loose-pillow couch. It's three in the afternoon, or thereabout. A weak December sun, slanting through the window, illuminates a faint column of dancing dust particles.

"You're not trying to squeeze out of this," I respond jokingly, but pursuing the question, "are you, doctor?"

"Mainly because I don't have an answer. With some stretch of the imagination, we could possibly see this as lending more credence to the angel thing."

"That might be a stretch," I concede, making a mental note. Then, going on: "If you were backed to a wall and had to offer an opinion, what would you say?"

"I'd have to say . . ." he begins indecisively, exhaling after a moment's thought, "you . . . tapped into some sort of cosmic energy."

This doesn't necessarily open him to rebuke for being an astrology nut or tarot-card-reading freak. Most of us know someone who's foreseen someone's demise or other calamity in a dream. Mothers know especially what it means to have 'a feeling' about a disaster befalling a child—miles away. Once we accept the scientific fact that electrons do indeed communicate—know what other electrons in very distant places are doing—we must necessarily accept that we ordinary humans occasionally tap into this reservoir of energy/wisdom without realizing it. To wit, the B-25 in my mind and then in the sky.

But again, what am I to make of this revelation?

This question causes Dr. Nolin to squirm noticeably. "I'm not too sure how the vision was structured," he proceeds ambiguously, begging the issue. "The obvious would be you're supposed to use this as a symbol—the manifestation of a visualization, if you will—to bomb cancer cells within your body. But that would seem overtly obvious. Hit your hand with a hammer and it hurts, kind of thing."

In that I'm a 'paying customer,' I can continue stalking this line of questioning, but don't. Figuring that since the aircraft did materialize—I'm comfortable with the fact I'd seen it—inevitably its message or purpose will make itself apparent in time. After all, Dr. Simonton, the one who got me into this in the first place, says it may take a few days for questions to unravel themselves.

Dr. Nolin seems far less troubled asking about my lack of hair, what this is doing to my self-image.

"First of all, doctor," I reply, "I see it as a step in the right direction. I don't look all that handsome, I know. But in me, I know the chemo's accomplishing something. That feels damn good. The drugs are tracking down all the little bad guys. Like cops and robbers."

Dr. Nolin, who I suspect dyes his thinning hair, seems mystified that this problem doesn't concern me more—this lack of hair.

"You see," I continue, "it's temporary. Other patients tell me—the woman at M.D. Anderson from the vice president's office, for one—that when the hair does come back, it'll be thicker, maybe even curly. I'll be somebody new. I have to confess, though—in church, people shy away. Think twice about sitting next to a guy with zero hair. Like I have some disease that might jump out and get them. But hell, I don't mind. Gives me more elbow room."

"Your sense of focus, Eric," Dr. Nolin offers, as though I'd energized him, "never ceases to surprise me."

"I don't see myself that way, doctor. But instead as a guy who's stubborn. That's who I am. That's what it takes to outwit this disease. In truth, I'm probably not all that complacent about being a chrome dome." The fountain in the koi pond beneath the slightly opened window is murmuring sympathetically. "Sometimes when I'm lying awake late at night, trying to believe in all this positive business, I get to wondering . . . if this chemo doesn't work . . . will I check out looking like this? Not a friggin' hair on my head? We're talking one unsightly corpse. My wife already accuses me of looking like Peanuts."

This causes the doctor to grin. "Have you given any more thought to retirement? Talked with Dr. Sloan about his ideas?"

"Still looking into it. Definitely. It's making more sense all the time, especially since the Mitotane has left me with little or no fight-or-flight response. Hell, most of my endocrine system is kaput. I'll be taking replacement steroids for the rest of my life for thyroid and adrenal function—and I'll still need testosterone shots every two weeks. Most of my energy and outlook on life comes from the drugs I put in my mouth every day . . . I don't know what the stresses I used to face would do to me now."

"I think," Dr. Nolin comments, uncrossing then recrossing his legs; he's wearing cordovan tassel loafers, "we have a pretty good idea."

Nodding in agreement, I take this opportunity to seek a pat on the back: "So you don't see me as a person who's over-reactive—a worry wart?"

"Heavens no! In fact, I hold you up to other patients . . . as an example. I have a feeling I'd handle things much like you. Or I hope I would."

"And before you bug me about it, I'm looking into the pet thing—the cat idea. Jane loves it."

"Give it a shot. You'll see that it helps—having a diversion, a second set of eyes around."

"You like this cat thing, don't you?"

"I recommend pets to all my chronically ill patients."

Weeks later: The final life-altering event—or vision—presents itself at a point roughly midway between the third and fourth chemo treatments, when I'm beginning to feel almost normal. Notice I say almost. 'Feeling normal,' in lay terms, means feeling good—when no part of your body's drawing attention to itself; when you're kind of suspended in a warm ocean of rapture . . . no aches, no pains.

It's the dead of night. Somewhere around 3:00 a.m.

For no detectable reason, I find myself instantly awake, as if there's a presence nearby. In me there's a sudden, overwhelming, swirling sense of elation—not unlike the forceful glow that overwhelmed me when Father Esperanza placed the Communion wafer on my tongue a few weeks ago.

It's the middle of the night, remember.

As I wake more fully and review my setting and body parts—I've become used to waking up in unfamiliar hospitals, seeing unfamiliar shadowy sights—the almost-full moon, a swollen blue pearl suspended over a glassy Pacific, captures my eye. A spirited shade of blue saturates the quiet bedroom, like a nearby neon light is illuminating it.

All of a sudden—again, for no obvious reason—I feel my body organs brimming with a wave of inexplicable ecstasy. Like the organs themselves are happy. I feel like crying out. I am that exhilarated. But . . . about what? And why?

This unbelievable sense of excitement—this radiance, this ebullience—is so filling it feels like my chest's going to rupture. Lying there, with only my eyes moving, hearing the soft lap of the surf on the beach, I began wondering—Is this some sort of self-fulfilling prophesy? Have I unconsciously *made* myself feel this way so I can believe I'm getting well?

Again I try addressing the B-25 image—in my mind. Eagerly, I've been waiting for this obscure symbol to 'become' whatever it's supposed to be—to me. Maybe if I combine these two visions, one answer will emerge. But again, the beefy aircraft just stands there, poised, doing nothing, engines silent.

Now I'm truly mystified.

I consider shaking Jane, telling her of this craziness. But she couldn't—probably no one could—comprehend this euphoric event.

Maybe, I deduce, this is a byproduct of the meditative routine I've developed for dozing off each night: I picture a broad beam of blazing light—not unlike a spotlight on an unlit stage—radiating down from above, inundating me, burning away specks of cancer in my body. This is my closing mental picture each night.

Nevertheless, lying there in the bluish, moon-lit bedroom, listening to the ocean, I conclude this exalted radiance is yet another explicit sign . . . a message from well, above, saying loud and clear: You're going to make it, kid!

The fourth chemo cycle proceeds as the foregoing three, not to downplay the barbarousness, the coarse misery in these treatments. Still, I have to keep both Zofran and Compazine within arm's reach for random bouts of nausea. A couple of weeks after the fourth treatment, an uncomfortable sensation begins creeping into my hands, my feet: Under certain conditions, they begin tingling, like they're asleep. Other times, they feel numb, dead.

Dr. Sloan says this is yet another side effect of cisplatin—progressive nerve damage. The condition's known as peripheral neuropathy, the partial or complete loss of feeling in your extremities.

"Are we talking forever with this feeling?" I ask.

Not responding right away, Dr. Sloan replies obscurely: "Sometimes it's temporary, sometimes not. Sometimes we see it leaving patients with a permanent loss of feeling. Hands, feet—and legs. With some patients . . . it can go on to become a permanent disability. I've known patients," he says, now getting into this subject, "who couldn't do simple things—like buttoning their shirt—because of it."

He cautions that if the neuropathy becomes too pronounced we'll be forced to terminate the chemo treatments. Then and there: I resolve to keep the progress of this neuropathy to myself: I don't want *anybody* taking away my crutch—these last-ditch chemo treatments. *Nobody.*

The weeks between chemo cycles drag by at a snail's pace. I'm wearing thin . . . feeling perceptibly more beaten down, cumulatively worse. Is it the chemo—or the damn cancer coming back? We're never sure. Fewer and fewer are the days when I feel even sort of good.

At the end of the fourth month there's yet another dreaded CT to endure. And then there's the issue of blood work . . . will this wearisome complication—elevated liver numbers—come to haunt me?

FINDING HOPE WHEN DOCTORS SAY THERE IS NONE

CHAPTER 73

TO WORK OR NOT TO WORK—
PONDERING AGAIN A MAJOR CHANGE IN
LIFESTYLE

A nasty on-shore wind is pelting the bedroom window. Now and then gusting beach sand hisses across the glass. Propped up on a pillow, I'm resting on the bed, eyes fixed on the stormy morning. The Pacific at this moment's almost white, churning wildly, looking like lemon meringue topping. Palm trees, those that I can see, are wagging like crazy metronomes.

Time at the beach today's out of the question.

Again I'm weighed down with concerns about my upcoming tests. This next CT and blood test can underwrite—or nullify—all the reassurance I've taken from my recent encounters: the wondrous late-night aura, the bizarre B-25 fly-by. Were these truly visions? Or wishful pipe dreams? Chemotherapy can do weird, weird, things to you. Has it scrambled my brain cells, my sanity?

Days later: As a diversion—with the blood test out of the way and the CT exam yet to come—I begin focusing on getting a pet. I follow up on this (Dr. Nolin's pet idea) because I want to, consciously, pursue all opportunities—proven and unproven—said to improve a patient's survival (meditation, a pet, shift in lifestyle, dietary changes, whatever). Admittedly, the camaraderie of a warm-blooded creature could be advantageous. But what species of 'prescription' pet to get?

Most often I feel too lousy to care for a bumbling puppy. So, mindful of Dr. Nolin's advice, I find myself leaning more and more toward a low-maintenance animal. A four-legged creature it has to be—no goldfish, no horny toads, no guinea pigs . . . *but a cat?*

How can I alter my negative bias toward these creatures? Dr. Nolin proposed that cats, being more arrogant than their canine brethren, make more suitable pets for cancer patients because they're relatively clean and they necessitate you coming to them, not vice versa—a therapeutic giving, of sorts.

Thus Nadia explodes on the scene. Well, explode may be overstating it. When I reveal to Jane that I'm considering getting a pet—maybe even a cat—she clutches her chest melodramatically. Fish, turtles and white rats, I tell her, are out of the question.

Days later: I'm on the front deck watering my prized chemo Ficus—which is doing beautifully, glistening new leaves everywhere—when Jane wheels in the driveway. With her is a bluish-gray, bug-eyed young cat, actually looking more like a terrified vampire bat. All of two months old, Nadia—according to the vet who sold her to Jane—was born in some deserted barn on the outskirts of town.

Wild-eyed, this skittish critter spends her early days cowering in the back corner of her dirt box—but curiously, purring loudly—or hiding in mysterious openings underneath the kitchen cabinets that only she, somehow, can locate instantly and slither into. When I telephone the vet, asking how to tame this wild thing, he says I'll have to spend time with her, each day, getting acquainted—stroking, feeding, and 'humanizing.'

Wooing the transient civility of a cat, I find, is a diversion, maybe even medicinal. I have to get up, physically saunter about the house, pandering to this indifferent little feline. She and I eventually become good buddies. She's even taken to sleeping with me—on my pillow, no less.

It is rejuvenating, when you're house-bound, feeling like the plague's taken over your life, to have a second living thing nearby, responding to your bellyaching. Frequently, when the mood strikes her, Nadia will punctuate my verbal complaints with a well-placed, poignant little cry.

As stated many times before, anticipating and undergoing a CT is never enviable, never a looked-forward-to experience. The bone-deep worries never change . . . whether you've been through this process ten times . . . twenty times . . . a thousand times. Once you witness what one of these soulless CT contraptions can do—alter your life indelibly—you live in gruesome fear of them.

This CT is no different.

I do, nonetheless, confess to feeling a shade more optimistic this go-round. The scan two months ago was favorable. With that to build on and a pair of emphatic visions that, outwardly, seem to be telling me I'm on the right path, I feel moderately safe as I lie in the scanner. If safe's the right word. Or . . . am I mellowing as a patient? For certain I'm not becoming indifferent.

"More terrific news!" a beaming Dr. Sloan says days later, breezing in the exam room, once again whisking the CT report before him like a kid proud of a good report card. "Your latest CT shows," he goes on fervently, "'a complete resolution . . . of the pulmonary density.' That's your pleural effusion he's talking about. There's apparently no evidence of it. That soft-tissue mass in the adrenal area—the one we've been hearing about—is still there, unchanged. He is saying it could represent a new neoplasm—a recurrence, but since it hasn't changed, I suspect we're seeing scar tissue."

"'A complete resolution,' you said?" I repeat disbelievingly, the radiologist's sweet words ringing in my head. "Meaning . . . I'm home free? We can stop these pesky chemo treatments?"

Aware that I'm being facetious, Dr. Sloan: "Don't go getting too rambunctious. We're trying to catch these bad guys while they're dividing, growing. Let's stick with our eight-month strategy . . . But this is extraordinary news. Oh," he goes on electrically, "and equally important, maybe more so, your blood work—your liver numbers and ACTH—are beginning to show signs of improvement. All and all, some pretty impressive results here."

Inside I'm bursting with excitement. But, having lived with long-term, deep-rooted worries in my soul, I just sort of sit there, encircled by amateur paintings of the sea, on the crankily table paper, stunned. I am grinning like a baboon, nevertheless. "ACTH is getting down there, too?" I manage to ask.

"Down from several hundred . . . to 37. Normal range is 10 to 52."

"That's wonderful," I comment, seeing again the mysterious B-25 rumbling across the clouded sky. Once more I try making sense of its strange emergence. "So many things . . . going right."

The numbness in my hands and feet, that mysterious prickly sensation, is becoming more pronounced. This doesn't alarm me as perhaps it should. As stated earlier, I don't want anything derailing this chemo regimen. So I don't address this subject.

"You're forcing me to say it again, Eric," Dr. Sloan replies, hand on door knob, "I don't know what you're doing, but keep it up. I'm truly amazed with this blood work. In 19 years, I've never seen—"

"Doctor," I interrupt, "there's something I've been wanting to ask. Why would you—or anyone for that matter—go into oncology? There's so little satisfaction—no cures—and so often everything seems like a dead-end street."

Pulling himself up, seriousness instantly seizes the doctor. "The rewards," he begins precisely, as if having given this talk before, "are, admittedly, few and far between. But they are there. Sometimes, when I see a patient—like you—coming from a seemingly impossible situation to one of promise . . . it all becomes worthwhile. There are many nights, though, when I lose sleep. A lot of sleep."

(Dr. Sloan's nurse, the vegetarian, told me there are times, when an HMO denies a patient a specific chemo or refuses to cover the cost of some needed medical procedure, Dr. Sloan will pay—out of his own pocket—for that patient's care. "That's the main reason," she explained, whispering, "that this place doesn't look more spiffy.")

"Don't mean to go on beating a dead horse, doctor," I resume, responding to his prior statement, "but again I have to say: My liver likes digesting fruits and vegetables better than it does meat."

Nodding dubiously, but affably, Dr. Sloan waves farewell. Physicians it seems—unless they're cardiologists scolding recent heart attack victims—don't put much faith in diet. (How is it—that diet can apply to one branch of medicine and not another? Aren't we all of one body? Seems that doctors just aren't trained in *preventing* disease . . . only treating and curing it.)

To reiterate: Each and every cell in your body—including the cancer-fighting cells of your immune system—is created from the foods we consume. How can it not make sense to put pure and wholesome foods in your mouth as a health measure?

But rather than beat my head against a solid wall, I don't argue the issue with doctors. This 'solution' to so many health problems is apparently too uncomplicated for the scientific mind to embrace as fact. They'll catch on . . . in due time.

With this excellent CT report under my belt, I'm sitting with the shrink at my subsequent session—like two buddies over a beer—and we're ticking off the reasons we think I'm doing so well against this cancer: the systemic chemotherapy, my change in diet, my return to spirituality—and maybe most important, he maintains, the elimination of work-related stresses.

"Okay, we've been talking about you dropping out—retiring," Dr. Nolin notes, pausing, breathing on his glasses, wiping them clean. "As an alternative, have you given any more thought to changing what you do for a living? A new career?"

"I feel so much better," I respond, "not having to deal with that nonstop tension, those jittery nights when I couldn't sleep because of work worries, the freeway skirmish twice a day."

"You're leaning more, then, toward not going back at all?"

"It all boils down to dollars," I explain. "Keeping busy isn't a problem."

"If not for monetary reasons," Dr. Nolin asks, "why even think about going back? You've seen how life is not working. You could do freelance writing. Put together a book on your experiences, maybe. Help others patients going through this."

"First, you've got to pay the mortgage. Will my long-term disability do it? The most immediate question, though, is whether the one person who has the ultimate say-so—Dr. Sloan—agrees. He has to originate the paperwork."

Something outside the office window—perhaps a bird-catches Dr. Nolin's eye. "Maybe, Eric," he says, resuming, "we should look beyond money—beyond dollars and cents. Your sole concern here should be health. That's job number one. So what if you have to live in a less desirable location. Can we put a price tag on life? Have you checked with Dr. Sloan? On any of this?"

"First, I'm putting all the facts together in my head—money, other issues."

"How do you think he'll respond?"

"Probably see things my way," I offer confidently. "He's implied as much. So, maybe."

"Still pursuing the diet? No meat?"

"Like a demon."

"Good. And what's the word on a pet? Still looking into that, too?"

"I meant to tell you—I got a kitten. A pot-bellied, scared-shitless little thing. If nothing else, she is a diversion."

"Perfect," the shrink replies, delightedly. Then after a pause: "Not to change the subject, but the other day I ran across something—letter to the editor or an opinion piece—and this person was putting another spin on what you and I were talking about the other day, claiming that sometimes ordinary people act as angels to help others through hard times. He equated this process to being deputized."

"In my case, the old guy didn't even exist—according to everybody at MDA. There may be deputies out there, but this fellow wasn't one of them," I reply, having decided not to tell the shrink about this most recent phenomenon—the late-night luminescence. People, even experienced therapists, can only absorb so many off-the-wall incidents without coming to question your veracity, your sanity.

Departing from Dr. Nolin's office I feel freshly focused. Jane, when she gets home that evening, builds upon Dr. Nolin's suggestions.

"You're 1000 percent easier to live with when you're not working," Jane offers as a shot of reality. "I hated those times. When you were working on those lousy deadlines, when you were so riled by the executives' inefficiency, their indecisiveness, their last minute flip-flops.

"You're so damn good at what you do, so meticulous. You're the one who got perfect grades in college, not them. And always they ended up going back to your original ideas. But that's beside the point. I'm thinking that your getting out's a marvelous idea. I care about you. We can make ends meet. I'll keep working, don't worry."

"I'm sure as hell glad," I say, hugging her, "the old Jane isn't around anymore."

"What old Jane?"

"Never mind—a slip of the tongue."

FINDING HOPE WHEN DOCTORS SAY THERE IS NONE

Chapter 74

No Stone Unturned—
The Radiologist and I Meet Face to Face

First and foremost, I'm thrilled with the outstanding CT results, the amazing blood news. Thrilled, but being a skeptic, there remains an element of doubt. In reading my copy of the CT report, there are still questions—especially about the make up of this dubious soft-tissue mass.

But still . . . can all this good luck be happening to *me*?

To be doubly convinced things are as they seem, I telephone and make an appointment to meet with the radiologist—that faceless being—who interpreted my films. The same guy who's done it the last several times.

The abilities of these 'invisible doctors'—like the other behind-the-scenes doctors, pathologists—are crucial to the outcome of your treatment. Their conclusions can literally redirect your life and your treatment plans. Yet these professionals often remain unseen . . . unquestioned. Primary-care doctors and oncologists, it seems, rarely have face-to-face relationships with radiologists or pathologists. It's a little frightening when you think about it. I'm a person who likes to see, to know the individual—albeit once removed—who's directing the flow of my life.

Dr. Elam, the radiologist, a hunched-over man with Nixon-like eyes that consciously evade mine, appears aloof, rushed, a bit exasperated at the idea of this meeting. He's wearing a blue and yellow striped tie, loose at the neck, a short-sleeve white shirt. We're in a very small, very dim, very muggy room utilized for film analysis, dictation. The inert air holds a yeastiness.

Briefly I explain my condition, the excursions to M.D. Anderson, telling Dr. Elam that I just want to see my films, first-hand. I vow not to take much of his time. Particularly, I want to see the latest films—where he mentions the alarming possibility that the soft-tissue mass is a recurrent neoplasm. This I need to see with my own eyes.

"Okay," he begins impatiently, "but I have to tell you: Patients regularly come in here wanting me to alter what I've written in my narrative. I won't do that. That isn't your intent is it, Mr. Scribner?"

FINDING HOPE WHEN DOCTORS SAY THERE IS NONE

For a second I'm taken back to earlier encounters with Dr. Zindler—my creepy primary-care doctor of several years back—and his cold-hearted greetings: "Well, Mr. Scribner, I see you're not dead yet, so let's have a look at you."

"Not at all, doctor," I reply calmly, reservedly. "I've seen many of my earlier films and want to compare. Reviewing x-ray film isn't new to me: I used to be a senior industrial x-ray film reader in the space program—a metals radiologist, if you will. So looking at films isn't entirely foreign."

Still eyeing me suspiciously, but now more acceptingly, he slides a thick stack of film from a green-edged manila jacket. With him positioning certain of these on the lighted wall, I mention I'd seen Dr. Norman, the local pulmonologist. We'd gone over my earlier films in detail. Just saying another doctor had yielded to a similar review seems to cut some ice.

Poking his half-glasses higher up the bridge of his nose, Dr. Elam commences circling suspicious areas on the films, talking. Glancing ahead, I indicate another area of interest—the crescent-shaped section adjacent to the left lung where the pleural effusion had been. Dr. Elam's temperament thaws considerably. Perhaps I do know my way around these films—at least enough to be conversant.

"Even I can see," I offer, "that the area's improved."

"You say," he asks vaguely, "you went to the Anderson Cancer Center?"

"They're the ones who decided I was a Stage IV—inoperable, after a thoracoscopy. I'm on chemotherapy now—obviously," I say, amused, running my hand over my hairless scalp for emphasis. "My first and second surgeries were done locally. At Anderson they were going to do a third, to eliminate this mass (I'm circling a small, gray region on the film) in the adrenal bed. But the effusion being malignant precluded that."

"I've been keeping an eye on that, the mass," Dr. Elam confesses, admitting to a bond of sorts. "Actually, I do know you—by your films. Are you going to have this biopsied? This soft-tissue mass?"

"They did at Anderson. Results came back negative, saying it's scar tissue, most likely. But they wanted to take it out regardless. Never can tell, they said, what it's going to do in the future. Better safe than sorry. While it may not show as malignant today—later on, who knows?"

"Valid observation. On film, that area looks like a neoplasm—a malignancy—to me."

"I know. You've said that in your last two reports."

"That's not to say," he goes on encouragingly, "the pathology wasn't correct. My phrasing is a legal imperative. This could well be scar tissue. See these surgical clips in the mass? That leads me to believe it could be scar tissue. But all the same, it's suspicious."

"They really seem to know what they were talking about," I put in, "the specialists at Anderson."

"My mother," the radiologist discloses, as though we're now contemporaries, "went there for therapy. Breast cancer. A while back, of course, but we were all very satisfied with the way she was treated. She's in West Palm Beach now. Living it up."

With this extemporaneous give and take, this doctor and I are now talking more easily. Nudging the door shut with his foot, he asks who established my chemo regimen, what it's expected to achieve.

"Well," I say, candidly, "the medical oncologist from Anderson—a real pull-no-punches sort of guy—forwarded it to my local oncologist, Dr. Sloan . . . You know him, right?"

"We've spoken a few times. By phone." A sign of moderation—Dr. Elam's got his hands folded on top of his head now.

"Anyway, this oncologist faxed Dr. Sloan the details. Not so much how to—Dr. Sloan already knew that. It's not an obscure protocol; they use for a lot of other cancers. It's only used as a last hope for people like me—Stage IV adrenocortical carcinoma patients."

"And the expectations?"

"If the drugs work at all—this is according to that Anderson oncologist—they look for a positive response in about 40 percent of the patients." I find myself verbalizing impersonally, as if my own plight weren't the topic of discussion—as if discussing some anonymous patient. Oddly, we're oftentimes more unguarded with strangers than with friends. "That response," I continue, "isn't likely to last beyond a year. That's the kicker. Then it's all up to me."

"Not the greatest of probabilities."

"Depends how you look at it. I've lumped myself in the 40 percent category—so, to me, it is going to work. Then, once the drugs have done their thing, I'll do my thing: Seeing that the response lasts as long as possible." I almost divulge I'm no longer eating meat, that I'm going to church again and meditating, that I'm thinking of retiring early for health's sake, and so forth, but decide why waste the words: this is a medical doctor, swayed not by common sense, but by scientific fact.

"A commendable outlook . . . I suppose."

"Lets me go to sleep at night."

"Yours is my first case," Dr. Elam reveals, "of adrenal cancer."

"Some will admit that, some won't." I think about telling him of my dubious adventures with local Drs. Crandle or Malone, but decide against it. These physicians—no matter what—stick together, and it isn't wise to bad-mouth any individual doctor. "A doctor at USC first told me about Anderson."

Eyebrows arched, Dr. Elam's once again searching my films: "Part of your left kidney, they took?"

"Upper pole."

"Your renal function's being monitored? Creatinine and so forth?"

"Every six to eight weeks I have blood tests. Why?"

"Because . . . the way the kidney's being 'illuminated' here (he circles the left kidney), I'm not sure it's functioning as it should. Could just be the way the film was processed, though."

Moving nearer, I look closely at the kidney. "You can *see* kidney function?"

"Sure," he says, once again pushing his glasses higher on his nose. "We can tell by the way the contrast is taken up. By the kidneys themselves." He points from one kidney to the other. "See the right versus the left?"

"One does look a little brighter," I note. "Apparently none of the paperwork that accompanied came along with these films said anything about previous surgeries or radiation therapy to that area?"

(In today's environment of do-it-yourself, mishmash HMO medicine, you can't ever *assume*—count on any once-removed doctor knowing anything about you or your prevailing state of health or treatment. This may seem incomprehensible, but it's *you* who must convey all information from one doctor to the next. You have to explain. And explain again. Then you know each doctor knows.)

"No. But I'm glad you pointed it out. Now I can make more sense of what I'm seeing. I'll be on the lookout for kidney function . . . .The left one looks okay, size-wise—with no discernible atrophy."

"The radiation oncologist said that kidney would shrivel up—quit working within a year. After he zapped me. Guess that hasn't happened."

"Now that I look more closely," Dr. Elam's employing an oversized Sherlock Holmes magnifying glass, "it may be just the way the film was developed . . . causing the kidney to look less illuminated. But I'll continue watching it in the future."

In all, I spend maybe a half-hour with Dr. Elam, personalizing my films with him, swapping relevant facts. Filling in blanks, as it were. Now, for him, there's an individual's face associated with these films.

Departing his tiny, darkened, yeast-smelling film reading room, I feel upbeat. By way of this face-to-face conference, Dr. Elam now knows my situation more intimately—and the suspected new neoplasm has been explained away. Sort of—at least for today.

I've now connected with all the doctors in the treatment loop. Everyone now has a face.

CHAPTER 75

FORGIVENESS = INNER PEACE

Month five of chemo treatments: I'm now—with a bit more confidence—looking toward to the future... concentrating on going more deeply into complementary cancer treatments: lifestyle, exercise, spirituality, meditation, fine-tuning my nutrition and so forth. Things that are going to nurture my life *after* chemo.

With the religion controversy long behind me, I now read the good book daily—to capture its 'centering' power. Communion I receive every Sunday. By way of my experiences with this lethal disease, I've gained a finer tolerance for what God is . . . and is not. The seasoned old guy in Houston seems to have been a turning point, setting me in the right direction. Now I more readily accept what some scholar or theologian more discerning than I once reasoned: Belief in the divine creator is not grounded in everyday logic—it's based solely on faith. Case closed.

For several months now I've been a strict vegetarian. Instead of seeing this as a form of denial, or torture, each meal I now see as a step forward, a declaration of my own healing. This no-meat policy's to be my permanent, self-administered 'chemotherapy.' Something I can accomplish for myself to deactivate cancer and maintain the positive effects of the cisplatin and VP-16. From my research, here are the main reasons meat should be avoided:

- Pesticides
- Hormones
- Bacteria
- Antibiotics
- Overworks the liver/pancreas
- Poor/slow digestion by humans
- Too much protein
- Too much cholesterol
- Too much fat
- Too much iron
- Dyes
- Parasites
- Mad Cow Disease (possible)

Still reading all I can on cancer and nutrition, I try merging my latest discoveries with my everyday lifestyle. I decide to begin juicing, fruits and vegetables, to more conveniently, more efficiently get a greater amount and assortment of these—raw broccoli, cauliflower, tomatoes, parsley, soy products, oranges, apples, sunflower seeds, and so forth—into my system three times a day. With the right juicer you can bring the health benefits of raw natural foods to any meal—including breakfast.

But what kind of juicing device should I buy? Most juicers separate the juice from the pulp, which you then toss out. Throwing away a major portion of the nutrients (and fiber) and consuming the juice alone is a flagrant waste. Thousands—perhaps millions—of health-giving phytochemicals (plant nutrients) are contained in a plant's skin, its pulp.

The complete fruit or vegetable, skin and all, is what I want.

Friends gladly demonstrate their juicers. All of these, though, are very inefficient machines—they isolate the juice from the pulp and take forever to dismantle to clean. No good. The equipment I want has to be easy to use and easy to clean.

One day a full-page ad in a health magazine, ballyhooing a "Total Juicer," catches my eye. The ad states that this device utilizes the whole fruit or vegetable in creating its juice. The brochure they send me compares brand-name juicers. The Vita Mix (this is *not* a product ad) is faster, very easy to clean (rinses clean in seconds—no disassembly), and uses less fruit/veggies to create the same quantity of fluid as other juicers. And it does *not* separate the juice from the pulp. Whatever you toss into the Vita Mix, you get back as drinkable liquid. Nothing is thrown away. Nothing.

Long story shortened: I cough up several hundred dollars for one of these babies. Admittedly, using it takes some getting used to—my first few drinks are like 'spinachy' purees. (For me, the Vita Mix is the best at creating whole, drinkable juice, quickly, in a near pre-digested form. This machine could be, quite conceivably, the reason I remain healthy today. See Appendix D for my basic anti-cancer juicing recipe.)

Once I purchase the Vita Mix, each morning I religiously prepare a 'brew' incorporating numerous raw organic—yes, organic *is* important—fruits and vegetables. Mine is a businesslike goal: I'm out to maximize the intake of cancer-fighting fruits and vegetables. I'm not striving to create a tasty smoothie-type beverage. Inspiration for this mode of eating comes from (1) Dr. Dean Ornish's healthy heart diet books, (2) anti-cancer writings of macrobiotic guru Kushi, (3) the AMA-scorned diet-oriented cancer doctor, Max Gerson, and (4) a *Newsweek* article on the NCI's Designer Foods program where the anti-cancer benefits of certain fruits and vegetables are being scientifically studied.

No one can label this form of complementary medicine—a meatless diet—as quackery. Many Americans used to eat this way before we, as a nation, began gorging on heavily advertised corporate potluck: over-processed convenience foods, frozen or canned with little or none of their original nutrient value.

Some researchers say our feasting on processed foods—with their ledgers of chemical additives, synthetic coloration, artificial sweeteners, partially hydrogenated this-and-that, MSG, tongue-twisting preservatives, hormones that mimic the human endocrine system, and God knows what else—is the driving force behind America's skyrocketing cancer rates. There's little argument that fresh certified organic foods, grown without chemical fertilizers and pesticides, have superior nutrient value and offer unquestionable health benefits.

An average morning in chemo month five: The day begins with me preparing a large raw fruit/veggie drink (see Appendix D), then storing half the mixture in the fridge in an air-tight container for lunch, and a sizable bowl of steaming organic cereal. After that, it's over to the waterfront to sit, to convalesce . . . to ponder things.

Today, steep, unhurried waves, looking to be in slow motion, slam the shoreline. A lively breeze is coming off the water, feeling like, well, life unspoiled. Random clumps of off-white froth, blown from atop the wave crests, tumble over the sand like balls of cotton. My naked feet, with much of their feeling now gone—peripheral neuropathy's worsening—are burrowed deep in the chilly sand.

A sense of rapture, sitting here—cradled in the sad clouds, the haze, the breeze. No dolphins cavorting today, though . . . no mysterious WWII bomber fly-by.

One of the physicists who determined that atomic particles in distant locations do indeed communicate with one another, concluded that we humans exist in a 'seamless reality.' All things in nature are interrelated. But this concept's nothing new. Many of the world's religions have, for thousands of years, seen all of mankind as part of one whole: We reside in the universe; the universe resides in us. In fact, in the Bible God talks of this connectedness, saying, "I am the vine, you are the branches." With my hand raking the cold sand, I'm reminded again of the body-mind concept in medicine.

As outlined in Chapter 8, science has isolated the proteins (chemicals) our bodies manufacture and use to carry out the process of communication between body parts. These chemicals, neuropeptides, were first thought to transfer information only within the brain. Researchers have since discovered immune system cells—those that attack diseases like cancer, throughout the body—also have receptors for these messenger chemicals.

Your immune system then is aware of any mental conversation you're having with yourself—your inner most off-the-wall reflections, whether they be joyous or dismal—and will react accordingly. It now becomes easier, then, to visualize your own mind-body connection—how your positive and negative thoughts are interpreted by our immune systems, affecting the way our bodies respond to disease—or don't respond.

This is why it's so important to release your negative thoughts.

It is said that all of our moods are self-induced. No external force is making you feel bored . . . exuberant . . . sad . . . or depressed. These are your reactions to some stimulus. Mood is how you choose—though perhaps unconsciously—to define the moment. Though you may not see yourself as doing this, being sad is a choice you make; being joyous, a choice you make. With training, you can modify this choosing process so your world's a more positive, a more joyous place. There's always something you can feel glad about.

You're still breathing, right?

Admittedly, freeing yourself of negativism can be very difficult, but not impossible. There are many effective techniques to reverse bouts of negative-itis. My second Bible, *You Can't Afford the Luxury of a Negative Thought*, explains how to spot negativism in its infancy and how to redirect those feelings in more healthful ways. This, so the immune system's not under a cloud of suppression.

Being aware that your immune system is influenced by these unpositive thoughts and attitudes should be enough motivation to get anyone—cancer patient or otherwise—headed in a more positive direction.

A true metamorphosis this was for me—like finally understanding how to live.

Sitting there in an aluminum chair, on this breezy beach—still abysmally fatigued by the snowballing effects of five long months of chemotherapy—I'm unexplainably in harmony with my convoluted thoughts, with the very real threat of cancer.

My fingers unconsciously rake the lifeless sand.

Glancing out at the ever-shifting Pacific, I'm reminded of how we humans are always changing—how the world's constantly evolving—even as we sit doing nothing. Never are we the identical person—mentally or physically—two days in a row. Not two minutes in a row.

A continual turnover of cells is constantly occurring within us, a renewal of who we are—or were.

We're each a transient stream of life, a shifting, fluid being, rather than a static fixture like a picture. It would seem, then, that we ought to be able to modify this ongoing process of re-creation so that, as new cells are produced, taking the place of the old, diseases like cancer aren't forwarded.

Would you, as a building consultant, for example, demolish a skyscraper and then rebuild it with the identical flaws found in the original? No. Noting the previous flaws . . . you'd see to it the new structure did not preserve (carry forward) any of these. You'd adjust the reconstruction process.

In a regenerating human, this is not so easy. Through forms of self-analysis (meditation comes into play), you must search out your nucleus, your core, your driving force, and modify, repair, or adjust that essence so your cells will regenerate themselves minus the former flaws (diseases).

Through this self-analysis procedure, I found several unresolved issues residing deep within, principally bitterness issues. Used to be I wasted a lot of mental energy on negativism—being pissed off. Deliberately. In a twisted sort of way, it seemed gratifying—dwelling on this misery. I relished the misdeeds of others, masterminding retaliation.

Looking at these issues with 'new' eyes—after seeing the harm they were doing to my well being—I heeded the guidance of Dr. Nolin and *Negative Thoughts* in forgiving everyone involved. Letting the misery go. This process is, admittedly, very difficult. But not impossible—not when you weigh jeopardizing your own health against the consequences of holding these corrosive thoughts.

Negative thoughts, especially bitter ones, over time, will make even a good immune system go haywire. Making you more susceptible to disease.

Earnestly putting into practice this forgive-everyone philosophy, I released (forgave) everything, everyone . . . Dr. Hubbard for slicing into the tumor . . . Dr. Malone for her non-aggressiveness in 'watching' the malignant effusion . . . even my body for bringing me this frightful disease. My youngest son for, seemingly, not caring.

I was finally free.

Granting an overall forgiveness sounds like so much psycho-babble, but not so. The hardest part is changing your life after the forgiveness—that rebuilding process—so you don't return to your old vengeful ways. In truly facing what you're dealing with—a merciless disease that can snuff out your life—forgiveness becomes an obvious alternative. When you finally come to understand you can accept something that's disagreeable without really approving of it, this makes forgiveness a lot easier to live by.

Advice: Relative to diet and not eating meat, never would I consider using this or other alternative treatments to replace traditional medical care. *Always* use alternative *and* conventional medicine in an integrated fashion. And always keep your oncologist abreast of any alternative treatments you're using.

CHAPTER 76

AN EXCITING DISCOVERY—A NEW CHEMO!

During the last two months of chemotherapy I'm finally beginning to accept myself as part of the 40 percent who do respond. But with the end of treatment in sight, I'm getting a little edgy: What'll I use as a crutch after the chemo's stopped? Just me, my body . . . no one intervening with potent drugs to arrest the disease.

The new diet and other alternatives are in place. But will they suffice?

Possessed have I become with doing all I can—leaving no stone unturned—to see this battle's won. If ever there comes another time when an oncologist tells me, 'Your cancer's back,' I want to be able to look at myself in a mirror, knowing I did everything within my power to avert this. No excuses. No thinking, 'I wish I would've done such and such.'

Dr. Drake, my initial oncologist, did preliminary research on ACC on his personal computer, turning up the fact that M.D. Anderson is an authority on this rare cancer. While he was an abrasive individual, he did at least open this door. At the local library, an accommodating reference librarian—a soft-smiling, salt-and-pepper-haired lady—takes an hour or so, clicking keys on a PC, showing me how to use the Internet.

Instantly, I'm hooked—anxious to expand my research with a home computer. After questioning computer-literate friends, I purchase a PC, hooking up with a regional Internet provider. A couple of how-to books get me started. With Nadia nesting warmly in my lap, purring soothingly, I find using the Internet simple and user-friendly.

This may sound sacrilegious, but accessing the Internet is like, well . . . tapping into the mind of God: Everything is there. There are, for example, what're called 'newsgroups' on just about every imaginable subject—including cancer-related issues.

Specialized groups like these open a whole new vista of immediate feedback on the newest cancer-related topics and therapies—a grand exchange of up-to-the-minute information among patients. I've linked up with numerous ACC patients via the Net. We now communicate regularly, exchanging treatment information, and helping new ACC patients get through the frightening jumble of misinformation on the disease.

Another means of gaining knowledge on cancer and its treatment on the Net is through an Internet Mailing List, an on-line cancer support group. Anyone with an interest in cancer can correspond. Subscribing is free (on the Net subscribing merely means you reply to a few questions and agree to become a member). I post a summary of my diagnosis, my treatment to date. While list members are sympathetic . . . none is an ACC patient.

Reviewing this group's daily postings—people like you and I talking back and forth—I learn how to access the National Library of Medicine (NLM) in Washington, D.C. That very day, from the comfort of my home, I'm exploring up-to-the-minute data on ACC in the NLM's Medline section.

Within in the NLM there's a section called CancerLit. Here you can read excerpts of contemporary and previously published articles relating to any specific cancer. (See Appendix E for Internet access information and web site addresses.)

The NLM provides the most up-to-date medical information on the planet—no waiting a year for published reports. There are volumes to learn about most any cancer. The National Cancer Institute (NCI) also has a web site (Appendix E) where you can easily search for nation-wide clinical trials by cancer type.

After several extended on-line searches of the NLM, I recognize a recurring theme: In numerous ACC articles, the pituitary hormone ACTH and its communication with the adrenal gland is the focus. ACTH, once released into the blood stream, stimulates the adrenal glands (or adrenal cells) to produce cortisol . . . or to propagate.

A light goes on.

If that's ACTH's function . . . then, in my case, conceivably, each cancer recurrence could correlate with—or was somehow promoted by—exaggerated levels of ACTH.

A potential cause and effect?

A library textbook on endocrinology explains that the pituitary, our so-called master gland, oversees and regulates all hormones in the blood. If too little of a particular hormone's detected, the pituitary will correct the situation by secreting a specialized stimulating hormone to that particular errant gland.

To illustrate: The hormone TSH is discharged when the pituitary wants to affect the thyroid gland. ACTH is released into the blood when the pituitary's urging the adrenals to react—produce more cortisol to satisfy some bodily need. And so on. In this manner the pituitary oversees and maintains the hormonal balance within the body.

In my excitement, this feasible cause-and-effect scenario becomes a possible stimulus for my recurrent ACC tumors. Granted this medical conclusion's simple in the simplest terms. But I'm thinking (and looking for a post-chemo crutch): Why not keep on taking a higher-than-necessary dose of Prednisone *after* the chemo—to deter the pituitary from secreting its stimulating hormone, ACTH?

The pituitary, in nonprofessional terms, by dumping an overload of ACTH into my system was, in the past, 'shouting' at my remaining adrenal gland—and any unattached adrenal cells within my blood stream—to (1) manufacture more cortisol, or more perilously (2) to grow. ACTH did its job—tracking down adrenal cells, wherever they were, telling them to propagate. In that these cells could not/did not secrete a sufficient amount of cortisol, they grew . . . became malignancies-tumors.

Could this conclusion be a case of doctors being aware of this basic endocrine interplay, but not seeing the forest for the trees?

Telephoning Dr. Sloan's office, I make a special appointment.

While he and I are on comfortable terms, he—appearing caught-off-guard, sitting back in his chair days later as I propose my reasoning—doesn't exactly light up with acceptance.

What I want to do, I explain, is continue taking Prednisone in sufficient doses to fool the pituitary—to keep that gland suppressed (deceived) so it won't release too much of its adrenal-stimulating ACTH. This, I tell him, may prevent unattached ACC cells—those released by previous malignancies—from being encouraged to develop into tumors.

"I've been doing a lot of reading lately," I offer innocently, "on the Internet. Poking around the National Library of Medicine." I couch this in such a way as to be conciliatory.

Adopting a standoffish posture, Dr. Sloan's reading the tiny advertisement inscribed on his ballpoint pen. "Let me see if I follow," he begins almost irritably. His look, his response, seems more knee-jerk than anything else. His eyes say: What could you, a patient, offer a highly educated and devoted doctor like me? "You're saying possibly your cancer . . . is somehow stimulated by the pituitary's release of ACTH?"

"Like the way . . ." I interject, feeling my anxiety germinating, "prostate cancer is stimulated by the hormone testosterone."

This nabs his attention, bringing his raised eyebrows down a notch.

"Looks to me," I continue hastily, but with caution, "like when the adrenals aren't doing what they're supposed to—producing the proper amount of cortisol—the pituitary, in response, dumps ACTH into the system to correct what it sees as a deficiency. In my case, cancerous adrenal cells could have broken free of the tumors and traveled anywhere in my body. When these loose adrenal cells came in contact with ACTH and its message, these cells did as ordered and grew—becoming recurrences."

Dr. Sloan is scratching his head above his ear with a single finger: "Hmmm. Can't say as I see a whole lot of medical basis for this—"

"Because ACC is so seldom seen," I go on, "I don't think many people—doctors—have considered this idea. The reading I've been doing lately on this adrenal—ACTH interaction seems to suggest this could work. 'Course it's just a wild theory. But," I say passively, watching Dr. Sloan's eyes, "I don't see how it'd hurt to try . . . for a while. I checked my records. Each time I had a problem—the original tumor and each recurrence—my ACTH was sky high. Like 50 times normal."

Here I hesitate—so as not to further step on any toes.

A new 15-inch stained-glass dolphin is dangling from a length of transparent fishing line in the window. Bright sunlight, passing through the dolphin flashes in dancing blues, reds, and yellows on the cluttered desktop.

"So, doctor," I resume carefully, "all I'm asking is that you allow me to remain at the higher-than-normal Prednisone dosage I'm now taking—after the chemo ends—to see if that holds my ACTH down. We could check it periodically. If it looks a waste of time, drop the idea. What do you think?"

"Again," he says, thinking, "I don't know of any medical basis for something like this." The impatience he exhibited moments ago seems to have given way to a mild sort of curiosity.

Sensing he may be getting miffed at my determination, or maybe he's just plain offended by my delving into his area of expertise, I resume delicately: "Well, how about this . . . Would you at least talk with Dr. Gleghorn? In Houston? To get his impression? Maybe he knows some reason for not doing this," I concede, afraid that any minute Dr. Sloan's going to raise his hand, saying no to this whole notion. I allow time for the hoped-for words to sink in. "The idea, I think, has some merit," I add.

Dr. Sloan, looking at me blankly, rolls his wedding ring. "Okay. I'll run it by him," he replies, moving to get up, to end our session. "I can understand your eagerness. The more I look at it, the more I can see at least a glimmer of logic."

At this, I'm lightheaded. "Thanks, doctor. That's all I can ask. We patients—as you know better than anyone—have to grab at whatever we can."

At our next meeting, Dr. Sloan, in relating Dr. Gleghorn's telephone conversation, seems almost exhilarated, as though he's accepted this ACTH suppression theory himself. "These academic types," he observes, nodding to himself, "really get into these experimental ideas."

Dr. Gleghorn, with due precautions, has gone along with my Prednisone-to-reduce-the-ACTH-output theory—saying it may have merit in some cases. Prednisone, he advises, should not exceed 10 milligrams a day. At this dosage, the long-term side effects can be minimized (immune system suppression, moon-faced appearance, loss of critical bone and muscle mass, creation of new areas of fat on the body, the heightened possibility of diabetes and glaucoma). These side effects, all of them serious, when weighed against the alternative—uncontrolled, deadly cancer—seem worth the trade off.

My post-chemo crutch is now in place. I feel safe . . . for the time being, at least.

Advice: This need, this yearning to have something to fall back on once your therapy is finished, is a widespread anxiety among patients. Once the professionals are finished with you, the ball's in your court. This can be quite disturbing for some patients, particularly those who have leaned heavily on their doctors during treatment. It's sink or swim time—a surreal turn of events for some.

FINDING HOPE WHEN DOCTORS SAY THERE IS NONE

CHAPTER 77

CHANGE AND MITIGATION OF THE SOUL— CHEMO IS UNEXPECTEDLY HALTED

I may have become too open, too truthful in revealing the extent of my increasing sense of neuropathy—the chemo-induced numbness and tingling in my hands and my feet. Dr. Sloan, growing less easy with this, puts in a call to Dr. Berger, the oncologist at Anderson, to get his take. A prompt response doesn't follow from Dr. Berger—he's away on business in Europe.

Following another clean CT (no change relative to the last one—the suspicious soft-tissue mass remains, however) and a good blood test (further declining liver enzymes numbers and a low normal-range ACTH level), I'm feeling pretty self-assured as I check into the hillside hospital for chemo session number seven.

One more after this one.

Ten o'clock Monday morning: Having completed the usual admissions paperwork, I'm sitting on a turned-back bed, in a hospital gown, in a reserved room overlooking the red-roofed town below. Everything's going according to plan. A young-ish chemo nurse, with IV syringe poised, is preparing to insert the needle, as the bedside phone rings.

Figuring the call must be a wrong number, I pick it up. "Eric." It's Dr. Sloan's voice, sounding nearly breathless. "Have they started your chemo yet?"

"The nurse is just about to," I reply, his sense of urgency immediately transmitted to me. "What's up?"

"Dr. Berger, in Houston, just got back from his trip," Dr. Sloan goes on, still sounding uncommonly anxious. "He's advising strongly that we go no further. Stop your chemo right here—at six cycles. This neuropathy, he feels, will only worsen, becoming unstoppable if we proceed. Believe it or not, my phone message to him was the first he answered."

I'm struck, instantly, with the enormity, the anticlimactic nature of what he's saying. Weird as it seems, I'm instantly infused with an inexplicable feeling—an overpowering, disturbing feeling—of being cheated: I'd geared up, mentally and physically, to suffer the full eight cycles.

That was what the original plan called for—to destroy the cancer. Two more cycles—this and the next—then I'll be done. Anything less . . . falls short. Many a night I'd fallen asleep ticking off the months: Eight of them in all.

"This fellow," Dr. Sloan resumes incredulously, bringing me back, "has been out of the country for weeks—I'm sure he's got hundreds of people nipping at his heels—and the first call he returns is here. Somebody out there, Eric, is looking out for us."

Not in my book, I'm thinking . . . the rock-hard phone jammed to my ear, in an open-back gown, in this lifeless cement-floor hospital room, eucalyptus branches scratching eerily at the window in an apathetic March breeze, a white-clad nurse ready to start the IV, her curious gray eyes watching mine—as Dr. Sloan's saying, dishearteningly, we have to stop. Everything. Right now. Chemo's over. Done. Kaput. No grand finale.

Staggering, I am, off a precipice . . . into a malaise of darkness.

"So," I ask redundantly, sounding despondent, I'm sure, ". . . that's it? No more of this chemotherapy?"

Reminded am I, as I speak, of the time when I was a kid, a terrified six-year-old, and my father threatened me, saying he's going to heave me off the end of the dock if I didn't learn to swim that week.

"Too risky," Dr. Berger is saying. "You could end up with little or no tactility left in your hands and feet, permanently." Dr. Sloan, perhaps perceiving my sense of defeat, my dismay, adds: "We have to, I really believe, go with the authority here. Hey, I thought this would be good news."

A whirling sensation. Am I happy? "It's confusing is all," I stammer.

Minutes later, sluggishly yanking on sweat pants and shirt, I dial up Jane. She's shocked to hear my voice.

"Honey, this means," she all but shouts, "you're through! Finished! No more feeling like you are dead. Your hair can come back! This is w-o-n-d-e-r-f-u-l news!"

Is she saying this to counteract the disappointment she's detected in my voice—or is she being sincere?

Later, with her at the wheel, I'm still feeling monstrously vulnerable, cut adrift. "To my way of thinking," I hear myself explaining, keeping an eye on the jagged purple high country in the distance, "I was all geared up—like the way you put on muscle for an athletic event—to go through the whole business . . . all eight treatments. Now it's like . . . unfinished business. I've fallen short, somehow." I stop, thinking. "Maybe the treatment should go the full eight cycles—to really do its thing. That was the original intention."

"Nobody knows more about this nasty disease than Dr. Berger," Jane contends, playing to my uncertainty. "And, besides, things change."

"All the same, I feel . . . abandoned. Scared, to be honest, about not getting enough cisplatin. Sounds crazy, I know, even masochistic . . . Like can these people inflict more hell on me?"

"Has this disease made you masochistic, Eric?" Jane jests, stopping at an intersection, looking at me over her clip-on sunglasses, her light hair looking particularly good in the sunlight. "You like them poking sharp objects into your veins?"

"You know what I'm talking about."

"All your tests . . . those weird liver numbers—the ones we were all so concerned about—are still coming back good."

"No sales pitches, please."

"And the doctors, they've agreed to try your ACTH idea."

"Jane," I go on sullenly, feeling a kind of hollow animosity, "when your heart's set . . . and you make all the friggin' preparations . . ."

"This worries me too. You're my life," she insists, squeezing my knee. "I've got to believe the Houston doctor knows what he's talking about. He's one of the few people in the entire world who's dealt successfully with this cancer. Relax." She looks at me, smiling genuinely. "If anything, you should be cheering. As of today, you're free!"

"But are they thinking first of cancer or first of the neuropathy. That's my concern. I can live with neuropathy. Maybe the chemo's only knocked out part of the bad guys," I persist, "not all of them."

"Are we supposed to be looking at the bright side or what? Isn't that what you've talked so often about?"

"Yeah, but there's all this murkiness now."

"Well, I'm sure Dr. Berger knows."

A motorcycle cop suddenly appears beside Jane's window, waving us over. With him off his motorcycle and advancing on my side of the car, I roll down the window. "You folks trying to outrun the next earthquake?" he asks, stooping over.

"We're just coming back, officer," I explain, preoccupied with my previous thoughts, "from the hospital. I was supposed to be getting my seventh round of chemotherapy, but things didn't work out. My wife's a little shook at the moment."

Through near-black aviator sunglasses, the cop's hard eyes are studying my polished head. "Well, next time," he growls, flipping shut his leather-jacketed ticket book, "let's watch it, okay? A lot of old people use this road."

"This decision, Jane," I resume, rolling up my window, watching the cop start his motorcycle, "moves things ahead, you realize."

"Things?" she echoes, easing back onto the two-lane country road.

"What to do from now on. You know, the rest of my life."

Jane reaches up, adjusting the mirror. "Should have seen that character. That was close. Frankly," she goes on, "I'm too damn happy to think about much else. Sorry, but some of us could just scream!"

"All these questions," I continue, now beginning to see my own dreariness as a burden, "now they merge."

"Relax, Peanuts," Jane jests. "Take some deep breaths, like you're always telling me. Let's pick up a bottle of champagne, shall we? Good French stuff, nice and cold. We need some afternoon delight. I'll take the day off."

Next afternoon: Dr. Nolin, too, tries putting a positive spin on this unforeseen shift in plans. He, too, sees it as great news.

"I'm just not mentally prepared for it, doctor," I explain. Part of me is now exhilarated with the chemo cancellation; part still doggedly wallows on the dark side. "I was all set to go the distance. Good God, now I'm sounding like some punch-drunk fighter."

"This whole process," Dr. Nolin begins deliberately, unconsciously pinching and releasing the faint cleft in his chin, "from the time of your first surgery, has been nothing but a physical and emotional battlefield. We're just looking at one more skirmish. And, realistically, your vote doesn't count. The big guys have decided. Your worry is for naught."

"So I should move on, you're saying?" I continue, weighing this notion. "In that case, I really have to come to grips with my employment."

"Eric, listen to you, sounding like a *Titanic* survivor, fretting over lost luggage. Remember the challenges we talked about?"

"There's some good news here, I suppose."

"I'm listening," he says, his thinning hair, catching the slanting afternoon sun, looks falsely bronzish-red.

"They *have* agreed to try my ACTH theory . . ."

"That ought to be enough to have you jumping for joy, a wonderful victory—a validation for your determination. You wanted something that didn't exist, and you went out and found it."

"Was a time," I divulge, feeling officially stroked, "when Jane—my wife—was all-the-time bad-mouthing my research. Dwelling on negatives, she said. She's come around, though."

"It's all come down to this," the shrink concludes, moving on. "Do you really want to transform your life as you've indicated . . . or, do you want to pussyfoot about and return to that hopeless regimen—that can-of-worms—you used to go to every morning? Do you really want to change your life . . . for good?"

My back's to the wall: Do I *really* want to get well? Do I *really* want to do what must be done to accomplish that? The ever-present koi pond, percolating effortlessly as if it were surely in my mind, submerges my thoughts momentarily. "No matter what," I resume, "money does dominate."

Dr. Nolin, amused, holding his half-glasses to the light, checking for dust particles: "You're copping out, Eric. What dollar-and-cents value shall we assign to your remaining days?"
"It's more complicated than that."
"Seems to break down pretty much that way," Dr. Nolin argues. "You've elucidated well enough for me, anyway, that your job and all the rain-dances you participated in were killers. These same stress factors—remember—contributed to your getting ill in the first place. And second. How much of a track record do we need? Recall how you felt after you returned to work? After the first surgery? And the second? How you said you could physically feel a burning in your chest, in your gut? Those relentless headaches. . . . Waking up in the middle of the night."
Clearly, the soundness of his theme's sinking in.
"All our lives, though, we're taught to move ahead, to achieve," I protest, trotting out the old work ethic. "Tossing in the towel seems like, well, admitting . . . they got me."
"Who got you? You doing this for you—for your health—or somebody else's?"
His blade's becoming keener. "I get you."
"At some point you have to step back, reflect on things from your point of view—quality of life issues, your health. The very real prospect of this disease cropping up again. It sounds, from all you've said, if there is another recurrence, that's pretty much it. Nothing more can be done."
"But . . . all those years in college," I continue. "Busting my butt to make the Dean's list and working so hard to get where I am."
Dr. Nolin, scrawling something on his note pad: "I give you—maybe a year," he offers bluntly, looking up, startling me with his openness.
"Easy to see which side you're weighing in on."
"Sometimes the truth is admittedly slippery."
"Such a gigantic step . . . backward. Take yourself out of the market. Entirely . . . forever."
"C'mon, Eric," he goes on unsparingly, "you could, if you wanted to, make money on the side. Little jobs. Didn't we have this entire dialogue before? Maybe twice?"
"I needed to hear somebody that I trust saying this. . . . " I reply, pondering aloud. "If Dr. Sloan doesn't go along, no matter what I decide doesn't matter."
"Stop wondering and ask. You're pussyfooting again. This isn't like you. You haven't exactly been on a hayride these past few years—with those gruesome surgeries, radiation that knocked you for a loop, this neverending chemo business. Most people couldn't have withstood half the treatments they've thrown at you," Dr. Nolin observes. "Dr. Sloan will see the light."
"I'm working on seeing the positive side here, but damn, it isn't easy."

"By the way," Dr. Nolin says, grinning, easing back, clicking his pen shut, "I spent some time thinking. On this bomber business."

"Ready, are you, to throw a Freudian spin on it?"

"Maybe just the opposite. The specter itself—now bear with me—might have been yet another means of contact. The old guy in Houston . . . maybe the fly-by was to underscore his message. I can't connect this lone B-25 in the sky with anything else. He would have been about the right age. During WW II, I mean, to pilot a B-25. God, listen to me, sounding like some right-off-the-bus gypsy."

"I think I can concoct something wilder than that, doc," I respond, chuckling, yet taking this occasion to see, to hear again the drone of the bomber in my mind.

Guffawing, Dr. Nolin: "Had you going for a minute, didn't I? Can't you tell when I'm pulling your leg? Try spending a few more minutes each day meditating. Anyway, promise me you'll talk to Dr. Sloan."

"It's time," I concede, "to fish or cut bait."

CHAPTER 78

INTO FIELDS OF LIGHT—
DR. SLOAN AGREES TO MY RETIREMENT

A month after my last chemotherapy treatment: My hair, surprisingly, has started coming back—a dark velvety fuzz showing on an abalone-pink scalp. From this budding image, a quirky inspiration springs forth.

The weekend preceding my big appointment with Dr. Sloan—the one where I'll broach the retirement idea—I find myself shuffling through community novelty shops, looking for a particular baseball cap: One having shoulder-length hair sewn in the band. An innocent prank, I'm thinking . . . to soften the gravity of the moment with Dr. Sloan—while pitching 'My life, Part II.'

The wiry mane looks eerily authentic, making me look like a well-seasoned flower child.

Concealing the overflowing cap in a plastic bag—I don't want any office folk catching on, forewarning the doctor—I reveal my intent to Dr. Sloan's nurse. Opening the bag, behind the closed exam room door, I show her the disguise. It looks curiously like a dead animal.

A warped impersonation, she laughs. A splendid idea. "I've got to see you in it first," she goads good-naturedly, folding her arms.

"How is . . ." I ask, turning away to pull on the disguise, "his disposition today?"

"Any day," she confesses, with a look that says being a cancer specialist's not fun, "he can use some cheering up." Giggling, vowing to keep my secret, the slender nurse slips quietly from the warm exam room, saying, "Darn if you don't remind me of one of those health-food store weirdos . . . with all that hair!"

Jane, thumbing an old *Field & Stream* and taking all this in through narrowed eyes, just nods. With the cap in place, I check my look in the small mirror on the back of the door. Sitting on the paper-covered table, fingers in motion, I'm actually nervous as hell. I can hear my own heartbeat.

Will he agree retirement is the way to go?

Soon, I hear my now-thick file being lifted from the plastic receptacle on the other side of the closed door. Swallowing, I'm ready. The door opens. Dr. Sloan's eyes, the second they come up from my file jacket, register shock.

"Doc!" I blurt out, dramatically flicking several long strands away from my ear, "how'd the surfing go this morning?"

Flushing, the doctor seems genuinely taken aback. "Whoa!" he exclaims grandly, glancing again at the file in his hand. "Seems I've got the wrong room."

"No, no, wait! It's me," I interrupt before he can depart, "Eric... Scribner." Tossing my stringy mane to exaggerate the point, I go on determinedly: "You said the hair would come back like gangbusters. I just didn't think it'd be this soon... or this much."

A reserved grin somewhere on the horizon. Moving nearer, cautiously—like a child reaching to pet a strange animal—he fingers the overflowing wig.

"For God's sake, Eric."

"Now, please, doctor," I petition kindly, "don't go laying some awful news on me. Not after this."

Outwardly pleased, but still maintaining a degree of professionalism, Dr. Sloan flips open my file. "Had me for a second," he admits with a grin. "No, it looks like everything's holding. Liver enzymes are now down into the normal range. In fact, one is low—normal."

"So," I ask, relieved, lying back, "how were the waves this rainy morning?"

"Too much for the likes of me."

"I thought you surfer dudes liked the monsters."

"That's my son. The big ones, I leave to him—and his friends."

"One sunny afternoon last month," I go on, unbuttoning my shirt, "I was sitting on the beach, in my trusty aluminum chair, catching a sea breeze, when a couple of gray whales cruised by. All I saw at first was the mist from their blow holes—half a mile out."

"I've heard it said," Dr. Sloan comments pensively, digging deeply under my arms for hints of swollen lymph nodes, "our coastal Indians—the Chumash—considered a whale sighting to be good luck."

"They thought the same of certain peregrine sightings, I've heard as well."

"Peregrines?"

"Just thinking out loud. Don't mind me."

I begin now, cautiously, launching into my rationale for retirement—as I'd done endless times before in my head. Dr. Sloan listens intently for several long minutes, as I go on. He's following, eyeball to eyeball, saying nothing.

"You needn't be so somber, Eric," he offers finally, as if he's somehow relieved. "I heartily agree. Bring me the paperwork. I'll get the ball rolling. This is the way to go, I think . . . if you're really serious about getting well."

Maybe, I'm wondering, this sentiment's evident to everyone—except me. My mind, the morbid side, is wondering: Since Dr. Sloan didn't hesitate in the least . . . is he saying, 'You had better smell the roses while you can . . . there isn't much time left?'

Letting sleeping dogs lie, I resist further questions.

Going on, Dr. Sloan says 'they' (the medical community) haven't yet learned the long-term consequences of aggressive chemotherapy—years down the road. After cisplatin . . . after VP-16, 5-FU, carboplatin, Tamoxifen . . . Mitotane.

"Most patients, unfortunately, don't live long enough for epidemiologists to put together a long-term sampling. And there are," he warns, "spin-off cancers to be watched for—as an aftermath of the chemo and radiation treatments.

"Also," he continues, "you have, among others things, chemo-induced Addison's Disease. Your adrenals don't work. You'll be taking steroids the rest of your life . . . like JFK. And you'll be coming back here every three months . . . for blood work . . . every six months for a scan."

"No let-up?"

"You know the answer to that. Over and over, you've heard—this cancer can come back any time. No five-year cure rates for you."

Buttoning my shirt, I comment, in disgust, that my HMO only recently paid my surgery bill with M.D. Anderson. "Six and a half months, it took them. Do they make you wait that long?" I ask knowing money is not his great motivator.

Shaking his head, Dr. Sloan grins. "You love baiting me, don't you? The other day I was reading an issue of *Time* or one of them, and some feature writer, talking about managed care, referred to HMO executives as . . . 'MBAs in limos.' I like that description."

"Accountant types . . ." Jane throws in unexpectedly, "educated well beyond their abilities—I've heard."

"You're making me repeat myself," the doctor goes on, growing more animated. "But how can this form of health care not be seen as a conflict of interest for physicians? I mean, how can a doctor withhold health care from a patient to save an insurance company money—often to make more money for himself—and not have this be a bald-faced conflict? . . .

"And let's not overlook the fact that HMOs are really starting to manipulate their prescription lists—their so-called formularies—the drugs they'll allow us to prescribe. These folks aren't talking about what's good for the patient—but what's cheapest. *Managed cost* is what we should be calling this. That's really what it is. Welfare of the patient's w-a-y down the list—if it's on the list at all."

"The roadblocks they throw up," I put in, fueling his ire, "to prevent people from getting the care they need. Each barrier is intended, by design—whether it's those time-consuming review-approval procedures or a slap-in-the-face denial of some accepted treatment or referral to a specialist—to make us throw up our hands and go away. Tragically, a lot of people do just that, particularly old people—and those less inclined to stand up for themselves. Most folks were brought up believing doctors were rock-solid in their word. Now we have to re-think all that

... and question everything, since we patients don't know if what we're hearing is from the HMO or the doctor himself."

"I've concluded," Dr. Sloan proceeds, taking my elbow, pointing me toward the door, "that HMOs should just do away with their whole administrative layer, the folks handling those frivolous reviews and approvals. We're talking a lot of wasted time and thousands of dollars in wasted salaries, some of them rather substantial. The already over-paid CEOs could still preserve their precious millions ... and at the same time, render decent healthcare. HMOs misspend an enormous amount of time and money attempting to keep patients from the care they deserve ... and have damn well paid for.

"Most distressing though," he goes on more seriously, now with us standing in the hallway, "is that there doesn't seem to be any rhyme or reason for the cancer patients they're taking away from oncologists. HMO primary-care doctors, while well-intentioned I'm sure, either don't react quickly enough to danger signals, or don't recognize them. By the time they do and the patient is referred back to me through that snail-paced Utilization Review process, it's often too late. But I'll keep writing letters.

"Know what we need to do?" he asks briskly, backing away, smiling. "We need to get someone like Jackson Browne to write us a song."

An uncertain but pleasing sensation—a grand release—fills me as Jane and I step outside, seeing rain clouds mixed with blue, on our way to the car. I've just taken a gigantic step, asserting my citizenship in a unfamiliar land: Finally I've made the move to confirm my own health, my own wellness. My own shepherd, I am now—no one taking my hand, leading me.

Traveling home, Jane says: "Sure gets going on HMOs, doesn't he?"

Everything after the morning rain looks clean, fresh—the soothing black roadway, the trees growing along side it, the cloud-flecked sky.

"He volunteers, did you know, one day a week on the oncology floor at the county hospital—gratis? We're talking somebody who's involved."

"Well, you did it," Jane offers perkily. "Brought up your retirement."

"Big step."

"You're not going to miss your favorite VP?"

"Haven't given it a thought."

"Oh, bull!"

"You do know me, don't you?"

"You noticed, I suppose," she goes on jauntily, after a few miles in silence, "that since a certain predestined soul came into your life . . . everything's been reprogrammed? For the better?"

"That again?"

"Have you—thought about it? The old guy who—" Jane clears her throat, "didn't exist."

"Could be a lot of reasons for how things are turning out. Chemotherapy being right up there."

"You said a month ago sometimes ordinary people get called upon to act as angels. Assisting others."

"That came from my mouth—yes, by way of the shrink."

"This is what I'm thinking," Jane says. "Someday people are going to be calling you that—an angel. Now wait before you jump in, saying I'm nuts—'cause I think that was the real meaning of the old guy's message. They're letting you hang around . . . to help others. That's your mission."

While I have no evidence to the contrary, this provocative thought awakens a sleeping body of images. "So, the old guy," I offer teasingly, "might have been an actor then?"

"Laugh now, but you'll see."

FINDING HOPE WHEN DOCTORS SAY THERE IS NONE

TODAY

After many years of struggling to stay ahead of this disease, I can look back and only attempt to categorize what's brought me to this point, this current cancer-free state. I still refer to myself as a cancer patient, however, but never see myself as 'being in remission.' (Remission, you remember, is an impermanent position).

What do I see as the main reasons for my good healthy today? A blend of things: some significant, some seemingly not so significant.

Diet is certainly a major factor in my current health. I've maintained my plant-based eating habits—that's the more acceptable way of saying vegetarian diet—since 1993. I haven't eaten any red meat, chicken, or fish. Truly, I believe feeding my body live enzymes—fresh, raw produce and fruit—has benefited me greatly. Never do I look upon this diet as denying myself something—I'm convinced that meat, as it is produced today, with all its hormones, pesticides and antibiotics—is a major source of various cancers. My blood work and CT scans continue to be good.

Also, as part of my self-fashioned chemo program, the doctors agreed to allow me to remain at a higher-than-necessary dose of Prednisone to keep my pituitary gland convinced that my remaining adrenal is doing what it is supposed to and, consequently, not overproduce ACTH.

And certainly retiring—changing my lifestyle from top to bottom—has proven to great benefit as well. No longer do I lose even a minute's sleep worrying about work schedules. Keep life as simple as possible, that's the motto I live by today. Keep everything in its proper perspective. I'm alive. . .I get out of bed each morning . . . that's the most important thing. Everything else takes a back seat when it comes to living a simple and uncomplicated life.

Psychologically, the forgiveness I bestowed upon everyone and everything during my chemo treatments still resides with me. Now I can find it within myself to genuinely forgive anyone almost anything. Not harboring feelings of resentment and anger is *wonderfully* cleansing, very liberating. I spend no time any more dwelling on retaliation or revenge—both of these contrary desires require that you create within yourself a destructive brew of negative energy.

In the realm of the spiritual, I still wholeheartedly attend church. This, in itself, relieves me of a lot of church-related guilt and has reconnected me with God. Being allowed to receive Communion and receiving the solemn sacrament of healing oils from a parish priest also made an immeasurable impact.

FINDING HOPE WHEN DOCTORS SAY THERE IS NONE

Each day I look forward to reading from the Good Book, and follow this with a 20-minute session of deep meditation. This meditation is often focused on what I have just read, or simply on nothing at all, or maybe I say a prayer for others who are suffering from cancer.

After seeing frail, hairless children being pushed about in wheelchairs and other maimed patients caught in the desperate grip of this life-altering disease at the Anderson Cancer Center, I was profoundly moved and decided to do something—recalling again the old crew-cut guy who reshaped my thinking about cancer and God at MDA—to return some goodness to those who need it most. After looking into several volunteer agencies, I signed on as a volunteer caregiver helping the aged—visiting with and driving the frail elderly to and from various destinations. Just doing what I can. (This, I admit, is a selfish endeavor—I, too, derive a good deal of inner satisfaction from volunteer work . . . helping those in need.)

Another positive move in my quest for recovery: I acquired a pet . . . a companion who is there day and night to console me with its silent understanding, its devoted company. While the acquisition of a pet may seem trifling, I assure you it is not. Making a pet part of your life if something I recommend to all cancer patients.

Of all the things I've undertaken (alternative treatments) and what the medical doctors accomplished (conventional medicine) to improve my health, looking back it is hard to say which did the trick . . . if, indeed, any one thing did.

To recap then, the top six contributors to my current health would have to be:

1. Aggressive chemotherapy
2. Increased intake of Prednisone
3. A strict vegetarian diet
4. Returning to a sense of spirituality
5. Understanding that forgiveness is the true path to inner peace
6. Changing my entire life—*and* outlook—by retiring

Assessing which of these was the *most* effective is impossible—was it all of them or just one? Today, many years after my last chemo treatment, Items 2 through 6 still play a major role in my daily life, my on-going state of good health.

Cheers!

I wish all of you the best of health, and remember—

No matter what your doctors have told you, there is always hope. I am a living example.

EPILOGUE

The secret of dealing successfully with cancer and HMOs—and other foes of your good health—is a deep-seated fighting spirit and constant vigilance.

After I'd gone two years without a cancer recurrence, my HMO decided I no longer needed the services of Dr. Sloan, the oncologist. My primary-care doctor, the HMO decided, was capable of managing my follow-up cancer care. (Never mind that, coincidentally, my primary-care doctor had, just weeks before, told me he was not qualified to oversee my unusual cancer care. "Your situation is too unpredictable, too rare," he rationalized, during a routine office visit. "I'd venture to say that most oncologists aren't too comfortable with you. You definitely present an uncommon situation.")

Pledging to fight the HMO's decision denying me the right to see an oncologist, I immediately drafted an itemized, point-by-point petition to the HMO's appeals group. When this was rejected I composed a letter to the local newspaper. Dr. Sloan, offering to assist my appeal in any way he could—even to the point of seeing me without fee—disclosed, in a moment of irritation, the amount of money that my HMO was saving by canceling his services for me.

"Twenty-three dollars per visit," he said with an understandable degree of outrage. "That's what they compensate me for each HMO cancer patient. I either accept . . . or they don't send any patients. Simple as that."

I was, at the time of the HMO's denial, only seeing Dr. Sloan three times a year for follow up. So, denying me the right to see him amounted to a *grand savings of $69.00 per year* for my greedy HMO. Dr. Bristol, long my ace in the hole, had mysteriously vanished. Rumor had it the HMO forced her out because of her 'softness.' No longer was there someone on the inside for me to confide in.

Days after the HMO's rejection of my written appeal, a honey-voiced customer service representative called to magnanimously suggest that I had the right, within HMO guidelines, to switch medical groups. She even offered to assist. Doing this, I knew, would essentially negate any further appeal—and would send me looking for a new primary-care doctor at the new medical group, an internist willing to refer me to an oncologist. No dice.

With the publication of my letter to the editor, my primary-care doctor called me at home—that day—telling me point-blank that he was severing our relationship. "I will only continue seeing you," he went on sternly, "until you find a new doctor."

"But Dr. Punjee," I argued, completely caught off guard, "that letter wasn't meant to implicate or denigrate you in any fashion. In fact, without referring to you by name, I said you were a first-class physician."

"Be that as it may, Mr. Scribner," he maintained curtly. "I can no longer continue seeing you."

"But doctor, just weeks ago, you yourself told me that I needed to continue seeing an oncologist. Remember?" I persisted, making an effort to retain this doctor, to make him see the light. "Are you reacting this way because the HMO's upset with me for fighting back?"

"This, unconditionally, is my decision, I assure you. You and I have experienced a break in trust."

"Doctor," I went on desperately, feeling cut adrift, seeing myself once again in the nameless ebb and flow of HMO medicine, "don't you ever stand up or fight for what you believe in?"

A uneasy pause. "Sometimes, Mr. Scribner."

"Only sometimes, doctor?"

"Because, Mr. Scribner . . ." yet another drawn-out pause, "I am a coward."

This undisguised response stopped me dead in my tracks. I had no comeback. A highly educated physician openly admitting he's *that* weak is, well, unsettling. The underlying message here, however, says reams about the shameless domination—the death-grip—HMOs hold over their core employees: the physicians.

In the end, I advanced my appeal to the supreme arbiter: the Social Security Administration (I'd become Medicare-eligible after two years of total disability). Spelling out that I must be granted ongoing follow-ups with an oncologist, Medicare officials compelled the HMO to re-refer me to Dr. Sloan (citing him by name) . . . until such time as he, the oncologist, feels that he no longer needs to see me. No matter how long that is.

The HMO concept in medicine is obviously an outgrowth of how accountants see health care.

For many people, managed care—with its many failings—provides a stop-gap measure to no health care at all. HMOs can be made to render skilled medical care through constant vigilance—if you're willing to buck the system whenever needed and never accept 'No' for an answer . . . and by always taking your case to a higher authority. Always speak with a manager or supervisor when dealing with an HMO. An HMO's first-line phone drudge is purposely inadequately trained and will most often say 'No' to any gray-area request.

Fight! Go to the newspapers . . . go to a court of law, if need be.

Satisfaction surveys of HMOs appear to make them look like a good choice for medical care. But if you look at who's being surveyed—HMO members who're generally young and in good health, not those needing catastrophic or costly ongoing care—you see that HMOs are nothing but an accounting smoke screen set up to harvest obscene profits (look at almost any HMO's annual report) at the expense of your health.

"Our problem is what to do with the money that comes in, not whether we have enough cash."

Director of Treasury Operations at a Colorado HMO whose cash position grows by $500,000 *a day* (*Wall Street Journal*, Dec. 21, 1994).

Recently a nationwide poll of HMOs, involving patient satisfaction, clinical care and customer service, revealed that:

- The top plans immunized 79.1% of children; the lowest less than 25%
- The best plans gave just over 90% of people with heart disease beta blockers, drugs that lessen the probability of heart attack. The worst-rated HMOs provided these medications to just over half of their members with heart disease
- The best plans gave mammograms to 80% of older women in the past two years; the worst gave these breast cancer screening tests to just 62.6%

For a first-hand review of HMO horror stories via the Internet . . . type: **http://www.harp.org**

FINDING HOPE WHEN DOCTORS SAY THERE IS NONE

THOUGHTS TO HELP YOU SURVIVE. . . .

- Stay in the moment: Don't let the past or future contaminate your 'now'
- Real strength isn't power, money, weapons—but deep inner peace developed through forgiveness
- If no one's survived your illness, you can be the first—No. 1! If only one person's survived your illness, you can be the second—*No. 2!*
- Don't think: "Sixty percent of the people treated with such-and-such a drug don't respond—I'm part of that 60%." Think instead, "Forty percent of those treated with the drug *do* respond—I'm part of that 40%!"
- I'm not a statistic! Statistical tables show only averages—they don't take into account facts of my life
- Surviving cancer patients realize their shortcomings and make a fresh start by changing their lives
- Try a little harder to connect with God—reach higher for His power, energy, spirit, solace, love
- Strive to know your essence through meditation and peaceful periods of silence
- Rid yourself of all toxins—in the environment, food, drink, emotions
- Throw off your need for approval
- Don't pass judgment on objects or people
- Find something to be grateful for each day, each hour, each minute
- Learn to relax: Be patient, enjoy the moment, the journey
- Learn to accept the world as is; you don't have to like or approve of all you see
- Never get upset: this exposes your limitations, inability to accept, your lack of patience, perseverance
- If negative thoughts appear say, STOP! and call up more pleasant times
- Fear is something to be moved through, not turned away from
- In times of anguish, imagine a pure white light enfolding you, cushioning you, sheltering you, cleansing you . . . healing you

FINDING HOPE WHEN DOCTORS SAY THERE IS NONE

APPENDIX A

NO-COST TELEPHONE RESOURCES FOR CANCER PATIENTS

There are some excellent *free* resources immediately available to cancer patients and their families over the telephone. One being the National Cancer Institute's Cancer Information Service at 800-4-CANCER. Once you're aware of the type and stage of the cancer you're researching, call and ask for information on that cancer—or ask for information on clinical trials for that cancer, if that's your interest. An information packet will be mailed to you within days, at no cost.

The M.D. Anderson Patient Network at 800-345-6324 is an excellent source of first-hand patient-to-patient information. Simply call, give them the details of the cancer you're looking into and, if there is a patient in their database with a like-diagnosis, they will have that person call you, usually within 24 hours. You can then discuss whatever you choose with that person—treatment types, success rates, side effects of drugs, surgery consequences . . . anything you want to discuss is open to conversation. And the Anderson Cancer Center pays for the call. In my own experience this network has proven invaluable.

A third source is the Block Cancer Foundation Hot Line at 800-433-0464. This is similar to the Anderson Network, however, Block obviously has a different database and therefore may have another like-diagnosed patient you can speak with. Block also pays for the call.

I urge you to try any or all of these free, no-obligation cancer information sources. Talking with another patient who has a like-diagnosis—who's "been there," so to speak—is incredibly empowering. Knowledge *is* power—the more you know about your cancer, the better equipped you are to beat it.

FINDING HOPE WHEN DOCTORS SAY THERE IS NONE

APPENDIX B

PREPARING YOUR PORTABLE MEDICAL HISTORY

One way of ensuring that you receive swift and accurate medical care is to have with you, at all times, an abbreviated medical record. Creating such a three- to four-page medical record is actually quite easy—most of it can be compiled from memory. It's easiest to use a home computer. What you don't remember, you can glean from copies of your medical record provided by your doctor.

Beginning on a single sheet of paper, simply list in chronological order all of your major medical events and their dates: surgeries, tests and results, chemo treatments and chemo types, and so forth. On a second sheet list *all* of the drugs and vitamins and supplements that you're taking and the frequency.

Now, when you're faced with a doctor unfamiliar with your medical history—because of an accident, out-of-town visit, or during a second consultation—you can simply hand him your highlights list and, in minutes, he knows you as well your personal doctor and can react accordingly. Following is a brief example of my own portable medical record:

E. H. SCRIBNER
Updated: JULY 2000
DOB 7/8/42

CANCER DISCOVERY & RECURRENCE RECORD
Diagnosis: Adrenocortical Carcinoma (ACC)

1989
10/89—CT discovered mass in left upper quadrant of abdomen
11/89—6-hr surgery to remove mass (20x13x9cm, 995 grms). Pathology: Adrenocortical carcinoma

1990
2/90—Began oral chemotherapy: 1grm/day Mitotane + replacement adrenal hormones
8/90—Began bi-weekly testosterone injections for (1) low libido, (2) low testosterone level, (3) gynecomastia

FINDING HOPE WHEN DOCTORS SAY THERE IS NONE

1991
1/91—Chemo: Mitotane 7grm/day
4/91—Called M.D. Anderson (MDA) Cancer Center (Houston). MDA doctors suggest Tamoxifen for reduction of breast tissue and tenderness.

(The chronology goes on from here. The above is presented so that you can get an idea of the general format and the abbreviated information that's needed to provide a new doctor with pertinent medical data so he can properly assist you quickly *without* guess work.)

Following is a listing of the prescription drugs and over-the-counter supplements I take. A list of this nature should accompany your medical history so doctors know exactly the medications you're taking and their frequency.

E. H. Scribner
Revised: June 2000
DOB: 7-8-42

Allergies: Keflex

PRESCRIPTION DRUGS
- Prednisone—8mg/day (5mg a.m.;1mg/noon; 2mg p.m.)
- Florinef—0.2mg/day (0.1mg a.m.; 0.1mg p.m.)
- Synthroid—0.1mg/day (a.m.)
- Calan SR—360mg/day (180mg a.m./p.m.)
- Zantac—300mg/day (150mg a.m./p.m.)
- Androderm Patches—5mg/day (a.m.)
- Aspirin—250 mg/day (Noon)

CHEMOTHERAPY (10/92 thru 3/93)
- Cisplatin—180 mg/4 weeks
- VP-16—540mg/4 weeks

VITAMINS (taken most days)
- Vitamin C—2 to 4 grms/day
- Natural Vit E complex—800 IU/day
- Multiminerals—1 tablet/day
- Selenium—250 mcg/day
- Beta Carotene—60 mg/day
- Vit A—25K IU/day
- Zinc—15 mg/day
- Milk Thistle (herb)—100 mg/day
- Omega-3 EPA—1000mg/day

APPENDIX C

THE PERFECT DOCTOR

The perfect doctor . . . isn't a doctor at all. He's going to be a bundle of sophisticated electronic components—a computer. Too often we patients see our doctors as possessing *all* medical knowledge. 'Walking medical schools,' if you will. But doctors, like the rest of us, forget things—or, God forbid, never learned them.

The approach I'm about to propose could revolutionize diagnostic medicine, yet make it a more precise science—and, greatly reduce *all* medical costs. I propose this: Instead of going to a doctor's office and having him/her physically look you over and listen hastily to your list of symptoms (Note: *Always* list most important symptoms first—doctors, being busy, only hear the first two or so) to determine your illness and its treatment, you simply sit at a computer keyboard at the medical clinic and answer a series of simple questions.

From your answers, the computer then scans its database (equivalent to an entire medical school), asking you a series of more specific questions relating to your symptoms. Using this more specific information, the computer then refines its search of its entire database (everything that your doctor learned in medical school *plus* the latest up-to-the-minute discoveries), coming up with a list of several probable diseases/conditions, in descending order of probability, for the physician to review with you based on your typed-in symptoms.

Added bonus: If this isn't your first visit to the doctor, the computer will have within its database all relevant information on you concerning your medical history—blood tests, EKGs, CT results and so forth—so that it can suggest specific tests and further refine its decision about your current condition.

This truly objective means of establishing your medical state will eliminate misdiagnoses by doctors who . . . forgot what certain tell-tale signs mean, who're too busy—or too lazy—to research your condition, who're erroneously impressed by your 'healthy appearance,' who only hear the first two symptoms you describe. Or who, because of 'physician indifference,' just don't care. This computer printout will also reduce the amount of time you spend with a physician because the computer has scanned *all* possibilities and presented them to your doctor for his review and application.

Example: In my case I presented my first doctor with these physical symptoms: bloating, frequent headaches, elevated blood pressure, prolonged constipation, night sweats, loss of facial color, weight loss, and unexplained tiredness. The family doctor who first saw me decided—because I *looked* young and healthy to her—that I had the flu.

It was actually several months before a doctor *really* began treating me for a rare cancer—adrenocortical carcinoma. If I'd sat before an objective computer—a machine that doesn't care how healthy I look—and typed in these symptoms, the printout would have advised the doctor to check for adrenal irregularities. The disease could have been diagnosed quickly—saving me a good deal of mental and physical anguish . . . allowing me to begin the cancer fight earlier . . . *and* saving the insurance company a considerable amount of money.

Benefits of this computer-as-diagnostician are many: (1) patients would be less 'shy' in telling a computer of their symptoms, (2) patients would be treated properly from the outset, (3) medical insurance costs would fall dramatically due to the elimination of erroneous misdiagnoses and the time spent treating them, and (4) doctors could see more patients per day.

Doctors, however, will probably object to this method—feeling it relegates them to the position of being technicians, those who *apply* medicine rather than those who *practice* medicine. In the long run, though, patients—and the medical community and insurance industry as a whole—will greatly benefit from this computerized system that rapidly accesses and utilizes the *entire* world of medical data. The most obvious immediate drawback to this method is financial: The creation of specialized programming for these computers, and of course, the cost of these smart computers.

APPENDIX D

FOOD AS MEDICINE

Eating like a gorilla

My dear friend Barbara at the Anderson Patient Network loves telling this true cancer recovery story: About 10 years ago a man was treated unsuccessfully for a virulent cancer. Returning home to Florida, he'd been advised there was nothing more that medical science could do. All the tools had been used. Some years later, alive and quite feisty, this fellow put in a call to the Network. An astonished Barbara asked how he'd accomplished this 'miracle recovery.' "When I got home," he explained spiritedly, "I started eating like a gorilla. Nothing but fruits and vegetables. And . . . *here I am.*"

Way back when, the founder of modern medicine, Hippocrates, acknowledged, "Let your food be your medicine and let your medicine be your food." Somewhere along the way we lost touch with this all-to-obvious tenet. *Our musculature, our circulatory systems, our skeleton—our entire bodies, are the by-product of what we swallow as food. It's that simple.*

The American Cancer Society calculates that more than 564,000 Americans will perish of cancer this year, up from 331,000 deaths in 1970. Another 1.2 million new cases will be diagnosed. Cancer researchers from the American Institute for Cancer Research and the World Cancer Research Fund concluded that as many as 4 million cases of cancer could be prevented worldwide each year if humans simply ate less meat and more vegetables.

"There's no question that largely vegetarian diets are as healthy as you can get," says Marion Nestle, chair of the nutrition department at New York University, in a recent magazine article. "The evidence is so strong and overwhelming and produced over such a long period of time that it's no longer debatable."

Our maturing awareness of and respect for the power of food is nothing new. Pharmacopoeias of ancient Egypt, Babylonia, Greece, and China were rooted in food. But an alarmingly few of our contemporary physicians grasp the connection between good diet and good health. The *Journal of Clinical Nutrition* says that fewer than 6% of the graduates from US medical schools are sufficiently trained in nutrition. . . .*What about the remaining 94%?*

FINDING HOPE WHEN DOCTORS SAY THERE IS NONE

According to the Intersociety Professional Nutrition Education Consortium—groups like the American Dietetic Association and the Americans Society for Clinical Nutrition—"Improperly trained doctors have left people deprived of the rapidly growing body of nutrition research." The consortium advocates a new medical field of study: Physician nutrition specialist.

Roughly 20 years ago science first openly accepted food as a weapon against cancer. Since then it's become indisputable, through research, that diet can either fight cancer—or advance it. As many as 80% of all cancers are due to known conditions, according to the National Cancer Institute, and are thus virtually preventable: 30% are due to tobacco use, and another 35 to 50% are due to quantity and type of foods we consume. Obviously, *an enormous number of cancers could be avoided with the correct diet.*

Premenopausal women, to illustrate, who consumed five or more servings of fruits and vegetables daily had a 23% lower risk of breast cancer than those who ate less than two servings per day. Vegetarians, it's been shown, have healthier immune systems. German researchers recently found that vegetarians have double the amount of natural killer cell activity—specialized white blood cells that attack and inactivate cancer cells—as do meat-eaters.

Investigators remain uncertain as to which phytochemicals ('phyto' from the Greek word for plant) in fruits and vegetables are responsible for cutting cancer risk. The everyday tomato, for instance, is said to have thousands of these compounds. These wondrous phytochemicals appear to prohibit certain cancers *and* limit the spreading of malignant cells—and, have also been shown to reduce cholesterol and control calcium depletion from bones. Phytochemicals fall into three classifications: antioxidants, detoxifiers, and phytoestrogens.

Antioxidants deactivate unstable oxygen molecules—free radicals—created by environmental contaminants and by the body's ongoing metabolic processes. Some detoxifiers have anti-bacterial traits; others bolster enzymes that clean up carcinogens and toxins. The most potent detoxifiers are found among cruciferous vegetables—cabbage, broccoli, cauliflower, and Brussels sprouts.

Phytoestrogens are estrogen-like compounds that bind with estrogen receptors in cells, reducing the effects of this hormone. A woman's lifetime exposure to estrogen is believed to play a role in her risk of breast, ovarian and endometrial cancers. Phytoestrogens, found in soy products, are reputed to be particularly good in fighting breast and prostate cancer. Another type of phytoestrogen, indoles, are found in numerous cruciferous vegetables.

One of the most promising cancer-fighting components yet cataloged is sulforaphane in broccoli. It demonstrates an extraordinary capacity to arrest the formation of tumors. Groups of rats fed sulforaphane developed 60% fewer tumors then rats not fed this phytochemical. Tumors that did form were 75% smaller, took longer to develop and grew more slowly than tumors in the non-sulforaphane-fed group. Broccoli sprouts—tiny 3-day-old plants—are the most potent source of sulforaphane. These sprouts, 20 to 50% richer in sulforaphane than mature broccoli, are available at most supermarkets.

Other lab studies disclosed that tumor cells function less aggressively in animals on low-fat diets than in those fed higher-fat meals. Plant-based fats have been shown to hinder cancer cell development. The phytosterol B-sitosterol, a fat profuse in vegetarian diets, strengthens an intracellular signaling system that directs cells not to divide. Researchers at the University of Buffalo showed a 28% inhibition of prostate cancer cell growth after being exposed to B-sitosterol for five days in vitro. This may support the hypothesis that vegetable fats—like olive oil—decrease the risk of developing certain cancers.

"The plant-based diet is a sure thing," relates Dr. T. Colin Campbell, professor of nutritional biochemistry at Cornell University, in a recent feature in *Better Homes and Gardens*. "In fact," he goes on to say, *"every cancer can be delayed or prevented to some extent by a plant-based diet* (italics mine)." Cancer researcher Gladys Block, previously with the NCI, in examining more than 200 studies, discovered that fruits and vegetables were allied with a decreased risk of nearly every type of cancer.

Not infrequently folks worry that giving up meat may short-change their protein needs. It's the contention of the American Dietetic Association that plant sources of protein alone—a vegetarian diet—afford ample amounts of basic amino acids when a diversity of plant foods are consumed.

Somehow, we Americans, conceivably through the ventures of groups like the National Meat Board, have come to accept that our bodies need a great deal of protein. But according to the World Health Organization, the Food and Nutrition Board of the National Academy of Sciences and the National Research Council, at the utmost, we need only 8% of our daily calories from protein. Most would concede that a mother's milk is nature's perfect food, intended for infants growing more swiftly than they ever will again. But, surprisingly, a human mother's milk delivers just 5% of its calories as protein.

Some people see nonmeat eaters as a freakish lot. As worldly beings, we all seem to have an undying passion to 'belong'. . . to be seen as conventional, a member of the old guard. As a consequence, some people eschew a nonmeat diet because they don't want to appear 'different'—even if it's scientifically proven to be in their best interest.

In our battle against cancer, we should, whenever feasible, seek out and consume only organically grown foods. An influential consumer magazine recently cautioned that the prevailing pesticide residue on peaches, pears, apples and spinach may be hazardous for young children. The Environmental Working Group estimated that 1.1 million children every day take in food that, even after it is washed, contains an unsafe dose of 13 pesticides, known generally as organophosphates. Remember this: Our primary interaction with the environment comes from the food we put in our bodies each day.

Today, antibiotics and vaccines maintain the health of animals in closely packed quarters, permitting a million or more chickens to grow to maturity, disease-free, in one cramped site. According to the *Kansas City Star,* 19 million pounds of antibiotics are fed to livestock each year. Unlike people, legions of farm animals are routinely given antibiotics whether they're infected or not. The Center for Science in the Public Interest is leading a push by 37 groups to prevail on the FDA to sharply pare down antibiotic use by farmers. Because of a growing human resistance to antibiotics, the CSPI maintains that drugs required for human well-being should be off limits to agriculture.

Nearly all of the nutritional advice our citizenry receives is financed by special-interest groups—the National Dairy Council, the National Meat Board, or even the American Medical Association.

Plain and simple: *Whatever you put in your body directly influences your freedom from disease.* If meat is the nucleus of most of your meals, excluding all of it right away may be too extreme. Try making moderate changes—it may take weeks or months to feel at home with a plant-based diet. It's best to look upon food as fuel—because, of course, we want nothing but the best *fuel* for our bodies. Should the USDA one day compel the meat and diary sectors to label packaging regarding the waste products fed to cows, chickens, pigs and turkeys, the number of vegetarians would skyrocket.

Prevailing wisdom holds that the robust person is the heavy meat-eater or the meat-and-potatoes guy. A glance at the animal realm contradicts this popular notion. The truly supreme animals *aren't* carnivores, but vegetarians and fruitarians. The elephant—a veritable giant in the animal world—eats fruits, leaves and immature branches. When we look at animals resembling us physiologically we observe vegetarians. The stalwart gorilla, not an animal to be taken casually, eats fruits and vegetables.

Some insist that a comparison of anatomies—that of humans and carnivores—distinctly shows that we aren't designed to consume meat. Carnivores have canine teeth and claws for cleaving flesh and tearing meat off the bone. While humans have teeth classified as canines, and fingernails, we're not skilled at slaying animals with these 'weapons.' And carnivores, unlike humans, have chemicals in their saliva that break down not only meat but bones as well. We also lack the enzyme necessary to properly digest uncooked meat.

Additionally, the digestive tract of a carnivorous animal is comparatively short, permitting that animal to dispose of waste matter quite promptly. The human digestive tract, on the other hand, measures some 30 feet in length, and appears designed for a fibrous diet, one that doesn't tolerate waste settling along the way. Concisely put, all meat is best avoided because it has:

- Growth hormones
- Residual antibiotics
- Insidious pesticides
- Sluggish digestion by humans, overtaxing the liver/pancreas
- Overlooked parasites
- Deadly bacteria
- Excessive protein
- Artery-clogging cholesterol
- Unessential animal fats
- Mad cow disease (potential)
- Excessive iron
- Unwanted dyes

Broccoli for breakfast?

In my own quest for a really sound cancer-fighting diet, one groundbreaking doctor's approach to cancer therapy caught my eye—Dr. Max Gerson. Spoken of by Dr. Albert Schweitzer as being one of the finest physicians he'd ever known, Dr. Gerson ministered to his cancer patients principally by way of nutrition, especially via freshly squeezed organic juices. Without endorsing this across-the-border cancer therapy, suffice it to say that I, in my on-going pursuit for alternative treatments, adopted some of Dr. Gerson's methods—the vegetarian and juice diet.

After a good deal of exploration, I purchased a rugged blender-like juicer. Nicknamed the Total Juicer, this machine does *not* discharge any of the vitamin-rich pulp as some sort of compost, as with other juicers. I wanted to get all the uncooked fruit and vegetables imaginable into my system at each meal. Everything put into this juicer comes back as an easily digested mixture of complete fruit or vegetable in a milk-shake-like consistency—and the device takes only seconds to rinse clean.

Every morning—I still do this religiously—I create a 24-ounce potion fashioned from assorted raw fruits and veggies, those thought to be especially effective cancer fighters. A piping hot bowl of whole-grain cereal—oatmeal, creamed rice or a ten-grain—accompanies this, to get as many grains as practicable into my system, as well. Half the juice preparation I drink for breakfast, the other half at lunch. Who else, I teasingly ask acquaintances, feasts on raw broccoli for breakfast? My uncomplicated formula for an organic chemoprentive blend:
- Into a blender pour a few ounces of organic carrot juice (as a fluid base)
- One whole orange (peeled of course)
- Several raw large collard green leaves

- Several slices of raw beets
- A whole raw tomato
- Several ounces of raw cruciferous vegetables (broccoli, cauliflower, etc.)
- A good-sized pinch of raw broccoli sprouts
- One tbsp. of raw sunflower seeds
- One tbsp. of ground flax seeds
- About 15 US-grown grapes (red or green)
- Several ounces of vanilla—or strawberry—flavored soy beverage
- Half a cup of ice (optional)

Run blender for about three minutes. To this basic recipe you can add all sorts of goodies—bananas, yams, apples, cantaloupe, turnips, garlic . . . well, you get the idea. Good flavor is *not* the goal here. Some days your drink may be a little *un*tasty—but that's okay. *The goal is to get as many fruits and vegetables into your body as possible.*

I emphasize: I'm *not* suggesting that you replace standard cancer therapy with a vegetarian diet—on the contrary. *This plant-based diet is in addition to the medical therapies your physician is using.*

Meat: the 'tobacco issue' of the new millennium
Studies have long linked the consumption of red meat with one cancer in particular—colon cancer. Researchers at Loma Linda University now say that even the previously thought-to-be-safe white meats—poultry and fish—can heighten colon cancer risk. "The strongest risk factor (for colon cancer) among the food variables . . . was found for total meat intake." This holds true regardless of whether the meat-eater favored white or red meat. Subjects who ate either red or white meat over four times a week had double or triple the colon cancer risk of those who did not. The researchers conclude that their results "suggest the presence of factors in all meats that contribute to colon carcinogenesis." Those ingredients, to date, remain largely undefined.

Our European neighbors understand hormone-laden meat can have disturbing health consequences. Most Americans are not aware of the fact that a good portion of Europe has for the last ten years prohibited the importation of US beef. The European Union, 16 autonomous countries—including France, Germany, Greece and England—suspended US beef imports because of the detected presence of six growth hormones.

The EU's Scientific Committee on Veterinary Measures says one of these growth hormones in particular, 17 beta-oestradiol, *"has to be considered as a complete carcinogen. It exerts both tumor initiating and tumor promoting effects . . . . Even small doses of residues of this hormone in meat . . . has an inherent risk of causing cancer."* (Italics mine)

The EU said it didn't have satisfactory details to make a conclusive finding for the other growth hormones used in US cattle. Today, an excess of 90% of US cattle growers feed FDA-approved hormones to cattle to force them to grow faster and bigger.

Time magazine, in a recent article on our health and the health of our planet in the new millennium noted, "Today's factory-raised, transgenic, chemical-laden livestock are a far cry from the wild animals our ancestors hunted."

Italian researchers, in the *Journal of Obstetrics & Gynecology*, report that eating beef may raise a woman's risk of forming uterine fibroids, the foremost justification for hysterectomies. Frequent beef consumption elevated the risk for fibroids 1.7 times higher than usual, researchers determined. They also found that a high frequency of eating green vegetables typically cut the risk of developing fibroids in half. Eating meat, they theorized, may boost a woman's estrogen level, a risk factor in developing fibroids.

In another portentous report, the Physicians Committee for Responsible Medicine, tallying US medical costs attributable to meat consumption for 1997, estimated up to $16.5 billion for cancer; $2.8 to 8.5 billion for hypertension; $9.5 billion for heart disease; $14 to 17 billion for diabetes; $2.4 billion for gallbladder disease; $1.9 billion for obesity related musculoskeletal disorders; and $5.5 billion for food-borne illnesses.

Sound chillingly familiar? Reminiscent, perhaps, of our head-in-the-sand tobacco industry discoveries of years past? The meat-based diet of today *will be* 'the tobacco issue' in the coming millennium. One US doctor has already gone on record saying that through marketing geared toward children, one of America's largest hamburger chains is fueling tomorrow's epidemic of costly meat-generated diseases.

Admittedly, 'eating like a gorilla' is no promise of perfect health. Even if we all eat the right things, some will still get cancer. . . . But fueling our bodies with the correct food in the fight against cancer is *definitely* a step in the right direction.

FINDING HOPE WHEN DOCTORS SAY THERE IS NONE

APPENDIX E

THE INTERNET AS A MEDICAL RESOURCE

A Beginner's 10-minute Tour
The Internet is nothing more than an immense electronic file cabinet. Don't let it frighten you. We're all familiar with the simplicity of file cabinets. Using a personal computer (PC) with a telephone hook-up (a modem) you can, in the quietness of your home, instantly track down an unimaginable profusion of state-of-the-art medical information.

Our doctors, it seems, are tremendously encumbered today. As a rule few of them have the time to scrutinize the innumerable new cancer therapies breaking on the horizon almost daily. This is particularly true in circumstances where the cancer is rare—where the disease is an orphan, so to speak—and there's only scattered data available. In this situation we patients—Internet users—can greatly assist our overworked doctors. *And* ourselves.

But beware: The Net's laden with deception. It can be a influential wellspring of wild, unfounded claims about every affliction and panacea that's ever been contrived. It's up to you to sort the good from the bad. It may be enticing to buy into a treatment rationale just because a substantial number of people profess to have been mysteriously 'cured' of a disease. So . . . watch your step.

With that said, there are innumerable competent Internet search sites you can readily access to investigate medical facts from influential cancer centers, universities, patient advocacy groups, support groups, and government agencies (the National Institutes of Health, for example).

No longer must we reckon with the unique (and often high-priced) expertise of medical researchers or our immediate medical team to amass life-saving information. Today, we can merely go to our computers and almost instantaneously unearth state-of-the-art news pertaining to virtually any medical topic—including any cancer.

If you're unversed in using home computers, you needn't be fearful of that flashing cursor. And don't think you're too old to learn. Home computers today are *intensely* user-friendly—if you make a error, simply click on 'Cancel' and go back to what you were doing.

Your home computer is a ponderous portal to the cost-free and unrestricted realm of Internet medical science. Not too long ago, patients, ordinary folk like you and I, had a difficult time gaining access to remarkable sites like the National Library of Medicine (NLM).

With a home PC (costing as little as $500) and telephone hook-up to the Internet (a connection that should cost about $19.95 per month or less) you can uncover up-to-the-minute medical discoveries that even your physician most likely won't be familiar with. Knowledge is absolutely power, and given that, it's incumbent upon us to avail ourselves of this exceptional instrument for intelligence gathering. Using the Internet is, well, like peering over the shoulder of a scientist or physician as he or she is putting pen to paper with respect to the newest treatment for a specific diseases—or a specific cancer.

Facts are *that* current.

If you don't have access to a home computer, most public libraries now offer free Internet access on their computers. And libraries customarily extend the bonus of having trained, hands-on assistance to shepherd you in your exploration.

Once your PC's linked to an Internet server, type **www.simplify.net** in the URL window. This is a comprehensive, multipurpose search site. Now, in Simplify's blank search box, type in whatever you're looking for. To illustrate, for news on renal cell cancer and Interleukin 2, you type those words in the vacant box where the cursor's blinking, then hit 'Enter.' A screen will quickly surface showing your phrase or word entered adjacent to the various "search engines." (These are free connections that allow to you explore places like the National Library of Medicine.) Just click on one of them to commence your search.

Some search engines, like Excite and Infoseek, permit you to search for a series of words, like "radiation treatment for lung cancer," whereas other search engines would turn up all references to "radiation," "treatment" and "lung" and "cancer" individually. Be sure to read the "search tips" for each search engine to further improve your searches.

Another outstanding location to initiate your cancer search is Oncolink. This comprehensive site—**www.oncolink.com**—is maintained and amended by the University of Pennsylvania Cancer Center. From here you can leapfrog to countless other sites pursuing 'links'—highlighted words on the screen—that capture your interest. Clicking on any of these links takes you directly to another affiliated site where you can read further applicable news.

Additional noteworthy reservoirs of cancer knowledge can be found among the free on-line cancer support groups. These furnish a marvelous wellspring of first-hand, patient-provided cancer facts. After subscribing (which is free) to one of these so-called **mailing lists**, you'll receive daily email in which any or all of the support group members are communicating about cancer-related topics. You can either just watch—read this exchange of email—or you can partake by emailing your inquiries, observations, and thoughts to the group.

To join one of these free on-line support groups, just open your browser and type: **http://cancer.med.upenn.edu/forms/listserv.html** in the location box and hit 'Return' on the keyboard. An alphabetical list of free on-line support groups should come into view. Countless groups will be outlined as you scroll down through them, and you'll be instructed how to subscribe and unsubscribe. The drawback to joining these groups is that they're inclined to spawn a lot of email. So if you're not up to scanning and deleting a lot of email, you might want to hold off joining one of these intensely active groups. But they're unquestionably worth looking into . . . and keep in mind, they're *free*.

More sites of interest to cancer patients
- Cancer Information Service of the National Cancer Institute (NCI): **http://rex.nci.nih.gov**
- NCI's Research Database: **http://cancernet.nci.nih.gov**
- American Cancer Society: **http://cancer.org**
- M.D. Anderson Cancer Center: **http://www.mdanderson.org**
- Medical Literature Searches (including free Medline search of the NLM): **http://www.cancernews.com/litsearches.htm**
- NIH Searches in general: **http://search.info.nih.gov/**
- Steve Dunn's cancer information page: **http://cancerguide.org**
- Medscape Drug Info Search Site: **http://www.medscape.com/misc/formdrugs.html**
- American Health Institute (the mind and cancer): **http://www.ahealth.com/**
- Doctor's Guide to the Internet: **http://www.docguide.com**
- Memorial Sloan-Kettering Cancer Center: **http://www.mskcc.org/**
- NIH's Office of Rare Diseases: **http://rarediseases.info.nih.gov/ord/index.html**
- Free Prescriptions for those who can't afford them: **http://www.themedicineprogram.com/**
- NCI's Investigational New Cancer Drugs: **http://dtp.nci.nih.gov**
- NCI's Clinical Trial Search Form: **http://cancernet.nci.nih.gov/trialsrch.shtml**
- CenterWatch Clinical Trials: **http://www.centerwatch.com/**
- Chemo Resistance Testing: **http://www.rational-t.com/**
- Cancer Information Sources from the NCI: **http://198.77.70.12/2_1.htm**
- Index of New Drug Approvals: **http://pharmacology.miningco.com/library/newdr98/blindxa.htm**
- The Vegetarian Resource Group: **http://www.vrg.org/**

- Center for Alternative Medicine Research:
  http://www.sph.uth.tmc.edu:8052/utcam/

Internet search engines
- Yahoo: **www.yahoo.com**
- AltaVista: **http://www.altavista.com/**
- Excite: **www.excite.com**
- Infoseek: **www.infoseek.com**
- Lycos: **www.lycos.com**
- Dogpile: **www.dogpile.com**
- Inference Find: **www.find.com**
- MetaCrawler: **www.metacrawler.com**
- Deja News: **www.dejanews.com**
- Liszt: **www.liszt.com**
- WhoWhere: **www.whowhere.com**

So . . . go ahead, give it a test run. The World Wide Web just might expose that one shred of information that could save your life . . . or the life of someone you treasure.

APPENDIX F

MEDITATION—HOW TO

"You must be the change you wish to see in the world."
—Mahatma Gandhi

The why and how of meditation
A crucial turning point in healing takes place the moment you, as a cancer patient, make a genuine and conscious decision to get well. Neuropeptides, the brain's chemical messengers discussed in Chapter 8, permit our emotions to communicate this positive get-well decision with the billions of defense cells making up our immune system.

Imagery is a way of accessing this power . . . of having the brain's neuropeptides instruct the body to act in a desired way. Employing your imagination to create pleasant mental pictures bestows emotional safekeeping, tranquility and fulfillment so your body can shift into a restful state where healing can begin. Once you consciously bring into being satisfying images and practice them, these images become permanent in the unconscious mind.

In various studies with medical students and nursing-home residents, meditation—the practice of connecting with something quiet, serene, and inspiring within us—was discovered to have immune-enhancing results: T-helper cells and natural killer cells, which attack cancer, were increased.

There may be all sorts of uncertainties eating at you and demanding resolution, but for the time being, meditation allows you to set them aside, to reside for at least a few minutes in the peace and serenity of your unruffled mind. Simply put: *Meditation provides a period of solitude for you . . . alone.* This empowering process is a healing strategy you can call into play yourself.

There are possibly as many ways to meditate as there are modern diets. In fact they're similar in many ways . . . some of us are forever pursuing the ideal diet, others are pursuing new and improved techniques to meditate. But there's nothing particularly enigmatic about meditation.

It's merely the procedure by which we clear or strive to clear all thinking from our minds to extend an awareness of inner peace and calming relaxation. Allowing the body to relax, meditation can cancel the effects of stress both mentally and physically. Meditation strives to go beyond the thought process, while many other types of relaxation—like reading a magazine or watching TV—enlist the thinking process.

Meditation takes practice. Our cantankerous minds are regularly off somewhere, thinking, doing this or that, or wallowing in some worrisome predicament. Meditation offers our minds a few minutes to breathe easy, to purge themselves of troubling thoughts. Some of the more frequently practiced methods follow.

First, set aside time each day—ideally twice a day—to meditate. Ordinarily about 15 minutes per session is satisfactory. Perhaps five or 10 minutes suites you better. But try working your way up to 15 minutes. Use a soft-toned alarm to inform you that the session's complete.

Go somewhere quiet, maybe a bit dark, and sit. A slightly uncomfortable chair's best in that you don't want to nap. Begin by mentally going through each body part, starting with the toes and working up to the brain, telling each part to loosen up, to relax. This process will take a few minutes.

Once you've subdued all body parts, begin your meditation by taking eight or ten comfortable but deep, unhurried breaths to further assist the quieting-down process.

Breath watching

One of the oldest and most widely practiced meditations is breath watching: You simply sit with your eyes closed (open is okay if you can avoid distractions) and either count your inhalations and exhalations (in—1, 2 . . . out—3, 4) or mentally say 'In' and 'Out,' watching each breath as it enters and exits the nose, or as it lifts and lowers the chest.

You can meditate virtually anywhere. It can be wonderfully consoling while sitting in a doctor's office, awaiting nail-biting news. This type of meditation's also a marvelous means of falling asleep at night when all else fails. Merely observe your inhalations in your mind as 1-2-3, and exhalations as 4-5-6. Doing this repeatedly will commonly bring sleep.

Distractive meditations

A distraction like the resonance of an air conditioner or a softly gurgling stream can be used as the focal point of your meditation. Just close your eyes and allow your mind to freely follow that sound alone. This will keep you in the now, yet render a restful mode of relaxation. You can, moreover, listen to taped recordings of a running stream, rainfall, or a choir doing Gregorian chants. Many times I alter my approach using sound tapes.

Walking and meditating can be brought together, as well. All you need do is engage one of the senses—sight, smell, hearing, touch, taste—focusing totally on that. For example, while walking along the waterfront I try focusing on the clamor of the waves and nothing more for an extended period of time. Though not easily accomplished, this practice will ground you—making you mindful of and in appreciation of your immediate surroundings, transferring your thoughts away from the negative aspects of life.

In different form of walking mediation, you can say to yourself, "Breathe in life," as you inhale, and, "Breathe out a smile," as you exhale.

Zen-type meditations
One of the more time-honored types of meditation seeks to empty the mind, to let what happens happen. Tibetan monks advise that as you commence this type of meditation you should effortlessly concentrate your mental attention on a shifting object—a flickering candle, for example—and then, once your mind calms enough to see the candle flame as unmoving, lightly transfer your thoughts to nothing. A blank wall, for instance. This sounds easier than it is. Our minds have a mind of their own . . . getting them to do what we want is like asking a ravenous, two-month-old puppy to sit still and stay.

With whatever type of meditation you use, as thoughts penetrate your mind there are practical ways to suppress them, to carefully set them to the side. First, heed what it is your mind's occupied with. Not infrequently it helps to pause meditating and jot down a list of what your mind's mulling over. That way, writing these issues down, your mind can disengage its concern, knowing you'll get back to the list later.

A further means of calming the mind is to observe what it's thinking, and see these objects or events as words materializing on a grand white screen: blood test results, CT results, kids' homework, surgery next week, balance the checkbook, paint the bathroom, and so forth. With the mind's preoccupations spelled out on this imaginary screen, you can then envision a beneficent paint roller coming along and covering each word with an opaque paint, obscuring not only the letters but the mind's interest as well.

As you meditate, as further concerns emerge, paint over these too so that as you carry on all you see is that vacant screen you've told your mind to center on. Applying this technique, you can better steer your mind into a fundamental meditative state. Here you can reflect on your desires—whether that be seeing your own well-being or envisioning yourself in a communal alliance with your Creator.

Mantra or chanting meditations
Another recognized sort of mediation makes use of a word or words—a mantra—recited over and over. This mental chanting needn't have meaning to you . . . it can be anything, a word you've fabricated, or you can repeat a condensed appeal like 'Jesus watch over me,' as a mantra. Probably the best use of a mantra's not one that's uttered within the mind but one that's listened to in the mind. At the

initiation of this meditation utter the word (your chosen mantra) a single time and then let your mind return to it, to perceive it, when out-of-the-way thoughts intrude.

A particular prayer, like the centering prayer, can also serve as focus for your chanting-type meditations—'Lord, Jesus Christ, Son of God, have mercy on us' . . . or 'Jesus, watch over me.' You can have this sort of prayer 'playing' at all times in your mind, albeit out of sight, and when you need to access it, the words can quiet your day, your mental state. You can call upon this meditative method while driving a car, enduring a CT scan, trimming a hedge.

Guided or visualization meditations

Contemplative praying falls within this category of meditative experience. Whether you're concentrating on your creator or the force or pure silence is not important. Your prospering from this presence is the goal.

Biblical stories can positively be exercised here. You can watch these themes as they reveal themselves as dramas played out in your mind, with you joining in as you wish. This becomes an exceptional means of involving yourself in both Old and New Testament narratives.

There are also visualization approaches to meditation: In your mind envision some arena that's particularly pleasurable and you go there mentally. Picture yourself many years from today, cancer-free, feeling great. See yourself looking the way you would like to look, doing things you would like to be doing, having spirited energy. Feel the euphoria, the happiness in this mental picture, and praise yourself for taking this unconditional step forward, this commitment to your improved health. This persuasive mechanism utilizes your mind to produce a positive outcome within the body.

In a more explicit form of this meditation, imagine a shaft of radiant white light, not unlike a stage spotlight, streaming down, outlining perfectly your body. Permeating all of you, the light subdues your anxiety. As long as you're in charge of your meditative processes—and you *are* in charge of all your meditations—you can imagine this light intensifying, growing more concentrated and burning away malignancies anywhere in your body.

Taped meditations (such as Drs. Simonton or Siegel or others) can be utilized to fulfill a targeted effect—guiding your imagery to see white blood cells as bombs, projectiles, or butterflies attacking cancer and ridding you of the disease.

What to expect from your meditations

Experiences while meditating will vary considerably from person to person. Relaxation, heightened consciousness, mental clarity, a sense of peace . . . these are the most prevalent rewards. There is no *right* meditative methodology for everyone. Some methods work better for some people . . . while others work better for others. The important thing is to find what works for you and use it daily.

On those occasions where you have a noteworthy meditative experience, you will naturally try to recapture that . . . but that experience may or may not reproduce itself. Take each meditative experience on its own.

One of the fundamental objectives of meditation, as one friend put it, is to derive 'the subtle healing benefits of plunking your butt down in a chair and closing your eyes for a period of time on a regular basis and getting in touch with who you are and your goals.'

There are times when I complete a daily meditation and feel I have accomplished something . . . other times things don't go as serenely. Either way, I know intuitively that my body/mind sojourned peacefully and worry-free for a good interval of time. And that's restorative.

While much has been authored about the enrichments of mediation, it is best to approach it without expectations. A sense of expectation during mediation will introduce uncalled-for exertion in the practice.

Failure to encounter soundlessness, tranquility or any other desired benefit of meditation isn't a sign that you're doing something wrong. Through repetition you'll acquire an enhanced comprehension and mastery of your preferred meditative technique.